KNOW DISEASE - NO DISEASE

Inventor: Prof. Dr. Aathi Jothi Babu

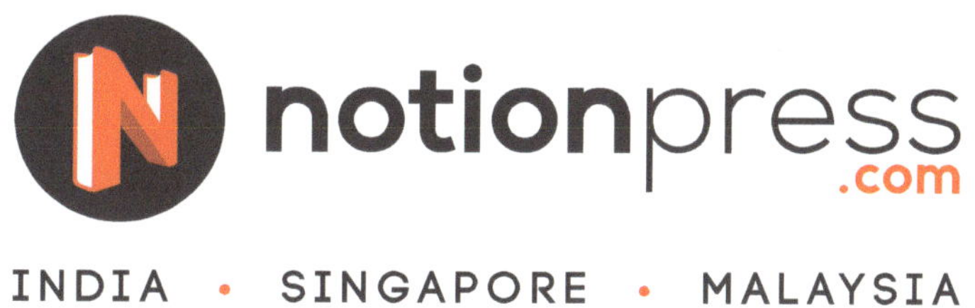

ISBN 979-8-88909-963-5

Contents

Acupuncture – Introduction

Acupuncture is a treatment method in which a needle, pressure or heat is applied to a particular point in the human body but with no use of medicines.

Chinese emperor, Huang Di was one of the pioneers, who formulated this rare art of treatment into a proper method and introduced acupuncture to the world in an organised form.

In the acupuncture treatment method, there is no need for diet, medicines, injections and laboratory tests on human stool or urine. The Pulse Diagnosis Method is used to diagnose any disease related to the body and the mind. Doctor Felix Mann was the first person to introduce an organised method to the world by which one could diagnose the disease, where the problem lies, which organ has been affected and whether it is occurring due to excess energy, less energy or a lack of energy in the affected energy channel, etc., and the accurate place of the point—either to store, create or eliminate specific energy—to cure the patient.

Dr. Fazlur Rahman and Dr. Siddiq Jamal from Tamil Nadu, India, created a milestone in the Pulse Diagnosis Method of acupuncture after the pioneer works of Dr. Wu—Wei-Ping and Dr. Mary Austin.

In the old Chinese method, the interconnection between the cosmos and the human body—the ***yin/yang*** energies, their inner five elemental energies and the creative as well as the destructive cycles that are created by these energies are well explained.

How these five elements are connected to the major twelve organs of the human body has also been explicitly explained.

The state and the interlink between these sixty points, twelve organs and the five elements are explained.

To diagnose these states, the pulse for twelve organs and four Chinese laws are given. The energy channels on the front and the back of the human hand and legs are very clearly stated. It is also stated that the central track runs through the centre of the body on the front and back side of the human body.

But the interconnections between the five element pulses, the related organs and the relevant energy channels are not explained or stated.

The organ diagnosis pulses and their places are stated. The interconnection between the five element pulses, their twelve organs and the energy channels is not stated.

Nothing is stated about the five elements pulses and the method to learn them. Diagnosing the interconnection between the five elements' pulses and the related organs, as well as the energy channels is not mentioned. How one can select the point of treatment related to the five elements and their organs has also not been mentioned.

Since the fire element is considered as two elements, it becomes six elements and the Pulse Diagnosis Method in which these six elements can be diagnosed has also not been explained.

The female and male energies of the five elements (six) are not systematically divided separately.

Amongst the elements, the fire element is divided into two kinds—**fire big** and **fire small.** The symptoms and organs for these two fires are stated.

But there is no explanation for how one can diagnose these two fires through pulses.

The second fire (small fire)-related point of selection is not mentioned in its energy channel.

Moreover, the points related to the second fire are not stated anywhere in any of the organ energy channels.

Hence, I, Professor Dr. Aathi Jothi Babu, after inventing the Five Element Pulse Diagnosis Method and the relevant points to treat people, have applied the points to almost sixty thousand patients and found that without medicines, exercises, severe diet control and hazardous side effects, one can cure the patient only with the help of the five elements present in the human body.

During this period, I could find that seventy-two points work concerning the six elements.

Beyond these seventy-two points, I could realise that every sweat pore acts as a point of any one of the elements and the energy channels, as well as the related organs, were shown to me by the grace of my Guru Gnanaparanjothi and the Lord.

Hence, I have named this wonderful treatment as ***Panchaboodha*** treatment in Acupuncture/Acupressure. I pray that the Lord may let this ***Panchaboodha*** treatment grow to its fullest with the capacity to cure all diseases and spread throughout the world to create a society without diseases.

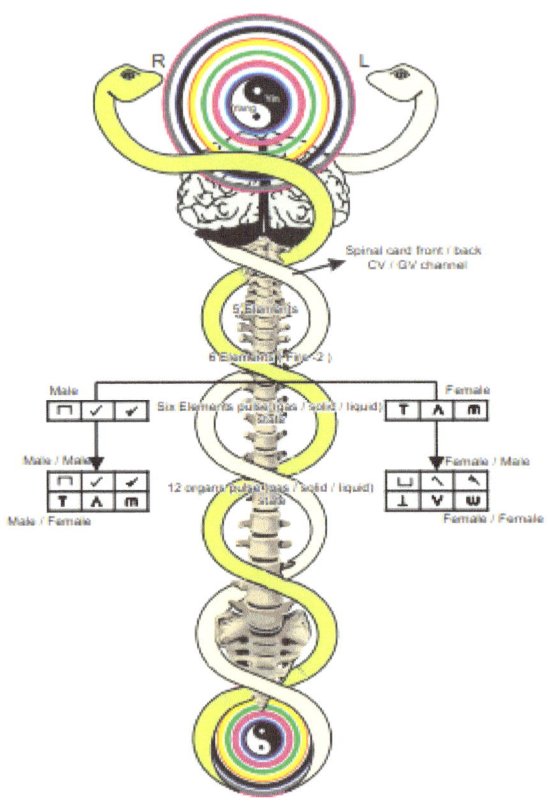

Diagram Spring of Wisdom

GNANATHIN VASANTHAM

Gurubiran Gnanaparanjothi Thunai.

The Invention of Professor. Dr. Aathi Jothi Babu — The *Panchaboodha* Treatment in Acupuncture/Acupressure

I, Professor, Dr. Aathi Jothi Babu, have been serving the people of Salem, Tamil Nadu, India, for the past twenty-seven years as an acupuncture doctor, and have acquired a diploma, a master's degree and a PhD, from the Open University for Complimentary Medicines and Alternate Treatments, Sri Lanka.

So far, acupuncture is considered a method by which pain in the human body can be eliminated. Since this great method of treatment was not applied properly, the hidden truths about this treatment could not be understood and realised by people.

The present state of the Acupuncture theory is not explained elaborately. The second fire element has been mentioned but the relevant pulses and the points of selection of that element are not mentioned.

During my doctorate studies, I invented the Five Elements and the sixth element, the energy cycles, five element points, as well as the energy channels in the field of acupuncture, which are neither mentioned nor explained in the existing acupuncture theory.

I have also synchronised the theoretical explanations and the practical application methods systematically. I have explained and synchronised the theoretical explanations of acupuncture, which were not connected at all. I have also given the practical applications of the existing theories. These inventions will enable people to understand the *Panchaboodha* Pulse Diagnosis Method and its applications.

Along with the above-mentioned inventions, I have explained how the two major energy tracts of the human body work harmoniously.

This invention of mine can diagnose the root cause of the disease/disorder of a patient and cure the disease/disorder without any medicine, strict diet, exercise, invasions or equipment. This treatment will help to diagnose the root cause of the ailments accurately. By touching on the relevant point based on the diagnosis, the ailment can be cured. Around two lakhs patients received benefits from me through this treatment. All of them had gone through either one or many schools of treatment but found no solution to their health problems. All of them got a proper and immediate cure/remedy from me.

I have registered my invention for patent rights in India. Australia has granted me a patent for my invention and thus, it has been proven that this is ***the first invention of its kind.*** This invention was also granted a patent from South Africa. This invention has copyrights from the United Nations in the US and India.

I have found that this invention in the field of acupuncture can cure diseases caused by genetics, food habits, wrong habits, sexual malpractices, immunity disorders, storage of excess energy, lack of energy, life force-related diseases, chronic diseases, etc.

In 2002, the additional commissioner of the Tamil Nadu central prison and the Tamil Nadu home ministry had given orders to treat the in-patients of the Salem central prison.

This invention of the ***Panchaboodha*** treatment in acupuncture/acupressure becomes imperative to systematise the existing acupuncture methods, elevate the status of acupuncture doctors, create proper acupuncture doctors in the future and on top of it all, create a disease-free world without medicines and the injection of drugs.

A Glimpse of the Acupuncture Treatment

The Acupuncture treatment involves the invasion of acupuncture needles, applying pressure on the points or heating a point.

The philosophy of acupuncture is that the *Panchaboodha* (five elements) energies, which are invisible and remain as visible things in the world are responsible for the creation and function of this universe. They are the energies that are responsible for the creation and function of the human body. These ***Panchaboodha*** energies are responsible for the life force existing as breathing and they create food and water for the human body to help it function. Hence, the imbalance in these energies is responsible for the cropping up of all kinds of diseases related to the body, mind and soul.

The medicines in this treatment are our ***Panchaboodha*** energies, which also exist as the invisible energies of the universe. When we balance these energies, all the diseases in the human body related to the body, mind and soul ***will*** be cured.

At present, the essential materials, which are needed to manufacture the medicines are becoming dear and so the prices of the medicines are increasing steadily. The WHO has acknowledged acupuncture as a traditional treatment—to enhance the medical support to the deserving.

This acupuncture treatment is a simple treatment, which involves no side effects. The Chinese acupuncture points are used by many doctors throughout the world. Many universities and medical schools are involved in research to find out more about the organised method of acupuncture and its uses.

For example, in Stockholm, Sweden the Karolinska Institute distributes the Nobel prize. In this place, they conducted acupuncture to relieve the pain in patients at the clinic since 1982. Through this method, one can get a remedy for the ill effects of diseases but not a cure.

The ***Varma*** treatment functions by stimulating a particular nerve, based on the acupuncture method. But this art of treatment has diminished because it has been widely used as a martial art. Teachers could not find properly qualified students. Thus, this type of treatment could not reach the world.

As explained previously, ancient India practised acupuncture in many forms. To protect people from the climate (a particular season), Indians practised walking on fire, piercing the cheek, tongue, back, legs, etc., with a metallic, sharp rod, by carrying the fire pots using bare hands, pulling the chariots of the gods, carrying ***kavadi***, etc. They also have the custom of piercing the nose and ears at a particular age, wearing bangles, anklets, toe rings, etc. All the above-mentioned methods are related to Acupuncture treatment. The tradition of tattooing one's body using herbs is also based on Acupuncture treatment.

All these points prove that acupuncture was practised in ancient India.

Since acupuncture is an ancient Indian technique, the West Bengal government has recognised this treatment and has granted permission to practice and teach acupuncture.

Acupuncture is implemented to treat insomnia, relieve pain in chronic conditions, treat paralysis, as well as help cancer patients who experience pain and other difficulties. It is also used to treat patients with circulatory disorders and those facing side effects of medicines.

Acupuncture could not get worldwide recognition because no one could understand and realise the scientific truth hidden in nature's secrets according to spiritual faith.

The following statements may explain that my invention may make acupuncture a unique subject and through it, any disease or disorder can be cured.

The Invention in Acupuncture

Professor Dr. Aathi Jothi Babu has invented his theory and the practical part of the Pulse Diagnosis method. He has compiled all the acupuncture theories together in an accurate manner.

Professor Dr. Aathi Jothi Babu has invented a Separate pulse for each element, and a Fine Technique to identify each element in the pulse, the related pulse for the energy channels, the element pulse for each organ and the points to be selected for the small (cold) fire. We shall discuss:

- The method to diagnose the diseases
- The method to find out the state of the diseases
- The method to find the condition of the diseases
- The *Panchaboodha* element cycles to cure the diseases

All the above inventions are very clearly stated simply.

Apart from the above-stated inventions, he has also invented a Fine Pulse Diagnosis method to find out the connectivity between the major two tracts of the human body, which run in the centre of the body alongside the spinal cord and the other energy channels.

The highlight of this invention is that this wonderful ***Panchaboodha*** treatment, which involves absolutely no medicine, is going to be spread throughout the world, from Salem, India.

To achieve this vision, Professor Dr. Aathi Jothi Babu has drafted a proper syllabus to conduct a Diploma, B.Sc., M.Sc. and P.G. diploma. He has named this course ***Panchaboodha - acu science*** and the institute received the affiliation from the Periyar University of Tamil Nadu, which has been awarded an A grade by the authorities for its services.

This is the only institute which offers all the above-mentioned certificates with the proper syllabus in acupuncture science.

The Vice Chancellor of Periyar University, Dr. C. Swamynathan, not only handed over the order to conduct classes with affiliation on 23-12-2014 but also took part in the opening ceremony as the chief guest. He introduced the patented invention to the public and the press. This opening ceremony was presided by Gurubiran Gnanaparanjothi Swamy.

All the above-stated patents were awarded by Australia and South Africa. The copyright obtained from the United States of America and India, along with the affiliation order from the Periyar University were all verified by the then Governor of Tamil Nadu, K. Rosaiya and his blessings were received as well.

Professor Dr. Aathi Jothi Babu has formed an excellent method to control and cure the glucose level of diabetic patients to prevent them from getting affected by the deadly disorder. By this method, one can not only control and cure the glucose level of the diabetic patient but can also maintain all the affected organs without any medicine or injection.

The *Panchaboodha* Treatment

A Non-Medicine Miracle Cure: Inventor, Professor Dr. Aathi Jothi Babu.

Prof. Dr. Aathi Jothi Babu, the acclaimed inventor of the ***Panchaboodha*** treatment has close to three decades of experience in the field of Acupuncture, Acupressure and Kundalini meditation. He is the founder chairman, professor and chief doctor of A.G. Cosmic Clinic and Research Institute, Salem, Tamil Nadu, India.

Professor Dr. Aathi Jothi Babu, born on 12th October 1971 to D. David William and R. Suseela in the Salem district of Tamil Nadu, India, grew up to be an M.D., PhD in Acupuncture/Acupressure from Sri Lanka University, Colombo and later, became an inventor. He is the only disciple to receive a Certificate of Completion after mastering the ***Kundalini Yoga*** from his mentor and ***Guru***, Gurubhiran Gnanaparanjothi.

He was a visiting professor for the Acupuncture/Acupressure Department of the Open International University for Complementary Medicine-Medicinal Alternative, Colombo, Sri Lanka.

Having mastered Acupuncture, Professor Dr. Aathi Jothi Babu strived to evolve a more comprehensive method of diagnosis and treatment using all six elements. That motivated him to invent this new method of treatment over and above the existing acupuncture methodology. He invented the six elements to devise the Pulse Diagnosis method of the six elements, their physiology, pathology and pathophysiology which highlighted a better way of understanding medical health.

He invented the Universal Cosmic Elements Pulse Diagnosis method to diagnose the root cause of all diseases and treat them without medicines. This will help him cure all types of non-curable diseases and disorders, including genetics.

To explain, first, he invented the five and the sixth elements and their pulse patterns to interconnect all the existing theories, laws, channels and points during his doctorate in acupuncture. This immense knowledge made him invent the growth and survival theories of micro as well as macro-cosmic energies of the universe and its elements of five, six, ten, etc. This is the first invention of two theories of the universe connecting all living things and the human body.

Professor Dr. Aathi Jothi Babu filed the patents in India and PCT (council for a hundred and fifty-two countries) in the year 2010 and he has been granted patent rights by Australia and South Africa. He filed for four patent rights in India for another invention, the Divine ***Vajra Brahma Gnana Maha Kundalini*** Meditation in the year 2022.

He has obtained three copyrights from India and one copyright from the U.S. Twenty copyrights have been granted by India for Spreading Global Awareness in twenty international languages against viral infections (including COVID-19) through the ***Panchaboodha*** Treatment. He has also acquired seven different trademark registrations for his other inventions and an institution.

He has treated four lakhs patients across the globe through his Unique Revolutionary Patented Non-medicine invention, ***The Panchaboodha Treatment***. He cured many non-curable diseases, such as Arthritis, lung diseases, pneumonia, diabetes mellitus, blood pressure, cholesterol, heart diseases, kidney failure, obesity, cancer, bronchitis, epilepsy, headaches, fevers, liver diseases, asthma, autism, allergic diseases, strokes, autoimmune diseases, insomnia, skin diseases, psoriasis, hair loss, lack of hair growth, gout, jaundice, Parkinson's disease, nervous, neurological diseases and disorders, multiple sclerosis, spondylitis, ENT, Alzheimer's disease, depression, ulcers, anxiety, bipolar disorder, schizophrenia, impotence, infertility, polycystic ovarian disease, stomach disorders, MND, cosmetic problems, myopathy, as well as brain and mental disorders.

Recognising and appreciating the twenty-five years of service to promote the health of society, Professor Dr. Aathi Jothi Babu has been conferred awards by many national and international organisations. The latest feather on the cap is the World Record Certificate conferred on 26th January 2022 by the World Records Union, which confirmed that the ***Panchaboodha*** Treatment is a one-of-a-kind, non-medicinal therapy. He holds special mention in the Asia Book of Records for his inventions with the title, ***Unique Patented Non-Medicine Treatment Therapy*** and was one of the top one hundred record holders of 2018 in the India Book of Records. The Global Health and Pharma, London, as well as the A. G. Cosmic Clinic and Research Institute, awarded him with the title, ***Best Alternative Medical Practice—2019.***He has also been conferred the Global Awareness Award by the Asia Book of Records and the India Book of Records for creating awareness about developing immunity against viral infections through the ***Panchaboodha*** treatment, especially during the COVID-19 pandemic. He is also the recipient of the Global Award for his revolutionary invention, the ***Panchaboodha*** Treatment. In recognition of Professor Dr. Aathi Jothi Babu's ***Panchaboodha*** non–medicine treatment, the Jetlee Book of Records conferred a medallion and a world record certificate for his achievements in 2019 followed by the World Achievement Award for his efforts to enhance world Health, Wealth and Peaceful Life in 2020.

Medicines aim to prevent diseases and prolong life. Professor Dr. Aathi Jothi Babu firmly believes that the ***Panchaboodha*** treatment can eliminate diseases and reduce the need for medicines. This defines the purpose of his life—to establish various educational institutions for sharing and spreading his knowledge. He aims to train a minimum of forty lakhs doctors throughout urban and rural India and one crore doctors throughout the world to ensure holistic health, using his unique techniques. Working towards accomplishing his mission, he supports establishing healthcare centres and organising awareness programmes related to health.

This keeps him focussed on accomplishing his mission—that people all over the world can attain good health, prosperity and wisdom, along with peace through the ***Panchaboodha*** Treatment and the Divine ***Vajra Brahma Gnana Maha Kundalini*** Meditation.

Phone Number: 98427 55935, 98427 55945.

Email id: agcosmicclinicgpt@gmail.com

draathijothibabu@gmail.com

Address: Head office: A.G.Cosmic Clinic and Research Institute,

94/C- 23, 5th Cross, Rajaram Nagar, Salem—636007.

Branch office: New No.34, Old No.19, 11th St, near Jessie Moses, 5th Avenue, Z Block, Anna Nagar, Chennai, Tamil Nadu 600040.

The ***Panchaboodha*** *Treatment in Acupuncture/Acupressure*, invented by Professor Dr. Aathi Jothi Babu.

The Emergence of the ***Panchaboodha*** *Treatment through Professor Dr. Aathi Jothi Babu—a Glimpse*.

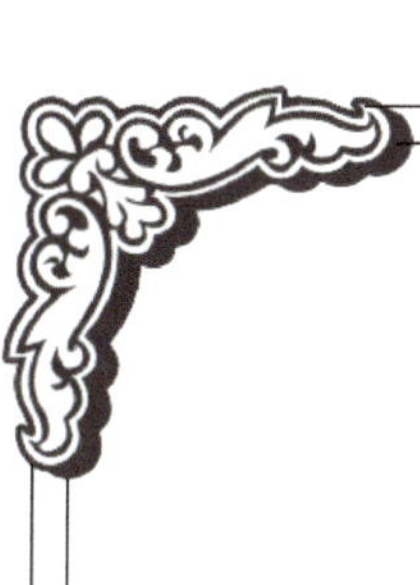

Part One

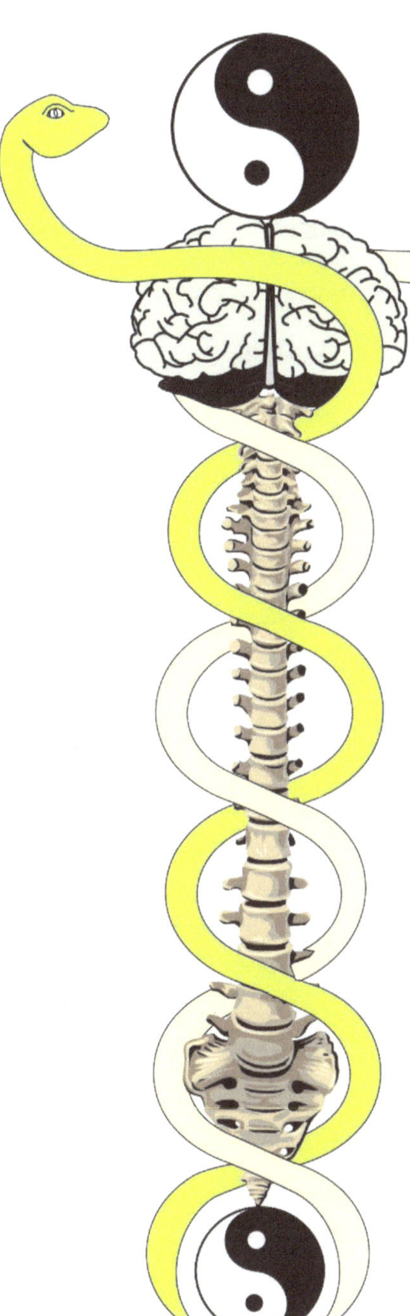

1.0. **The history of the invention of the *Panchaboodha* treatment by Prof. Dr Aathi Jothi Babu**

1.1. ***Yin-Yang* philosophy**

1.2. **The creative and destructive cycles**

1.3. **The six cycles apart from the creative and destructive cycles of the elements**

1.4. **The effects of the six cycles and the cause of disease formation**

1.5. **Explanation of the formation of six cycles**

1.6. **The relativity between the four Chinese laws and the five cycles**

1.7. **The organs of five elements and the Pulse Diagnosis Method**

1.8. ***Panchaboodha* (six) acupuncture points—seventy-two**

1.9. **The reasons for the formation of diseases**

1.10. **The dreams, insomnia and the symptoms of diseases**

1.0 The Emergence of the Sixth Element

- The Spring of Gnana
- The History of the Invention—The *Panchaboodha* Treatment
- With The Blessings of My *Guru*
- Gurubiran Gnanaparnjothi

I, now known as Aathi Jothi Babu, was named, D. Babu Charles by my parents, D. David Williams and Mrs. R. Suseela. I was born on 12th October 1971. When I received my secondary school education, I was affected by pimples and acne. During my teenage, it was a great problem for me, and to cure it, I started consulting allopaths, homoeopaths and all other schools of medicine. I was also taking all the medicines internally and externally.

At that juncture, I came to know that a ***siddha*** doctor in Salem was curing all sorts of skin diseases and hence, I went to him to get rid of my pimples and acne. After diagnosing my ailment, he prescribed internal ***siddha*** medicines and medicines for external application for about a month. He had also asked me to consume ***siddha*** medicines to help clean my bowls.

The liquid medicine, which was in a bottle had to be shaken well before consuming it and while doing so, the cork of that bottle flew up to the roof of my house. Seeing that, my mother, who was the daughter of a traditional folk doctor, cautioned me by stating that the medicine was very strong.

But I did not take it seriously and started to consume the medicines and applied the external ointment. Exactly on the third day, I started getting reddish boils all over my body. I also started passing bloody stool fifteen to twenty times a day. My mother was very upset when she saw my problems and felt worried. My maternal uncle, who was a teacher near Chennai, came home. He was a school teacher and had knowledge of homoeopathy. He prepared a herbal oil for me After applying it, the red boils on my body vanished but the bloody stool did not stop. From the mouth to the anus, the whole digestive tract became ulcerated—which could ***not*** be cured.

To cure my ailment, I consulted all types of doctors—from allopathy, homoeopathy, ***unani***, ***Ayurveda***, to ***siddha*** but all in vain. Nothing could change my hazardous conditions.

With each passing day, the condition worsened. I could eat none of the food that consisted of any of the six types of flavours. I could live only on the water which was filtered from the cooked ***Thur dhal*** and the white, cooked rice.

From 1988 to 1995, my life was a living hell—with this condition. Every doctor would try some medicines on me and stop them without showing any positive results. That would make my life worse. Then, the point came when there was no solution for my condition—except death.

At that time, my uncle, Dr. Oshomani suggested that the doctor brothers, Dr. Siddhiq Jamal and Dr. Bazlur Rahman could probably cure my condition. They were doctors from the allopathic discipline and had experience in homoeopathy and acupuncture. They used the method of ***feather-touch needling***. When I heard that, I did not have faith in them since all the disciplines of medicine had failed me. But my uncle insisted that I meet them.

Meanwhile, he also suggested that I should learn meditation from my *guru*. After giving me a brief introduction he taught me ***Kundalini*** meditation for almost thirty years. He resides in Yethapur, my village and home. He also assured me that with meditation and the feather-touch needling treatment, my ailment would get cured. So, I went to his residence with him and the ***Thavalayam*** of Gurubiran Gnanaparanjothi at Perumal thottam, Thumbal Road, Yethapur. Here, I would like to mention that, till that moment, I was brought up as a Christian.

I longed to meet pastors, such as D.G. Dinakaran, as well as Thuthi Shankarand who had a strong belief in Jesus. Not only that but till then, I had the opinion that only Jesus is God and the Holy Bible is the only spiritual book. I had the principle that I would kneel only to my Lord, Jesus and not in front of any human being.

When we entered the ***Thavalayam,*** the ***Guru*** was sitting there.

My uncle introduced me to ***Guru Gnanaparanjothi*** and fell at his feet to receive his blessings. I just wished him and stood there. He casually told me that people fall at one's feet at their wishes and will and are not compelled to do so.

Then, I was made to sit inside the meditation hall and I was given the first stage of my initiation. After that, within a month, I was given the second and third stages and the title, ***Guru***, which meant that he gave me the authority to initiate others in the three stages.

At that point, one of my ***Guru***'s disciples, named Ramanan, who was a grandmaster in the art of ***Reiki*** visited him. I maintained the habit of visiting my ***Guru*** in the morning before starting my day and back then, I was doing a wholesale business—selling eggs. When I visited him on that day, I was told that my ***Swamy (Guru)*** was talking to one of his disciples named Ramanan on the first floor of the ***Thavalayam***. I was waiting downstairs and talking to others. I could see that from right upstairs, my ***Guru*** and Ramanan were looking at me and Ramanan was talking about me by pointing to me before the ***Guru***.

Then, my ***Guru*** called and introduced me to Ramanan and told me that he wished to teach me ***Reiki*** after seeing something behind my head. Although I was not interested in learning another art, since I was practising meditation, my *Guru* insisted that I learn ***Reiki***. Along with me, around forty persons were taught ***Reiki*** on that day.

After the class, everyone was asked about their experiences. I felt a light entering me and my whole body felt a mild vibration. My body was floating and some energy was running throughout my body. Hearing that, Ramanan expressed his thoughts and shared his experience. In his fifteen years of teaching students, he had a very wonderful and unique experience after teaching that art to me.

We were given instructions which stated that for fifteen days, we had to practice the ***Reiki*** methods by applying pressure on certain points and touching our bodies. We were asked not to give therapy to anyone else as we had learnt only the first step of the art with which the therapy could not be given without touching.

The next day, I went to the nearby area called ***Umayalpuram*** to distribute the eggs to a shop. A few blocks away, in front of a house, people had gathered as a group.

My eldest brother, Thomas was with me then, and one person from the group informed us that an elderly man from that house lost consciousness and he was on his deathbed. My brother asked me to use the art of ***Reiki*** on the elderly person to help him survive.

Despite my protest—that we should not treat anyone and that too, a person in the dying stage—my brother insisted that we help him. Reluctantly, I prayed to the Lord, Jesus and my ***Guru*** and wished that the eternal power would enter that patient through my hands. Immediately, I could realise that a power entered my body and through my hands, it reached that elderly person. After a while, his mouth opened and closed. A peculiar sound came out of his throat. I was scared and wondered whether I had done something wrong. I went to him and checked his pulse, which was stable. After asking his family to clean him with a wet towel, I went home along with my brother.

The next day, an elderly man came to my house to thank me. Though at first, I could not recognise him, later, I understood that it was the same elderly man whom I had treated the previous day. He told me that he suddenly passed urine and stool at night and then felt hungry. After that, he became completely alright. That was my first experience as a successful healer.

After that incident, my uncle, Dr. Osho Mani, asked me to go with him to meet the doctor brothers in Chennai. He informed me that ten other people would accompany us. He also told me that the elder brother, Dr. Siddhiq Jamal heard the patients' problems politely but the younger one would straightaway diagnose the pulse and would not hear the symptoms. So, I was praying that the elder doctor brother would become my doctor since I had a long list of health issues which needed to be told in detail.

But when I arrived at that hospital, the younger doctor's brother was on duty. I became very upset and thought that I might not have anyone to hear about my health problems. But to my surprise, Dr. Fazlur Rahman came to my bedside and examined my pulse. Then, he asked me about my symptoms. I was very happy and started telling him everything from a long list of my health issues in a single breath. He listened intently and asked if I had left out any of the symptoms.

I assured him that I would tell him if my memory came across anything new. He smiled and asked me to lie down on my stomach. He selected a point at the back of my knee and touched it with a small needle. Then, he asked me to get up after five minutes. When I asked him about my diet, he simply opened his palms and told me that everything could be eaten—there were no restrictions. I told him that I feared I would immediately pass bloody stool. But he was confident and assured me that I would be taken care of by him.

Then, I ordered a paper roast and ***poori masala***, all the while ignoring my mother's advice—of eating soft, cooked food. I mention the menu here because, for seven years, all that I could eat was cooked rice with filtered water from the cooked ***dhal.*** After eating my meal, I waited for two hours in the hospital. The doctor came and enquired whether I felt any disturbance, such as a burning sensation or loose motion. When I told him that I was comfortable and sat without any adverse effect, he smiled and asked me to depart. He assured me that nothing would happen if I ate proper food.

He also asked me to return if I started experiencing the symptoms on the way back. But I never had any of my problems from then onwards.

All my seven years of suffering came to an end on that day within just a few minutes. That experience inspired me to have a new ambition—to learn the art of acupuncture, serve society and help patients have a healthy life.

After returning home, I narrated the entire incident to my family and expressed my wish to become a doctor. My ***Guru*** customarily asked all his disciples about their health issues and their ambitions. So, I told him about my ambition of becoming an acupuncture doctor to help people get relief from their health problems since I did not want anyone to suffer like me because of ill health.

I wanted to learn more about that treatment from the doctor brothers only. I went to them every month for follow-up. I requested my ***Guru*** to recommend me as a student to the doctor brothers as my ***Guru*** was well acquainted with the doctor brothers.

Meanwhile, my ***Guru*** took me to Attur, a nearby town for a meditation programme. There, he took me to a house which was owned by Mr. Viruthagiri—where the meditation programme was intended to take place. There were almost forty to fifty meditators of both sexes seated in the room. Usually, Mr. Subramani went with my ***Guru*** to such programmes to help him in training the disciples. On that day, he did not accompany us. My ***Guru*** asked me to touch the disciple's ***Ajna chakra*** on the forehead—between the eyebrows and sat in his seat. My ***Guru*** had the habit of repeating the command twice but that day, he told me that only once and after a while, he began the meditation. All the people were meditating and I was sitting in front of my ***Guru*** with women on my right side and men on my left.

Though my ***Guru*** had asked me to touch all the disciples after commencing the meditation, I was not sure about touching them as it could disturb them while they were meditating. I remembered the ***Reiki*** classes that were taught by Mr. Ramanan and then, I memorised the faces of all the meditators in the order of their seating arrangement.

Then, I meditated on my ***Kundalini***, located on my forehead, received the cosmic energy through ***Reiki*** and together, we prayed to the Eternal Energy mentally to go to each of the disciples' ***ajna chakra***. After completing that with the disciples, I saw that the ***Guru*** was there too. I was confused about whether to do the same thing with the ***Guru*** too—or not. I opened my eyes and saw my ***Guru*** sitting peacefully. Then, I closed my eyes to see him through meditation but to my surprise, I could not see him. Instead, I saw a big image of ***Karpaga Vinayagar* with a huge garland and a sparkling golden aura.** I thought that it was my imagination and opened my eyes to see my ***Guru*** who was sitting there in deep meditation. Again, I closed my eyes and tried to see my ***Guru*** during meditation and again, I saw ***Karpaga Vinayagar*** only. I kept quiet and meditated. The meditation session came to an end. Both of us kept quiet and to my surprise, my ***Guru*** did not enquire anything regarding the ***retouching***. Just as he had the habit of insisting (twice) that we do the task, he also had the habit of confirming the results. With this experience, we came back without discussing it.

My ***Guru*** made me realise that in the state of deep ***Kundalini*** meditation, God existed within him.

After that, we both went to the doctor brothers twice for treatment and returned but my ***Guru*** never recommended me to them so that I could learn acupuncture. When I inquired about that issue for the third time, my ***Guru*** simply said that he had forgotten about it, which made me feel angry.

Another disciple of my ***Guru***, Mr. G.M. Ramachandran reminded me that I had accepted my ***Guru*** as my Lord. He also spoke about his doubt—that maybe I learnt the art of acupuncture without the help of the doctor brothers.

He also mentioned that only I, amongst all the senior disciples, could get the vision that my ***Guru*** is none but God Himself. So, he suggested that I should get true knowledge from him.

Immediately, I apologised to him and my ***Guru*** for my ignorance and drove the car to my hometown. From that day onwards, I was made to meditate continuously for fifteen days by my ***Guru's*** holy powers. During that period, I came to understand a lot about all these ***Panchaboodha*** energies and their functions in the form of cycles, the points to be applied to cure someone and the specific pulse for the elements.

Just a day before that incident, I received books on acupuncture from my uncle and got subtle knowledge about acupuncture. Based on that knowledge, I could learn about the findings in a proper way.

To be accomplished and enhance my educational status, firstly, I did my diploma in acupuncture and then an M.D., under the guidance of Dr. Joseph Paul. Then, I completed the course to become a professor in this discipline under Doctor Abdullah Sehu. To find the relationship between the pulse, elements and the point of selection accurately, I became a research student and invented all my findings during my PhD.

During that period, I also realised that the basic energy in the human body is the ***Kundalini*** power which travels throughout the body and only from this, the five elements or the ***Panchaboodhas*** and the relevant internal and external organs emerged. I realised that with the blessings of my ***Guru*** during my ***Kundalini*** meditation practice.

I realised that the pores of the skin are as important as our breath—for humans to live. Because only through the skin's pores, the eternal energy can enter the human body as elemental energy and the unwanted energies get out of the body through the skin. Hence, the ***Panchaboodha*** energies become the basic energies for the human body—for them to live and survive.

1.1 Yin-Yang Philosophy

According to ancient Chinese treatment, Yin and Yang are two entirely different and opposite energies which complement each other. Human health is determined by these two vital energies only. Based on the imbalance in their energies, diseases emerge.

These Yin and Yang energies depend on each other and complement each other in their functioning. Yin and Yang cannot function independently. In a healthy body, there will be a small existence of Yin in Yang and Yang in Yin. When any disease affects a human body, either of the energies becomes excess and the other energy will be found in lesser amounts.

New Approach

The Yin present in Yang is an equal amount and Yang in Yin also exists equally. Likewise, the positive exists in the negative and the negative present in the positive also share an equal amount, unlike the old concept.

Page 1 Figure. 1.1.

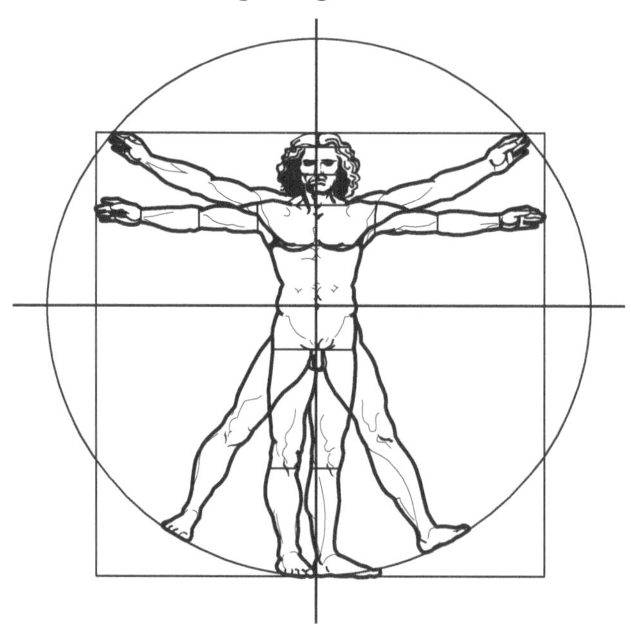

In the figure, the right side is male energy *Yang* (Yang).

In the figure, the left side is female energy *Yin* (Yin).

In the figure, the right top portion is female in male, that is, *yin* in the *yang*.

The right-down portion is male in male, that is, *yang* in *yang*.

The left side upper portion is female in female, that is, *yin* in *yin*.

The left side down portion is male in female, that is *yin* in the *yang*.

Five Elements

According to an ancient Chinese book called ***Noijing,*** the human body consists of five element energies namely, ***wood, fire, earth, metal*** and ***water***. These are the basic energies for the whole world.

Amongst them, **fire** is divided into **fire big** and **fire small**.

Fire big represents **the heart** and the **fire small** represents the **pericardium**.

Wood	**Wood**	**Wo**	**(I)**	**(T)**	**(┴)**
Fire	fire	F	(✓)	(✓)	(^)
Fire Big	hot fire	IF	(✓)	(✓)	(^)
Fire Small	cold fire	HF	(✓)	(✓)	(^)
Earth	Earth	E	(/)	(Λ)	(V)
Metal	metal	M	(\)	(┌┐)	(└┘)
Water	Water	Wa	(—)	(m)	(ω)

Elements	**Related Yin organs**	**Symbols**	**Related Yang organs**	**Symbols**
Wood	Liver	LIV	Gall bladder	GB
Fire Fire big	Heart	H	Small intestine	SI
Fire Fire small	Pericardium	P	Triple warmer	TW
Earth	Spleen	SP	Stomach	ST
Metal	Lung	LU	Large intestine	LI
Water	Kidney	K	Urinary bladder	UB

These five elements work through a creative cycle (*Shen*), and a destructive cycle (*Ko*).They also complement each other. They make each other an excess, as well as dominate and suppress each other. The life source functions only along with the arrow mark.

These are the creative and destructive cycles of the five elements.

Figure 1.2.

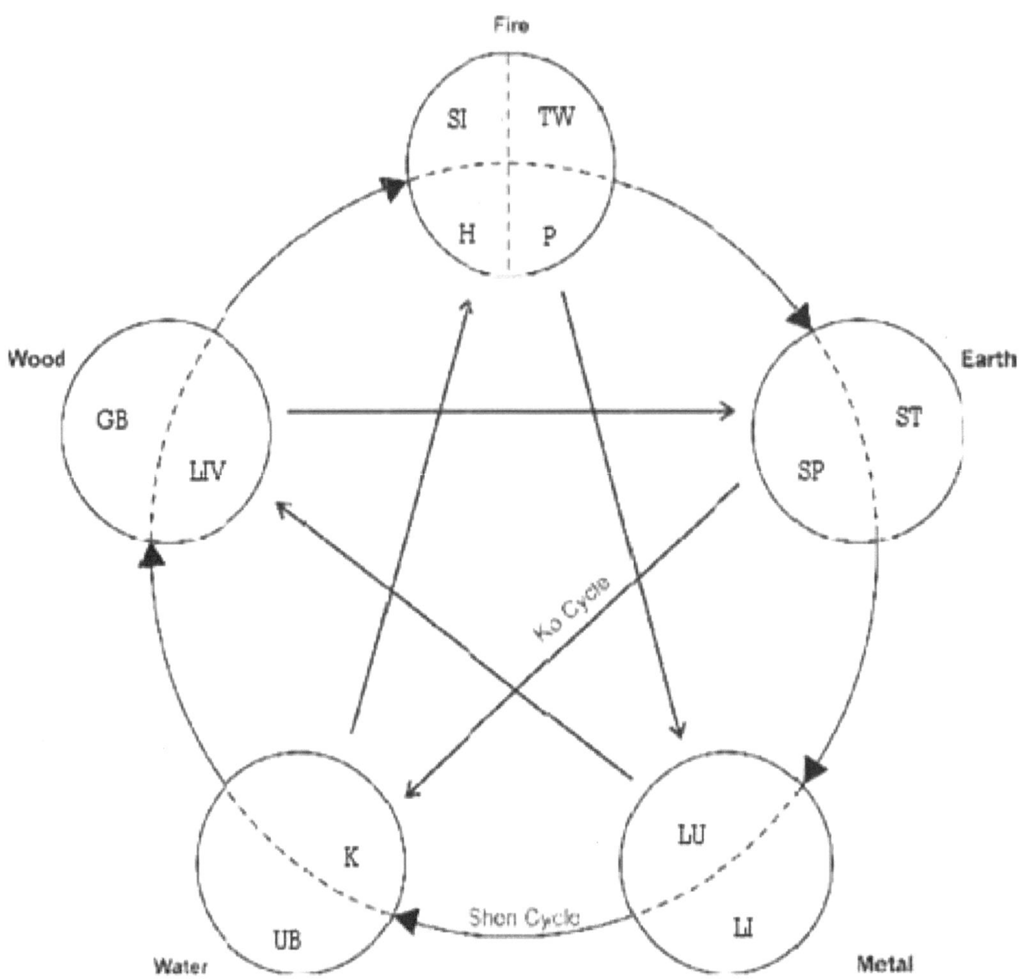

***Shen* Cycle—Creative cycle (generative). *Ko* Cycle—Destructive cycle—An explanation of the creative and destructive cycles:**

Creative cycle

Mother element	Function	Effects	Son Element.
Wood	By burning	Fire	The wood creates fire.
Fire	After burning ashes remain.	Earth	If we consider ashes as earth, fire creates earth.
Earth	Metal is formed under the surface of the earth.	Metal	The earth creates metal.
Metal	When it melts, we get a liquid. When compressed, it creates gas.	Water	The metal creates liquid or, in other words, water.
Water	The water helps the wood to grow.	Wood	The water creates wood.

Destructive cycle

Five elements	Function	Efforts
Wood	Excess growth	Encloses the earth.
Earth	If its energy becomes excess	Drains the water.
Water	If its energy becomes excess	Put off the fire.
Fire	If energy becomes excess	Melts the metal.
Metal	If energy becomes excess	Cuts the wood.

The Invention

1.2 The Six Cycles of the Five Elements and Their Correlation With the Creative and Destructive Cycles

Diagram (or figure on page 5) 1.2.

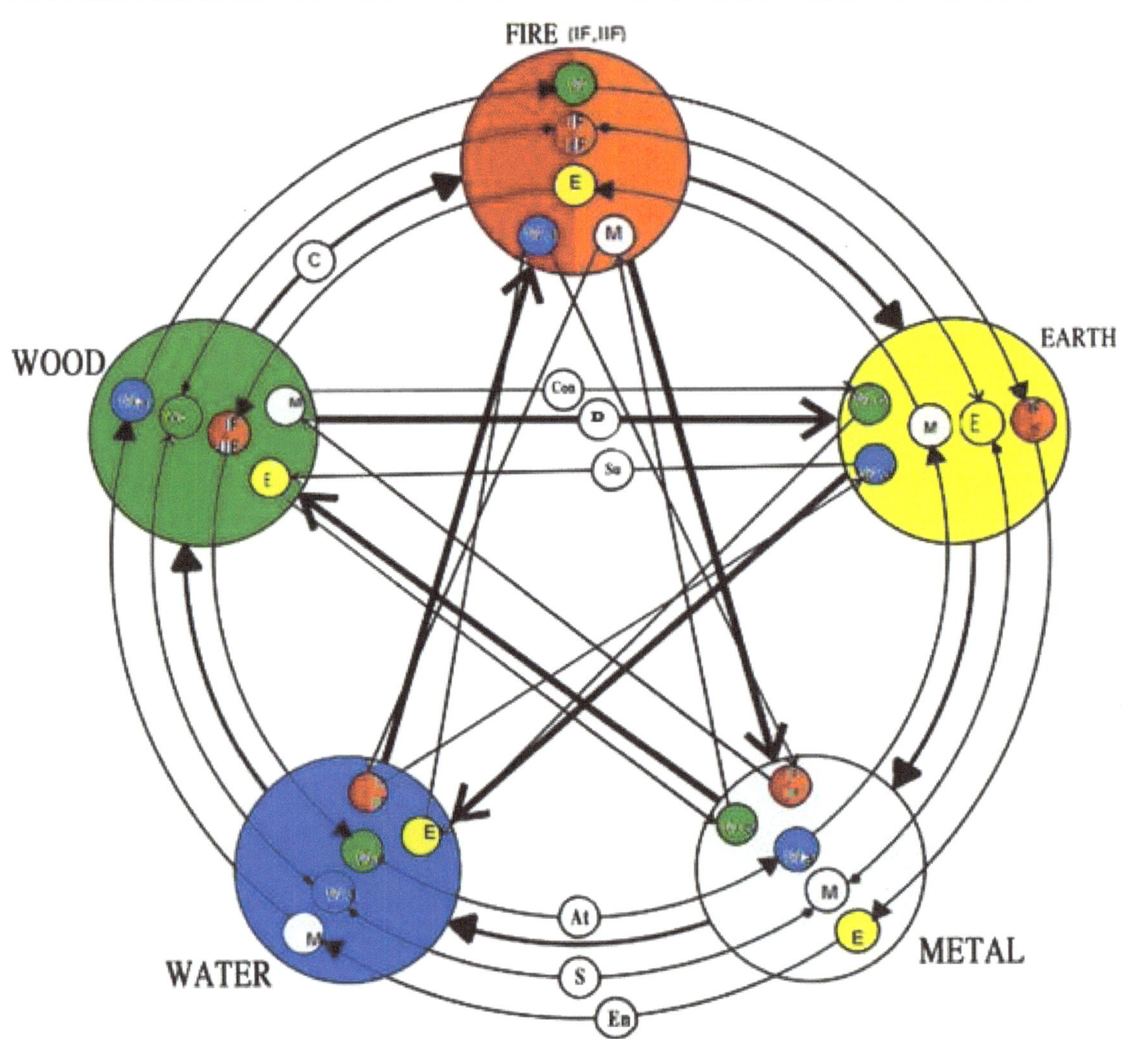

1	(C)	I (C)	Creative Cycle
2	(D)	II (D)	Destructive Cycle
3	(S)	1(S)	Self Energy Cycle
4	(En)	2(En)	Enlargement Energy Cycle
5	(At)	3(At)	Atrophy Energy Cycle
6	(Con)	4(Con)	Control Energy Cycle
7	(Su)	5(Su)	Suck Energy Cycle
8	(Ba)	6(Ba)	Balance Energy Cycle

In this (S), (En),(At),1,2, and 3 are related to the creative cycle.(Con),(Su),(Ba), 4,5, and 6 are related to the destructive cycle.

1.3 Six More Cycles Apart From the Creative and Destructive Cycle

Apart from functioning as creative and destructive cycles, the five elements or the ***Panchaboodhas*** (elements) also create other cycles with their presence in every element, that is, each of the elements will be existing in all the elements.

Each of the elements has a self-energy cycle, an expanding or enlargement cycle, an atrophy cycle, a controlling cycle, a suck or draining cycle and a balancing cycle, apart from the two stated creative and destructive cycles.

When these cycles function in a normal state, there will not be any disease or disorder.

If these cycles become excess or less, the symptoms will start to appear, which gets converted into diseases and ends up in organ failure or disorder.

Self-energy Cycle

Each element and its organ has got the nature of creating its energy for its own need. This is called self-cycle. If this self-energy cycle does not work, then that energy and organ will not function. Also ,it cannot receive or give energy to the other elements and its organs.

Enlargement Energy Cycle

Each element, along with its organ gets the energy from the mother element to expand. If this energy cycle does not work, then that element and its organ cannot expand. If this expanding energy cycle becomes excessive, then the element and its organ expand excessively and become enlarged.

Atrophy Energy Cycle

Each element, along with its organ gets the energy to shrink from its son element. If this Atrophy energy cycle does not work, each of the elements and its organ cannot shrink. When this Atrophy energy cycle functions excessively, then that element and its organ will get extremely shrunk.

Control Energy Cycle

Each element and its organ gets the controlling energy from the element and the organ which destroys those elements. When the second set of elements and any organ's destructive energy becomes excessive, then the relevant element and the organ will get destroyed.

If this controlling energy cycle does not function properly, then the concerned element and its organ loses control and works without any control.

When the controlling cycle works excessively, then the concerned element and the related organs will get excessively controlled and the self-energy cycle of this element and organ will get destroyed.

In short, if the controlling cycle is excessive in an element and its organ, then the self-energy cycle of that element and organ will get destroyed.

Suck/Drain Energy Cycle

Each of the elements, along with its organ gets the energy for its suck/drain energy cycle from the element which is controlled by this element.

When this suck/drain energy cycle becomes excessive, then the element which is controlled by that element and its organ will destroy that element.

When this suck/drain energy cycle does not function properly, then the energy which must be drained will become stagnant and that element and its organ will get destroyed.

Balancing Energy Cycle

When all the five elements do the cycling in the concept of five energies, the controlling cycle and the suck/drain energy cycle complement each other. Then, each one of the elements will be equal when in contact with the other element and will function in a balanced way with neither excess nor less energy. This is called the balancing energy cycle.

The suck/drain energy cycle and the controlling energy cycle will get affected when this balancing energy cycle faces imbalance, and the relevant organs will get destroyed.

- **The six cycles**
- **Their effects on the human body**
- **And the emergence of diseases**

Let us see how the six energy cycles namely, the Self-energy cycle, Enlargement energy cycle, Atrophy energy cycle, Controlling cycle, Suck/drain energy cycle and the Balancing energy cycle become excessive over each other, and affect the other cycles as well as the pattern by which they affect them (control the cycles of the opposite elements) initially and later it can destroy the opposite cycle.

How these are related to the creative and destructive cycles to form acute and chronic conditions of diseases are discussed below.

Moreover, how these energy cycles (through their three levels of functions, namely, the natural state, excessive state and diminished state) disturb the energy channels and the exact location where they are affected are discussed.

Amongst these six energy cycles, three are connected to the creative cycle and the other three are connected to the destructive cycle.

The Three Energy Cycles Related to the Creative Cycle

- **Self-energy cycle.**
- **Enlargement energy cycle.**
- **Atrophy energy cycle.**

When these cycles are affected, then the relevant organs also have chronic diseases.

The Three-Energy Cycles: Related to the Destructive Cycle

- **Control energy cycle.**
- **Suck/Drain energy cycle.**
- **Balance energy cycle.**

When these cycles are affected, then they affect the relevant organ which causes acute diseases.

The Creative Cycle

The Self-energy Cycle

Normal state: When each of the five elements and its organ remains in the normal state of the self-energy cycle, then there will not be any disease. This is because the other four energy cycles will remain in their cycles. When this self-energy cycle becomes excessive or less, then diseases occur.

Excessive state: When each of the five elements and its organs in the excessive self-energy cycle gets connected with the destructive cycle namely, the control energy cycle or the suck/drain energy cycle or both, they will get affected and will not work. This will create an acute state of disease.

When this self-energy cycle gets connected in its excessive state, then it will affect the related enlargement and/or the atrophy cycle and stop it from working. This will create a chronic state of diseases.

Diminished State: When the self-energy cycle in the diminished state gets connected with the control energy cycle of the suck/drain energy cycle (of the destructive cycle), then either these two energy cycles or any one of them will work excessively. This will cause an acute disease condition.

When the self-energy cycle in its diminished state gets connected with the enlargement and/or atrophy cycle of the creative cycle, then this will make it work excessively and cause chronic diseases.

The Creative Cycle

The Enlargement Energy Cycle

Normal state: When each of the five elements and its organs remains in the normal state of its enlargement energy cycle, then there will not be any diseases/such conditions for the person.

This is because the other four energy cycles will also remain in the normal state of their cycles.

Only when these energy cycles become excessive or less will they create certain diseases.

Excessive state: When each of the five elements and its related organs remains in an excessive functional state in the enlargement cycle and they are all in connection with the destructive cycle, then those cycles, namely, the control energy cycle and/or the suck/drain energy cycle get damaged and do not function properly. This leads to an acute disease condition.

When the creative cycle-related energy cycles namely, the self-energy cycle and/or the atrophy energy cycle are connected to the excessive state of the enlargement cycle, then it will lead to a chronic disease condition.

Diminished state: When each of the five elements and its related organs remains in a diminished functional state in the enlargement cycle and is in connection with the destructive cycle, then those cycles, namely, the control energy cycle and/or the suck/drain energy cycle get damaged and do not function properly. This leads to an acute disease condition.

When the creative cycle-related energy cycles, namely ,the self-energy cycle and/or the atrophy energy cycle are connected to the diminished state of the enlargement cycle, then it will lead to a chronic disease condition.

The Creative Cycle

The Atrophy Energy Cycle

Normal state: When each of the five elements and its organs remains in the normal state of the atrophy energy cycle, then there will not be any disease, since the other four energy cycles also will stay in their normal states. When this atrophy cycle becomes excessive or less, then the diseases will occur.

Excessive state: When each of the five elements and its organs in the excessive Atrophy energy cycle gets connected with the destructive cycle, namely, the control energy cycle or the suck/drain energy cycle or both, they will get affected and will not work. This will create an acute state of disease.

When this atrophy energy cycle gets connected in its excessive state, then it will affect the related enlargement and/or atrophy cycle and stop it from working. This will create a chronic state of diseases.

Diminished state: When the atrophy energy cycle in its diminished state gets connected with the control energy cycle or the suck/drain energy cycle of the destructive cycle, then either these two energy cycles or any one of them will not work. This will cause an acute disease condition.

When the atrophy energy cycle in its diminished state gets connected with the enlargement cycle and/or the self-cycle of the creative cycle, then this will make either one or both work excessively and cause chronic diseases.

The Destructive Cycle

The Control Energy Cycle

Normal state: When each one of the five elements and its related organs is in connection with the normal state of its control energy cycle, then there will not be any disease because the other related four energy cycles will also function properly. Diseases occur only when these energy cycles become excessive or diminished from their normal states.

Excessive state: When the control energy cycle becomes excessive from its normal function and gets connected with the destructive cycle, then the related suck/drain energy cycle gets affected and stops working. This will lead to acute disease conditions.

Whereas, if the control energy cycle becomes excessive from its normal function and gets connected with the creative cycle, then the related self-energy cycle and/or enlargement energy cycle and/or the atrophy energy cycle or all three energy cycles will stop working. This will lead to a chronic disease condition.

Diminished state: Whereas, if the control energy cycle becomes diminished from its normal function and gets connected with the creative cycle, then the related self-energy cycle and/or enlargement energy cycle and/or atrophy energy cycle or all three energy cycles will start working excessively. This will lead to a chronic disease condition. If the control energy cycle becomes diminished and gets linked with the destructive cycle and its organs, then the related suck/drain cycle will start to function recklessly, which may lead to acute diseases.

The Destructive Cycle

The Suck/Drain Energy Cycle

Normal state: When each one of the five elements and its related organs is in connection with the normal state of its suck/drain energy cycle, then there will not be any disease because the other related four energy cycles will also function properly. Diseases occur only when these energy cycles become excessive or diminished from their normal state.

Excessive state: When the suck/drain energy cycle becomes excessive from its normal function and gets connected with the destructive cycle, then the related control energy cycle gets affected and stops working. This will lead to acute disease conditions.

Whereas, if the suck/drain energy cycle becomes excessive from its normal function and gets connected with the creative cycle, then the related self-energy cycle and/or enlargement energy cycle and/or the atrophy energy cycle or all three energy cycles will stop working. This will lead to a chronic disease condition.

Diminished state: When the suck or drain energy becomes diminished and is in contact with each of the five elements and its organ, then the control energy cycle of the destructive cycle will work excessively. This state will lead to an acute disease condition.

When the suck or drain energy becomes diminished and is in contact with each of the five elements and its organ, then the self-energy cycle of the creative cycle and/or enlargement energy cycle and/or the atrophy cycle or all three may work excessively. This will lead to a chronic disease condition.

The Destructive Cycle

Balanced Energy Cycle

Normal state: When each of the five elements and the related organs gets connected with the control and suck/drain energy cycles, becomes the balanced energy cycle and functions in its normal state, then there will not be any disease. Only when these energy cycles work excessively or less, do diseases occur.

Excessive state: When the balance energy cycle of each of the five elements and its related organs becomes excessive and gets connected with the destructive cycle, then it will affect either the control energy cycle or the suck/drain energy cycle or both. This will make these cycles inactive. This causes an acute state of the disease.

When the balance energy cycle of each of the five elements and its related organs becomes excessive and gets connected with the creative cycle, then it will affect either the self-energy cycle and/or the enlargement energy cycle and/or the atrophy energy cycle, or all the three cycles and make them inactive to cause chronic disease conditions.

Diminished state: When the balance energy cycle of each of the five elements and its related organs becomes diminished and gets connected with the destructive cycle it will affect either the control energy cycle or the suck/drain energy cycle or both. This will make these cycles inactive. This causes an acute state of disease.

When the balance energy cycle of each of the five elements and its related organs becomes diminished and gets connected with the creative cycle, then it will affect either the self-energy cycle and/or the enlargement energy cycle and/or the atrophy energy cycle or all the three cycles and make them inactive to cause chronic disease conditions.

1.4 Explanation of the Diseases Caused by the Six Energy Cycles

Self-energy Cycle

Amongst the five elements in the human body, fire is related to the heart. When the element, fire, works excessively, the heart also starts to work excessively. Because of this, the body temperature becomes excessive and the water content of the body becomes less.

Because of this, blood circulation-related diseases, heat abscesses and a burning sensation while urinating may occur.

When this element, fire, works less, then the related organ, the heart also works less. Because of this, the temperature of the body becomes less and water becomes excess. Since this function is related to blood circulation, this will create a feeling of numbness. Since the water is not excreted properly, kidney-related problems may start to appear.

Enlargement energy cycle

In the human body, the heart represents the fire element. This fire element gets the energy to enlarge itself from its mother element, **wood**. When this enlarging energy becomes excess in this fire element, then the related organ, the heart also becomes excessively enlarged, thus leading to the condition known as *the enlargement of the heart*. This may also create high blood pressure. When the fire gets less supply of the enlarging energy, then the related organ, the heart gets affected. Cardiomyopathy may occur and problems related to blood circulation occur. The consequence of this may be neuro disorders, paralysis, etc.

Atrophy Energy Cycle

In the human body, the kidney represents the water element. This water element gets the energy to shrink from its son element, wood. Because of this, the kidney also gets the energy to contract.

When this energy becomes more excessive than is needed, then the muscles of the kidney are unable to function normally and this can result in oedema of the body, irregular breathing, loss of appetite and lead to kidney failure.

When the element, wood becomes less than the needed amount in the water element, then the energy of wood will be very less in the kidney too. Because of this, the kidney cannot contract and excrete urine. Because of this, the energies which must be controlled and filtered from excreting cannot be controlled. This is the reason why polyuria, semen discharge and/or albumin in urine appears. Since all the necessary life energies get excreted in the urine, it becomes fatal to the person.

Control Energy Cycle

In the human body, amongst the five elements, the earth element is related to the stomach and the spleen. This earth element is controlled by the wood element and its organs, the liver and the gallbladder.

When this controlling energy becomes excessive, then the bile secretion becomes excessive in the stomach and creates excess bile-related diseases and ulcers in the stomach.

When this becomes extremely excessive then patients have a swollen stomach, jaundice, a swollen spleen, anaemia, etc.

When this controlled energy becomes lesser than the amount that is needed, then indigestion, gastritis, a bulging stomach, less appetite, etc. ,occur.

Suck/drain energy cycle

Amongst the five elements in the human body, the wood element and its organ, the liver and the gall bladder suck/drain the energies from the earth element and its organs, the stomach and the spleen, and make the elements' energies as well as the food energies into the needed energies and all this is given to the body.

When this suck/drain energy cycle becomes excessive(more than the needed amount), then the liver and the gall bladder start to suck/drain the energies that are produced and/or stored by the stomach and the spleen. Because of this, the person will have very excessive hunger and immediately becomes tired as well as shivers with weakness. Patients can also feel nauseous, have a burning sensation in the stomach, have dizziness, etc.

When this suck/drain energy cycle does not work as is needed, then the person becomes underweight, might faint, will have excessive weakness/fatigue, have very less hunger and have excessive cholesterol, as well as have diseases related to the spleen, the stomach, the liver and the gall bladder.

Balance Energy Cycle

Amongst the five elements present in the human body, the earth element is related to the organs, such as the spleen and the stomach. This earth is controlled by the wood element and gets sucked/drained by the element, water. The stomach and the spleen get controlled by the gall bladder and the liver, and they get sucked/drained by the kidney and the urinary bladder. The changes in these functions may lead to excess bile in the stomach and related diseases. This may also create ulceration of the stomach. When the bile becomes excessive in the stomach, it will cause jaundice, a swollen stomach, a swollen spleen, etc. When the water energies get linked with this, it may cause symptoms ,such as drooling, water-related jaundice, indigested food, along with water coming out through the patient's mouth, etc. Because of this, shivering, fatigue, burning sensation in the stomach or dizziness may occur.

1.5 Explanation of the Formation of the Six Cycles

Self-energy Cycle

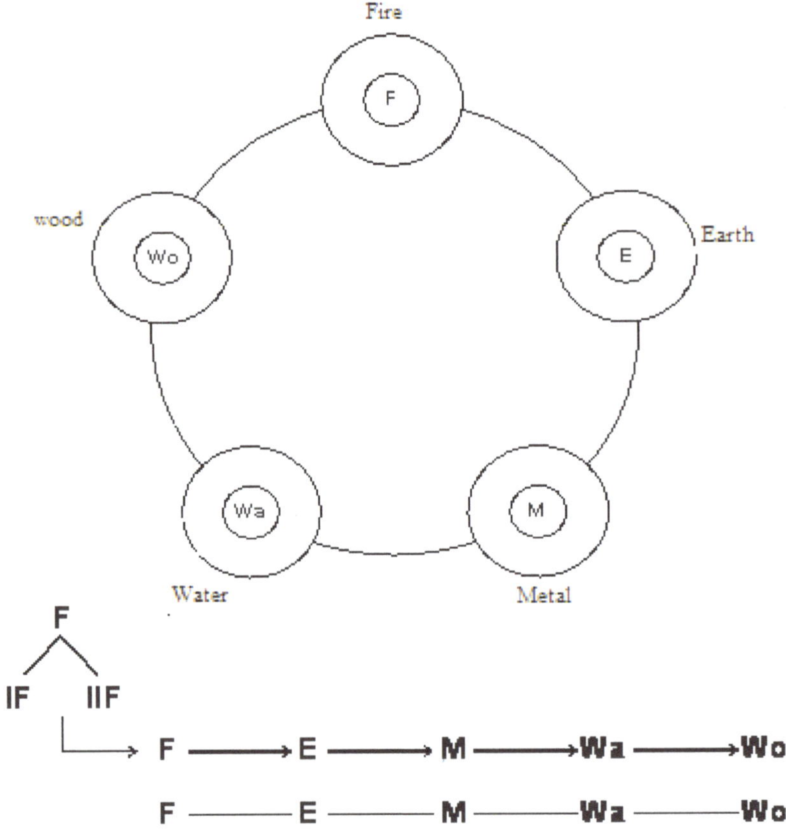

Figure on page25. 1.4.

When each of the five elements creates its needed energy cycle, it is called a self-energy cycle.

In this self-energy cycle, the energy of each element will be retained in the same element:

- **Hot Fire in Fire.**
- **Cold Fire in Fire.**
- **Metal in Metal.**
- **Water in Water.**
- **Wood in Wood.**

Enlargement Energy Cycle
(Mother Energy Becomes Excessive)

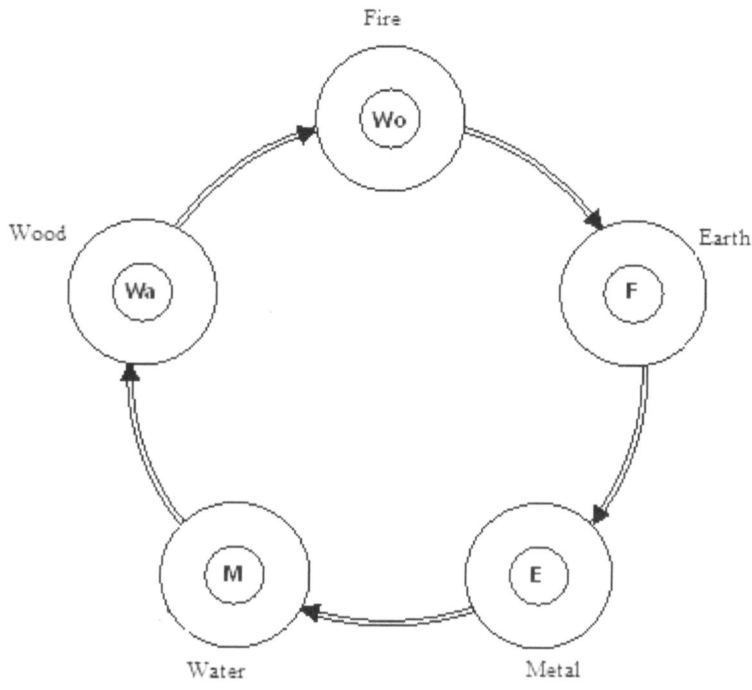

Figure 1.5: Page 26.

The mother element's energy of wood becomes excessive in the fire to make the fire element and its organs enlarged.

When the mother element, fire becomes excessive in its son element, earth, then the earth and its organ become enlarged.

When the mother element, earth (of metal) becomes excessive in metal, then the metal and its related organ become enlarged.

Metal is the mother element of water. When this mother element becomes excessive in water, then the water and its organs get enlarged.

When water, the mother element of wood becomes excessive in wood, then wood and its related organs become enlarged.

Atrophy Energy Cycle
(Excessive Energy of the Son Element)

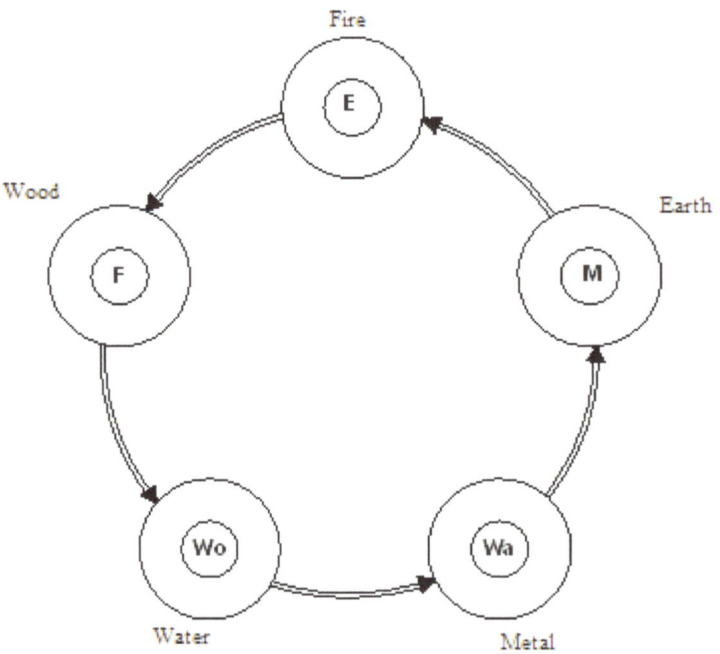

Figure as on page 27, figure 1.6.

When the son element, earth becomes excessive in fire, then the fire element and its organs shrink.

Metal is the son element of earth. When this son element, metal becomes excessive in earth, the earth element and its organs are shrunken.

Water is the son element of metal. So, when the son element's energy becomes excessive in water, then the metal and its organs will shrink.

The wood element is the son of water. When this son element's energy becomes excessive in water, then the water element and its organs will shrink.

Fire is the son element of wood. When this son element becomes excessive in the wood element, then the wood element and its organs will shrink.

Control Energy Cycle
(The Destructive Cycle Becomes the Control Energy Cycle)

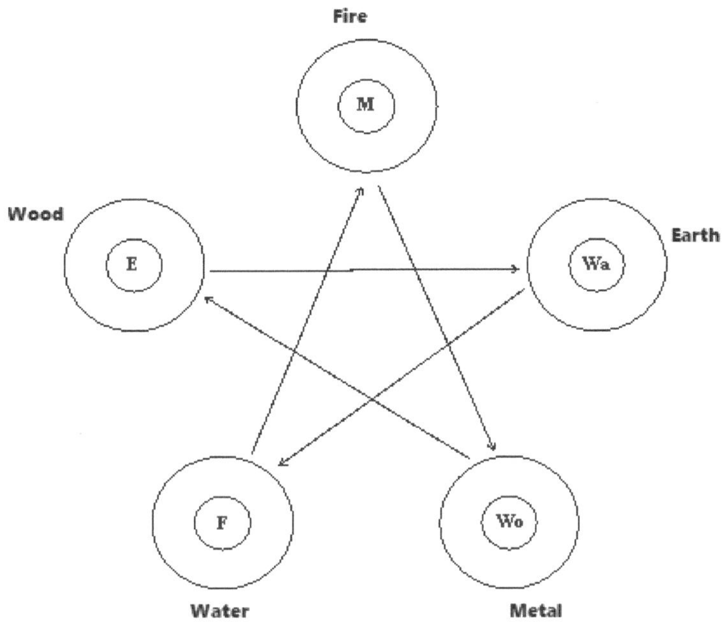

Figure as on page 28. Figure 1.7.

Because of the controlling power of the element, fire, the metal element's energy is controlled.

Because of the controlling powers of the element, earth, the water element's energies are controlled.

Because of the controlling powers of the element, metal, the wood element's energies are controlled.

Because of the controlling powers of the element, water, the fire element's energies are controlled.

Because of the controlling powers of the element, wood, the earth element's energies are controlled.

Suck/Drain Energy Cycle

(The Destructive Cycle Becomes the Suck/Drain Energy Cycle)Figure as on page 20. Figure 1.8.

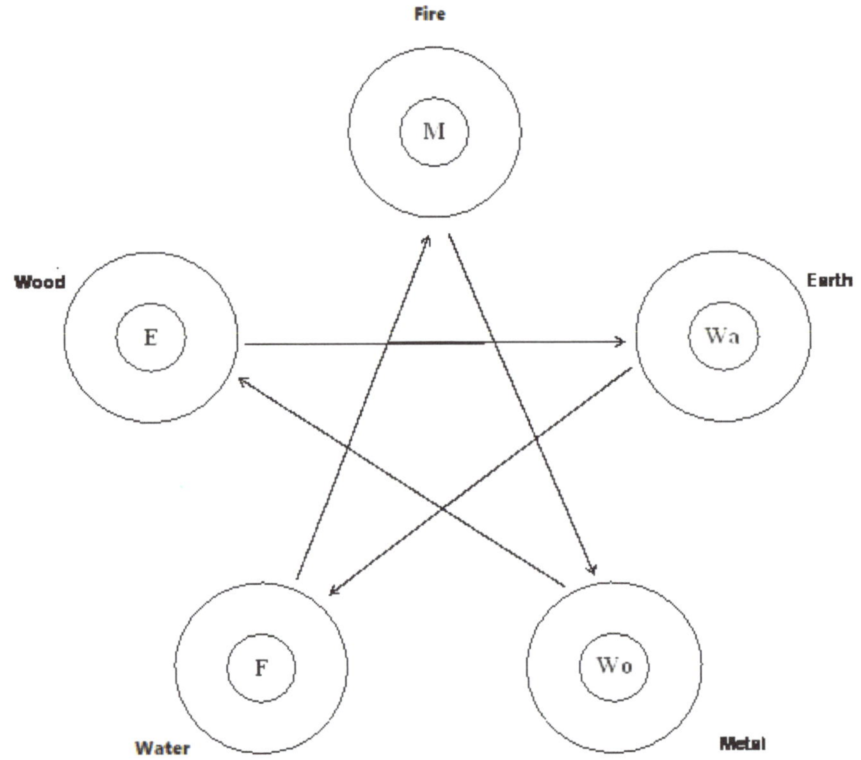

With the sucking powers, the fire sucks the energies of metal.

With its sucking powers, the earth sucks the energies of water.

With its sucking powers, the metal sucks the energies of wood.

With its sucking powers, the water sucks the energies of fire.

With its sucking powers, the wood sucks the energies of earth.

Balance Energy Cycle
(Controlling Energy and Suck/Drain Energy)

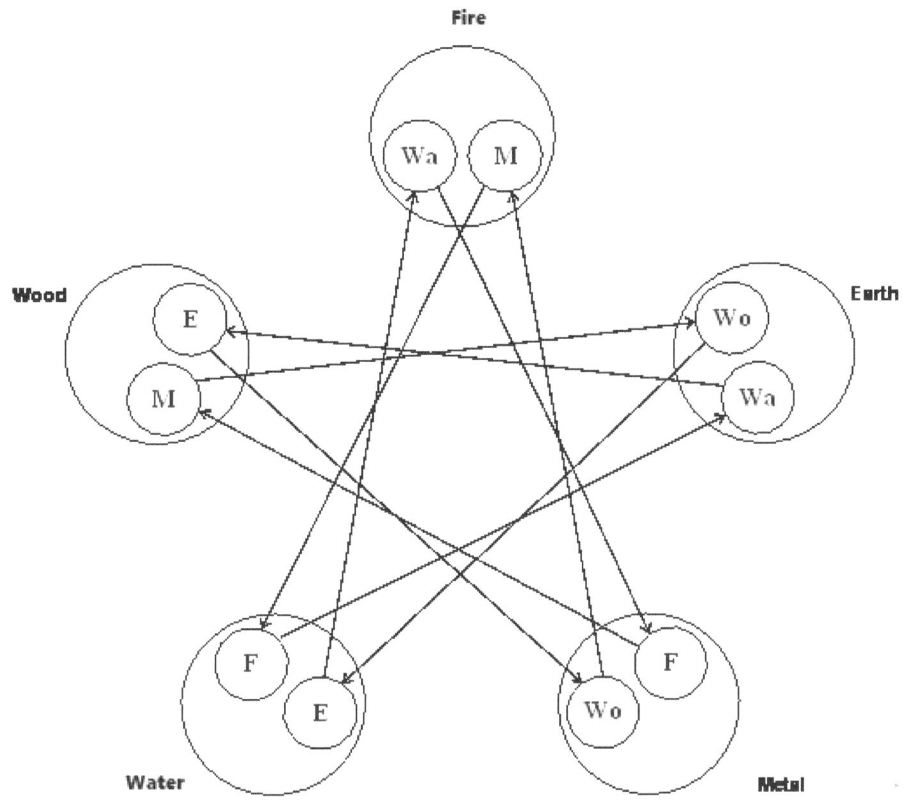

Because of the fire element's balancing energy cycle, the metal energies are neither controlled nor sucked/ drained excessively.

Because of the earth element's balancing energy cycle, the water element's energies are neither controlled nor sucked/drained excessively.

Metal—Because of this element's balancing energy cycle, the wood energies are neither controlled nor sucked/ drained excessively.

Water—Because of this element's balancing energy cycle, the fire energies are neither controlled nor sucked/ drained excessively.

Wood—Because of this element's balancing energy cycle, the earth energies are neither controlled nor sucked/ drained excessively.

1.6 The Connectivity Between the Four Chinese Laws and the Five Cycles

- **Law of Five Element Philosophy.**
- **Law of Mother and Son.**
- **Law of Husband and Wife.**
- **Law of Midday and Midnight.**

(I). The Law of Five Element Philosophy

In this law, the creative and destructive energies are related, because

Creative cycle (page 31) as on page 12.

Mother Element	**Action**	**Impact**	**Son Element**
Wood	Burning process	Fire	Wood creates fire
Fire	After the burning process, ash is the only thing that is left	Earth	If we consider ash as earth, fire creates earth
Earth	Things under earth	Metal	We can consider metal creates earth
Metal	From the melting process, we get water (liquid) because of pressure or air produced, condensation.	Water	If we consider liquid as water, metal creates water
Water	Due to the nutrient's property, water grows	Wood	Water creates wood

Destructive cycle(page 32) as on page 12.

Five elements	**Action**	**Impact**
Wood	Rapid growth	Cover earth
Earth	If Power increase	Sucks water
Water	If Power increase	Extinguish fire
Fire	If Power increase	Melting metal
Metal	If Power increase	Cut trees

(II)The Law of Mother and Son

The life energy is imparted from the mother element to the son element. When the life energy (force) is found to be less, either in a particular energy channel or in an organ, then the mother element of that organ must be kindled or aroused.

In the same way, if it is found that the life force is in excess, then the son element energies must be aroused or kindled. Thus, the enlarging capacity of the mother element will get reversed.

According to this law, the enlargement energy cycle and the atrophy energy cycles are connected.

Mother	Son
Liver	Heart
Heart	Spleen
Spleen	Lungs
Lungs	Kidney
Kidney	Liver

Mother	Son
Liver	Pericardium
Pericardium	Heart
Heart	Spleen
Spleen	Lungs
Lungs	Kidney
Kidney	Liver

Midday Midnight Law (Law of Midday Midnight)

At a particular time of the day, a particular energy channel and specific organs receive more energy. To treat a particular organ or channel, time can be utilized to get better results. This law is connected with the self-energy cycle. Because at a particular time, a particular organ gets more energy, it indicates that the organ's energies are working more.

Time	Organ
3 am–5 am	Lung
5 am–7 am	Large intestine
7 am–9 am	Stomach
9 am–11 am	Spleen
11am–1pm	Heart
1 pm–3pm	Small intestine
3 pm–5 pm	Urinary bladder
5 pm–7 pm	Kidney
7 pm–9 pm	Pericardium
9 pm–11 pm	Triple warmer
11pm–1am	Gall bladder
1 am–3 am	Liver

The Law of Husband and Wife (Husband and Wife Law)

The pulse of one hand is related to the other hand's pulse. This is called the husband-and-wife law. Based on this, the opposite energies of the husband-and-wife law-related organs are all related to the destructive cycle.

This cycle is connected to the control, balancing and suck/drain energy cycles.

1.7 The Organs Related to the Five Elements and the Pulse Diagnosis Method

According to the acupuncture treatment, the following table shows the element and their related organs.

Fire big	Heart, small intestine. (H) (SI)
Fire small	Pericardium and triple warmer. (P) (TW)
Earth	Spleen, stomach. (Sp) (ST)
Metal	Lungs, large intestine. (Lu), (LI)
Water	Kidneys, urinary bladder. (K), (UB)
Wood	Liver, gall bladder. (Liv), (GB)

In acupuncture, the pulse and the related element are described as follows:

Left wrist

Upper layers	Small Intestine (SI)	Gall bladder (GB)	Urinary bladder (UB)
Lower layers	Heart (H)	Liver (LIV)	Kidney (K)

Right wrist

Upper layers	Large Intestine (LI)	Stomach (ST)	Triple Warmer. (TW)
Lower layers	Lungs (LU)	Spleen (SP)	Pericardium (P).

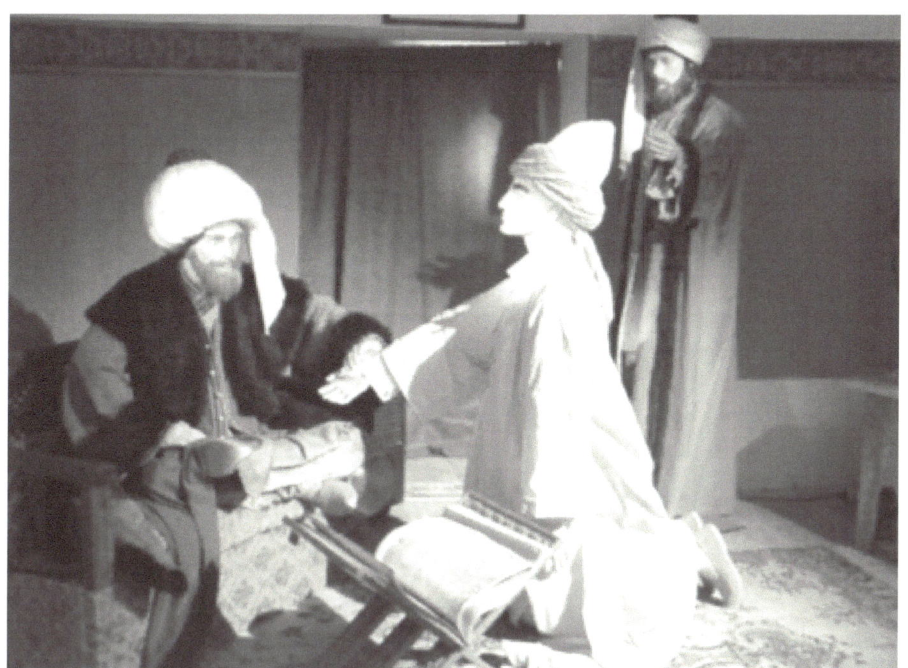

Picture

Ivory Status revealing the ancient Chinese Pulse Diagnosis method.

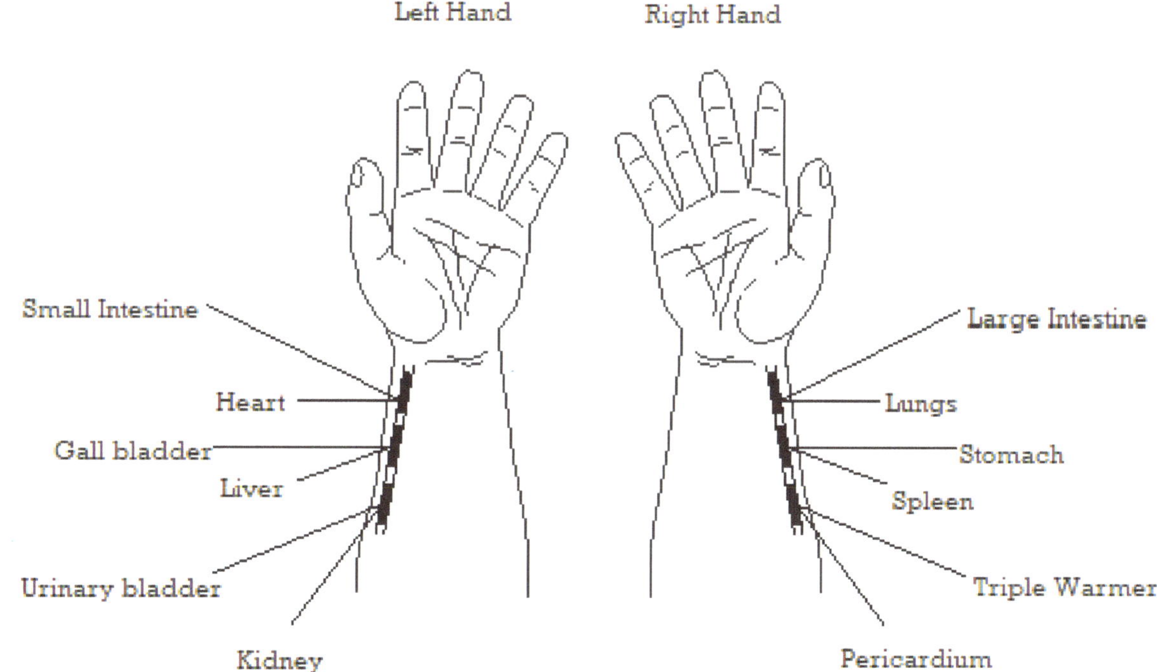

Picture2: (Hands).

The places where the five element organ pulses are diagnosed, according to the acupuncture method

Amongst these, the upper layer pulses help to diagnose the state of these six organs (SI, TW,LI, GB, ST,UB) and diagnose the diseases that occur in their energy channels.

Amongst these, the lower layer pulses help to diagnose the state of their six organs (H,P,LU,LIV,SP,K) and diagnose the diseases that occurred in their energy channels.

The upper layer pulses are related to the ***yang*** energy channels and their organs. Amongst these six pulses, three have the nature of ***yang*** in ***yang*** and the other three have the nature of ***yin*** in the ***yang***.

The three energy channels of ***yang*** in ***yang*** are on the outer side of the hand. They represent the energy channels of SI, TW and LI.

The energy channels of ***yin*** in ***yang*** are on the legs. They represent the GB,SI and UB organs' energy channels.

The lower layer of pulses represents the state of six organs namely H,P,LU,LIV,SP and K. Their energy channels and diseases occur due to the imbalances in their energies.

The lower layer pulses-related organs and their energy channels represent ***yin*** energy.

The three organs and their respective energy channels, representing ***yang*** in ***yin*** run along the hands. They are H,P and LU.

The three organs and their energy channels, representing ***yin*** in ***yin*** run along the legs. They are LIV,SP, and K.

The ***yin***-natured six organs and their energy channels as well as the ***yang***-natured six organs and their energy channels run along the sides of the right and left hands as well as the legs.

The central tracks which unite all the twelve energy channels run through the centre of the body. One is placed in the front and the other at the back. The track which runs along the front centre of the body is called the Conception Vessel and it is of ***yin*** nature. Hence, it stores all the energy.

The energy track that runs along the back centre of the body is called the Governing Vessel which is of a ***yang*** nature. Hence, it utilises the energies and takes them to the whole body.

Through the Pulse Diagnosis method, one can tell a lot about the mind's and body's state (of any patient) without the patient's statement since the ***panchaboodha*** or the five elements present in the human body are also connected to each and everything present in the world. One can analyse which of these elements have problems in the human body with the help of the patient's statement, such as his dress or skin condition. Because each of the elements or ***panchaboodhas*** and its related organ has its colour, taste, smell, dream, imagination, mental state or emotions, feelings, timing, season, day and star, when a particular element and its organ gets affected, then its entire nature, as has been mentioned above, will also get affected.

A person does everything based on his likes and dislikes. Based on this, his needs and diseases are caused. This is because if a person states that he likes a particular food item, thing or colour, then it means that his six ***yang*** organs and their energy channels are affected. In the same way, if a person states that he does not like anything or a particular food or colour, then it means that one or more of his six ***yin*** organs and their energy channels are affected.

Pulse Diagnosis Method

When the upper and lower pulses are diagnosed, then one can diagnose the state in which each of the five elements exists, the function of its organ and the energy state—whether the energy is present or absent.

If the pulse is absent when the organ pulse is diagnosed, then it means that the energy transaction of that organ is not occurring properly or the energy of that organ would have increased and affected the opposite energy channel. In turn, its energy channel would have gotten affected. Or, that specific organ would have gotten affected by the energy which would affect this organ and energy.

When there is excess energy in an organ pulse, it may be due to the excessive energy of that organ.

Or the controlling energy must control this energy would have got affected .Hence, this energy is excessive without control.

Or this organ would have gotten affected and that may also reflect through the pulse pattern not occurring properly, as a result.

If one of the upper layer pulses is excessive, then it indicates that the ***yin*** energy of that organ is spent through the respective ***yang*** organ. This is because the upper layer pulses represent the ***yang*** energy and the ***yang*** spends energy. This indicates acute diseases/conditions. If any one of the upper pulses has a lesser feeling of a sense of energy, then it indicates that the respective ***yin*** energy is not spent from the body but stored as stagnant energy. This is because that ***yang*** organ is not working properly, but it spends energy.

If the energy is in excess in the lower layers, it indicates the presence of either excess energy or stagnant energy. This is because the lower layer pulses are ***yin*** energy pulses, which store the energy. This condition leads to a chronic state of disease. If the energy is less in the lower layers, it indicates that the energy of that specific organ is spent or utilised excessively. This also leads to chronic diseases.

When the pulses are diagnosed as ***panchaboodha*** or the five element pulses in a properly described manner, then each of the elements and its organ will be diagnosed accurately and the linked or disconnected element and its organ from this element and its organ can be analysed immaculately. This not only indicates that element and its organ but also clearly renders the state of other elements and their organs. Through this, the root cause of the disease and the cycle to cure it will be found accurately. The pulses can be diagnosed in any structure, apart from the upper and lower layer method.

The New Pulse Diagnosis Method with Four Layers

The ***yang*** energy channels are situated on the right and left sides of the human body (on both sides of the hands and legs.)

In the same way, the yin energy channels are also situated on the right and left sides of the human body (on both sides of the hands and legs.)

The pulses are diagnosed as the upper and lower layer pulses. On each hand, six organ pulses are diagnosed, which sums up to twelve organ pulses. But there are twenty-four energy channels on both sides of the hands and legs.

If a problem arises on the right side, it is believed that the left side energy channels should be treated and vice versa.

But in the four layers, using the Pulse Diagnosis method, the diagnosis can be done immaculately and each limb's energy channel can be diagnosed separately.

Besides this, the energy level of the affected element is related to the organ, whether it is high or low and the cause for that can be diagnosed accurately through the four layers pulse diagnosis method.

Thus, one can diagnose the accurate, root cause of the health problem.

This method also would indicate the side of the body, whether it is the right or the left, on which the treatment should be done.

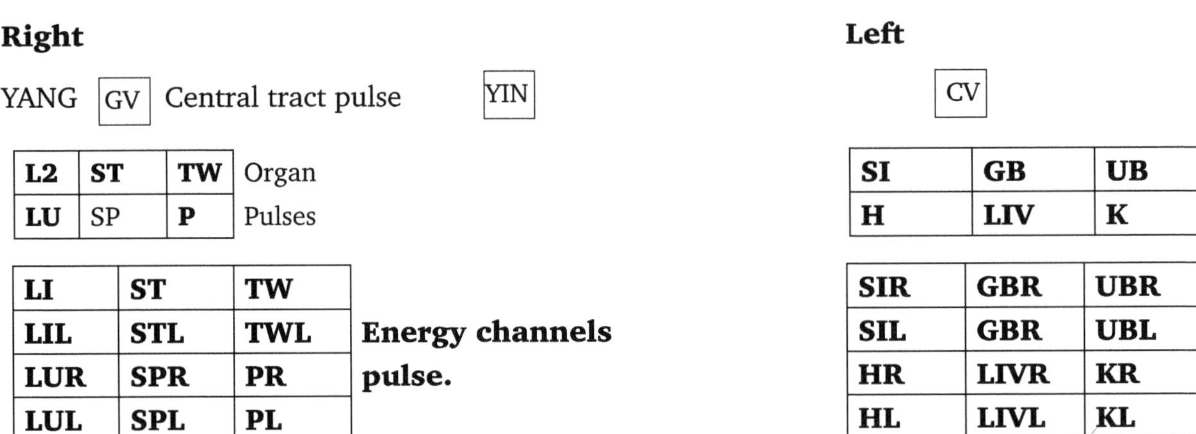

Right **Left**

YANG GV Central tract pulse YIN CV

L2	ST	TW	Organ
LU	SP	P	Pulses

SI	GB	UB
H	LIV	K

LI	ST	TW
LIL	STL	TWL
LUR	SPR	PR
LUL	SPL	PL

Energy channels pulse.

SIR	GBR	UBR
SIL	GBR	UBL
HR	LIVR	KR
HL	LIVL	KL

Left wrist

Upper layer of upper layer	Small intestine pulse (SI) R	Gall bladder pulse (GB) R	Urinary bladder pulse UB R
Lower layer of upper layer	Small intestine pulse (SI) L	Gall bladder pulse (GB) L	Urinary bladder pulse UB L
Upper layer of lower layer	Heart (H) Pulse R	Liver pulse R	Kidney pulse (K) R
Lower layer of lower layer	Heart (H) Pulse L	Liver pulse L	Kidney pulse (K) L

Right wrist

Upper layer of upper layer	Large intestine pulse (LI) R	Stomach (ST) R	Triple warmer (TW) R
Lower layer of upper layer	Large intestine pulse (LI) L	Stomach (ST) L	Triple warmer (TW) L
Upper layer of lower layer	Lungs (L) L	Spleen (SP)R	Pericardium (P) R
Lower layer of lower layer	Lungs (L) L	Spleen (SP) L	Pericardium (P) L

The upper part of the superficial layer of the right wrist helps to diagnose the energy channels of the organs LI,ST and TW of the right hand.

The lower layer pulse of the upper layer of the right wrist helps us to diagnose the energy channel of the organs LI, ST and TW of the left hand.

The upper layer of the lower layer of the right wrist helps us diagnose the energy channels of the organs H,P and LU of the right hand.

The lower layer of the lower part depth (layer)of the left wrist helps us diagnose the energy channels of the organs H,P and LU of the left hand.

The upper layer of the upper layer of the left wrist helps us diagnose the energy channels of the organs GB,ST and UB of the right leg.

The lower layer of the upper layer of the left wrist helps us diagnose the energy channels of the organs GB,ST and UB of the left leg.

The upper layer of the lower layer on the left wrist helps us diagnose the energy channels of the organs LIV, SP and K of the right leg.

The lower layer of the lower layer of the left wrist helps us diagnose the energy channels of the organs LIV,SP and K of the left leg.

Note

One can diagnose all the twenty-four pulses in the same place, that is, the left pulse which can be diagnosed in the right pulse's place and the right side pulse can be diagnosed on the left side.

1.8 Panchaboodha (Six Elements) Acupuncture Points—72

Element points		Wood	Fire small	Fire big	Earth	Metal	Water
Three *yin* energy channels on the hands.	Lung LU	Lu11	Lu10	LU9.5	LU9	LU8	LU5
	Pericardium P	P9	P8	P7.5	P7	P5	P3
	Heart H	H9	H8	H7.5	H7	H4	H3
Three *yin* energy channels on the legs.	Spleen SP	SP1.5	SP2.5	SP2	SP3	SP5	SP9
	Liver LIV	LIV1	LIV5	LIV2	LIV3	LIV4	LIV8
	Kidney K	K1	K2	K3	K6	K7	K10

Element points		Metal	Water	Wood	Fire small	Fire Big	Earth
Three *yang* energies on the hands.	Large Intestine LI	LI1	LI2	LI3	LI4	LI5	LI11
	Triple warmer TW	TW1	TW2	TW3	TW4	TW6	TW10
	Small Intestine SI	SI1	SI2	SI3	SI4	SI5	SI6
Three *yang* energies on the legs.	Stomach ST	ST45	ST44	ST43	ST42	ST41	ST36
	Gall bladder	GB44	GB43	GB41	GB40	GB38	GB34
	Urinary bladder	UB67	UB66	UB65	UB62	UB60	UB54

In the acupuncture theory, only sixty points are said to be the five elements' points. Amongst these, the point for the fire small of each element is not stated. When conducting the research as per the above-stated table, the stated points are found to represent the fire small. Hence these points are stated as fire small.

Five elements	Internal organs	Emotions	Colour	Taste
Fire big	The small intestine, heart	Happy, without happiness	Red	Bitter
Fire small	Triple warmer, pericardium	Frustrated, hatred	Orange	Astringent
Earth	Stomach, spleen	Worry, no worries	Yellow	Sweet
Metal	Lung, large intestine	Anger, no anger, irritation	White	Spicy
Water	Kidney, urinary bladder	Fear, fearless	Black	Salt
Wood	Liver, Gall bladder	Weeping, without weeping, sorrow	Green	Sour

Reasons for the Onset of the Diseases

External reasons

- No proper ventilation.
- Excess ventilation or air.
- Chillness
- Summer heat
- Wetness
- Dryness

Internal reasons

- Excessive happiness
- No enthusiasm
- Deep disconsolation
- Deep sorrow
- Fear
- Panic/horrors
- Insomnia
- Excessive sleep
- Excessive anger

- Excessive weeping
- Excessive frustration
- Excessive hatred
- Excessive worries
- Excessive panic

Other reasons

- Injury
- Related to food (excessive hunger or anorexia)
- Liquor
- Less hygiene
- Excessive brain work
- No exercise
- Excessive sex
- Excessive excretion of urine, sweat and faeces
- Insufficient excretion of urine, sweat and faeces

1.9 The Reasons for the Formation of Diseases

The State of Diseases

The Cause of Diseases.

***Zang* organs(also known as *yang* organs)**

The Heart and pericardium

- It regulates the functions of the mind. Hence, it cures mind-related diseases.
- Controls blood circulation.
- The heart is connected to the tongue. Hence, it cures diseases related to the tongue.
- The heart (*yin*/female)forms a pair with the small intestine (*yang*/male) so the heart channel may help to rectify small intestine-related diseases.
- The pericardium—yin (female)forms a pair with the triple warmer—yang (male). Hence, it helps to balance the body temperature.

The Lungs

- Controls breath
- The lungs' external opening is the nose.
- Balances the skin and the hair on the body.
- The lungs (*yin*/female)form a pair with the large intestine (*yang*/male).
- This lung channel helps to cure ENT problems.

The Spleen

- Balances digestion.
- Water-related metabolism is balanced.
- Controls the blood circulation in the blood vessels.
- Controls reticuloendothelial system. (Production of blood cells).
- Protects the soft muscles like the heart muscles.
- The external opening of the spleen is the mouth.
- This pairs with the stomach.
- Helps to control the excessive production of water in the body.

The Liver.

- The liver secretes bile.
- Protects the tendons and endocrine glands.
- This is related to the eye.
- The liver is paired with the gall bladder.
- This has an important role in the growth and the dimensional growth of body muscles.

The Kidneys.

- Related to the ear.
- Responsible for the skeletal system and its growth
- Related to the growth of the hair on the head.
- Related to the genitals.
- The kidneys are paired with the urinary bladder.
- Has an important role in diseases related to the water in the body. Responsible for excreting excessive water from the body.

Fu Organs.

- Stomach.
- Small intestine.
- Large intestine.
- Gall bladder.
- Urinary bladder.
- Triple warmer.
- These organs are responsible for the assimilation of food and the excretion of unwanted things inside the body.

Classical System of Meridians and Acupuncture Points

There are approximately seven hundred acupuncture points in the human body. Amongst them ,three hundred and sixty-one points exist in fourteen special channels and the others are placed near them.

Explanation of the fourteen channels.

Six channels are on the hands.	**Six channels are on the legs.**
Amongst these, three belong to *Yin*.	**Amongst these, three belong to *Yin*.**
The other three belong to *Yang*.	**The other three belong to *Yang*.**

The three channels belong to *yang* and *yin*.

The ***yang*** channels run on the outer side of the hand. The ***yin*** channels run on the inner side of the hand.

It works the same way on the legs where the ***yin*** and ***yang*** channels are situated.

The rest of the two tracks are situated in the middle of the trunk. In the front, it is called the Conception Vessel, and at the back, it is called the Governing Vessel.

Through the upper side ***yang*** channels of the hand, the life energy enters through the fingers and reaches the face.

Then it reaches the chest through the leg-related ***yin*** channels from the face.

From there, it travels through the ***yin*** channels of the hands, which starts from the chest and reaches the fingers. A part of the Chinese people follow this philosophy—that each of the ***yang*** channels combines with the ***yin***, becomes paired and spread like a net across the body.

The Paired Channels

- Heart with Small Intestine.
- Lung with Large Intestine.
- Pericardium with Triple Warmer.
- Spleen with Stomach.
- Liver with Gall Bladder.
- Kidney with Urinary Bladder.

The appropriate path on which the life energy travels.

LU—Lung channel—LI Large intestine channel

SP— Spleen channel—ST Stomach channel

H—Heart channel—SI Small intestine channel

K—Kidney channel—UB Urinary bladder channel

P—Pericardium channel—TW Triple warmer channel

LIV—Liver channel—GB Gall bladder channel

Apart from these twelve important pairs of channels, there are eight separate main tracks, which include the Conception Vessel and Governing Vessel.

Motor Gate Theory

The G-1 and G-2 entering points of the backbone get closed because of the onset of diseases, such as paralysis and polio. Acupuncture helps to open or kindle them and thus, helps the nervous system work properly.

Gate Control Theory

Substantia gelatinosa in our spinal cord has a part through which the feeling of pain is transmitted to the brain. Using the acupuncture method on this point, we can make this point numb or stop the transmission of pain to the brain.

Endorphin Explanation

According to Mr. Bruce Pemorang, the pain gets reduced through acupuncture due to the secretion of endorphins. This acts as morphine and like other opiates, the impulses are transmitted through the transmitters in the muscles to the brain, where the pituitary gland secretes the endorphin. This endorphin, along with other opiates, stops the impulses of pain.

The Diseases and Symptoms Based on the *Yin*and *Yang*.

***Yin* Type**	***Yang* Type**
Cold diseases.	**Heat diseases.**
***Xu* diseases. (Chronic diseases) (*Shi*) long duration diseases**	***Chi* diseases.(Acute)**
Chilliness of the body	**Excessive heat.**
No thirst	**Thirsty**
Pale face	**Bright face**
Excessive phlegm in the lungs	**Dry cough with thick phlegm**
Difficulties in breathing	**Rapid breathing**
Diarrhoea	**Constipation**
Pain reduces if pressed with pressure	**Pain increases if pressed with pressure**
Excessive urine without colour	**Less urine with difficulty**
Shallow pulse	**Fast pulse**
Pale tongue with white coating	**Red tongue with dry white/yellow coating**
Lethargic	**Anxious**
With heat, the pain reduces	**With chillness pain reduces**
Likes hot food	**Likes cold food**
Less bleeding for more days during menstruation	**Frequent, excessive bleeding during menstruation**
Clear watery white discharge white in colour	**Thick yellow-white discharge with bad odour**

Five Elements Acupuncture Points

These five-element acupuncture points are situated in every channel. These are also called the five ***Shu*** points. Generally, they are located on people's hands—between the tip of the fingers and the elbow as well as located in the area between the toe fingers and knees on the legs.

According to the general philosophy, the mother point must be strengthened and the son point does not need to be strengthened.

Example.

1. **Gall Bladder:** The gall bladder energy channel is the wood element according to the five element principles. The mother element of wood is water. Hence, we must strengthen the GB 43—the water print in the wood channel. The son element of wood is fire. So, we must do **Tonification** on GB 38, which is the fire point of G.B.
2. **Stomach:** If the stomach pulse energy is less during the Pulse Diagnosis, then the mother element of the stomach should be strengthened. The mother element of earth is fire. Hence, fire must be strengthened, that is, ST41.

Clinical Examination.

- Diagnosis of one's pulse, checking one's body temperature, examining the nails, the eyes, the neck, boils on the skin or any change on the skin and examining the throat.
- Systematic examination of the stomach, the throat, the heart, the muscles, the bones and the nerves through the conditions of the related organs.
- Doctor's examination of the patient by observation.
- Examining by touch and tapping.

Special clinical test: After diagnosing the symptoms, giving special importance to certain tests, such as a proto scope can diagnose colon cancer, etc.

Investigation

- Laboratory tests on sputum, blood, urine, ECG, EEG, blood count, urea and cholesterol in human blood, and specific tests, such as VDRL and widal tests can be done to diagnose illnesses.
- Diagnosis through biopsy.
- An autopsy to help diagnose the reason for which the person died.

Diagnosis Based on the Chinese Method to Diagnose the Root Cause of the Disease

There were many diagnosis methods to help diagnose the patient's illness or to identify the root cause of the disease in ancient times when there was no modern equipment.

Inspection: Observing the patient by standing in front of him.

Auscultation: Before the invention of the stethoscope, the doctors listened to the sounds produced by the body of the patient, by pressing the doctor's ears on the patient's body.

Smelling: Diagnosis based on the odour of the patient.

Case history: Probing the patient to talk about the history of the illness.

Percussion-Palpation: Diagnosis through the pulse beat.

Laboratory: Diagnosing through the tests conducted in the laboratories (on the faeces, phlegm, urine, blood, etc., of the patient.)

By diagnosing the ears: Specific points on the ears will get affected and become reddish and inflamed. The doctor will compare that point with its relevant organ and diagnose accordingly.

There is an occurrence of frequent cysts or boils.

Family history can be obtained through conversation with the closest relative of the patient, such as parents, an uncle, an aunt, a wife, etc.

Diagnosis Methods

Modern Diagnostic Methods

Case history: The suffering of the patient, duration of his/her occupation, his/her income, circumstances, previous health history and family history.

Systematized Diagnosis Method of Acupuncture

- One can apply all the modern methods of diagnosis.
- Can touch and see the sensitivity of the ***Ah-shi*** points/alarm points.
- Can use the point detector after examining the ears.
- Before starting the acupuncture treatment, the doctor must diagnose the patient through the Pulse Diagnosis method.

Zang–Fu Philosophy

According to the ancient method, ***Zang*** refers to solid organs and ***Fu*** refers to shallow organs. (Organs which have grooves in them.)

The ***Zang*** organs have the ***yin*** nature of storing the life energy (H,P,LIV,K,SP and LU).

Whereas the ***Fu*** organs have a ***yang*** nature through which they use up the life energy or even discard or waste the energy. (SI, TW, GB, LI,UB and ST).

1.10 The Insomniac Condition and Dreams Are also Symptoms of the Diseases

Let us discuss sleep as well as dreams during sleep and how they are related to the disease.

An average human must sleep for an average of eight hours and that sleep must be a deep and peaceful sleep. The meditators can sleep for six hours.

During this deep sleep only, the food and water eaten by the person get converted into blood and energy.

All the organs in the body get refreshed.

The whole body gets energised and the body is restored with vital energy, health, stamina and strength.

The best time considered to sleep is from 9pm to 5 am or from 10pm to 6am.

Sleep during these hours indicates the healthy condition of the body. Sleeping at other times of the day indicates that they are a symptom of diseases/conditions since the twelve important organs of our bodies continue to work constantly for twenty-four hours per day.

Large Intestine:(5 am to 7 am)

Though all the organs work throughout the day, there are specific times for the specific organs when they work their best. The large intestine works at its best from5 am to 7 am. While we sleep at night, the consumed food and water get digested and absorbed by the body.

The undigested food and the waste from the consumed food after assimilation will be pushed to the large intestine. Thus, the large intestine becomes ready to eliminate the food and waste from our bodies in the morning. By excreting the faecal matter, all the other organs also get ready to do their work for that day. Patients with defects in the energy of the large intestine cannot wake up early in the morning. They will always have their minds set up to sleep further and cannot get up from bed in the morning. This will make them sluggish and lethargic throughout that day and the person will be in active. If this condition continues, it will lead to constipation. Due to the weakness of the large intestine, parasites and germs will affect it. Because of these germs and parasites as well as their contamination, it will create sinusitis, cough and phlegm.

Some patients will get dysentery or diarrhoea with stomach pain within these two hours of the time taken for the large intestine to be active (5 am to 7 am). In chronic conditions, this will continue even after 7 am for some hours.

Hour of Need for a Good Transformation

Some of us may have the desire to wake up early in the morning. But due to fatigue and excessive pain in the body and limbs, some of us cannot get up from our beds. Even if people wake up, they cannot stand or walk immediately. Slowly, after the senses on their limbs are activated, their bodies will become normal. Usually, these patients get scared of such fatigue and will not get up in the morning.

Because of the contamination in the large intestine, which in turn affects the sinus glands, asthmatic patients will experience nose blockages, sneezing, watery eyes and runny noses, at the time of the activation of the large intestine, that is, between 5 am and 7 am. They may become normal at other times of the day.

All these symptoms and problems can be removed, just by strengthening the large intestine. We can completely cure the patients with the above-mentioned symptoms without the need for any test that identifies the parasites or germs, which affect the large intestine or the application of any medicine. This is achieved by strengthening the large intestine using acupuncture treatment. Just by strengthening the large intestine, the energy and blood circulation can become normal in the large intestine and hence, the LI will become healthy. Thus, immunity will be restored to help the body fight against infections.

Constipation, asthma and sinusitis will start to diminish.

The sluggishness and tendency to fall asleep during the day will disappear.

Acupuncture can create such wonderful changes.

The same patients will feel pain in the lower lumber area during the LI time, around 5 am. This indicates the weakness of the large intestine. A particular acupuncture point in that area becomes paralysed, causes that pain and makes the patient wake up and even get up from bed.

For this pain, patients are advised to undergo traction treatment and are advised to use tools like the hip belt. However, the pain can be easily cured by strengthening the acupuncture point.

Dreams

Dreams occur due to the weakness of the large intestine—mostly related to the faecal and urinary matters. In the dreams, the patients defecate in public and try to hide it. If such dreams involving faeces occur often, it indicates the weakness of the large intestine's energy. Dreams related to anger also indicate problems with the large intestine.

Stomach

7 am to 9 am: These two hours are the prime time for the stomach's energy to be activated. If we eat during this time, the food will get digested and assimilated well by the whole body and gives energy to the organs. That is the reason why we eat our breakfast between these hours.

If the stomach does not function properly, then the loss of appetite will occur initially. These people will not eat breakfast at all. This habit of avoiding eating breakfast will make the patient weak.

Every day, at 8 am, some people will have a sort of weakness, such as tremors. The body will have extreme weakness, and one's eyesight will be diminished. Then, automatically, everything will become normal. These symptoms indicate that the stomach region is weaker and without enough energy. According to acupuncture, nervous weakness would occur.

Some people have the urge to excrete urine and stool immediately after eating food. They may feel the urge to use the restroom every ten minutes after eating food, unfortunately. They will have this symptom from 7 am to 9 am. They will be forced to spend time in the toilet and hence, they cannot concentrate on other activities. This indicates the inefficiency of the stomach. This disease is called IBS and can be cured very easily with the help of acupuncture.

Dreams

When the stomach is affected, the related dreams will be about the death of very close relatives, loss in the business, worms in the stomach, as well as being unable to eat, even if there is surplus food. These dreams will disturb one's sleep. They may also have land-related dreams and in general, dreams which make patients feel sorrowful.

Spleen: 9 am to 11 am.

We get energy and become brisk immediately after eating. This is because of the good condition of the spleen.

Contradicting to this state, if a person feels heaviness, belching, phlegm formation in the throat or sleepiness, it indicates that the spleen is not functioning properly and the energy is blocked.

Every morning, at 10 am, persons with such problems with their spleen energy will become extremely sleepy without having any control over their sleep patterns. Even in the office, such patients work while experiencing sleepiness. Though others think that these people are lazy, the real problem lies in the changes in the nature of the spleen.

Dreams

Excessive eating, phlegm in the throat and coughing in sleep are some symptoms amongst patients. This cough will disturb one's sleep. If the cough occurs along with dreams, then it is due to the inefficiency of the spleen. Land-related dreams and grief-related dreams are often seen by such patients.

Heart: 11 am to 1 pm

Between these two hours, the heart functions with full energy. People who have less energy in their hearts will not like these two hours. They cannot come out in the sun. People get sun strokes during this time because of their weak hearts. They feel very sleepy during these hours. Their body temperature may rise and they may feel feverish. This may happen every day or on an alternate day during these two hours.

These people can sleep only if they have many pillows under their heads and necks. These patients, for sure, cannot sleep using one pillow. Some will sweat while they sleep to such an extent that the pillows will get wet.

Dream

Fire and fire-related dreams are mostly seen by such patients. They get dreams as though they are caught in a fire accident and are not able to escape. They may also feel as though they are not able to move their limbs when they want to go to a place in the dream. This indicates the paralytic condition of the limb, which would occur later. They also dream of someone chasing them. They sweat profusely and wake up with a jolt. They can never sleep peacefully. The dreams will start immediately after they fall asleep. These dreams will continue till the person wakes up from his sleep.

Acupuncture very clearly explains that these continuous dreams, till they wake up, occur because of the reduced energy in the heart.

Their Dreams will be happy dreams—agriculture-related dreams.

Small Intestine: 1 pm–3pm

We feel hungry in the afternoon, only after the twelve feet long small intestine absorbs all the food from the stomach. The small intestine works at its best only during these two hours. If the SI does not work properly, then one will not have an appetite or feel hungry in the afternoon.

They will feel as though their breakfast is still inside their stomach and feel extreme heaviness. Because the food is not digested and assimilated in the small intestine, unwanted gases will be produced and bloating will occur.

Gastric problems, burping, stomach upset, a sour taste while burping, chest burning, as well as mouth ulcers will occur. The abdomen will look like a pot. Many people sleep for at least half an hour after eating.

Those who work actively in the afternoon after eating lunch, have a small intestine which is in good shape.

If the acupuncture points of the small intestine are strengthened, all the above problematic symptoms can be solved immediately.

Dreams: Fire-related dreams and dreams related to their desire.

Urinary Bladder: 3 am–5 pm

Patients with an ailment in the urinary bladder will have back pain while lying down and sleeping at night. They cannot lie on their backs for a long duration. They toss and turn on the bed while they sleep. They cannot have a good posture while they sleep due to back pain. They cannot stretch their legs and sleep. The back muscles of the legs may feel like they have cramps. They will be disturbed constantly by neck pain too. While sleeping, the back of the head, the nape and the neck, may feel numb or may experience pain—as if they are being pulled sharply with a hook.

All these problems can be immediately cured by strengthening the urinary bladder with acupuncture treatment.

Dreams: Water, waterfalls-related dreams, Fear-related dreams.

Kidneys: 5pm–7 pm

If a person says that he/she becomes very tired after 5 pm, feels fatigued, feels like sleeping or has tremors in the limbs after 5pm, this indicates that his/her energy flow to the kidneys is repaired.

Asthma patients can be categorised based on the time of the attack. If their problems are aggravated between 5pm and 7pm, then asthma is caused by the kidney's energy in a faulty condition. If it is between 9 am and 11 am, then it is caused by the spleen. If it is aggravated between 3am and 5am, then it is caused by the lungs.

Hence, the reason for having asthma is identified and cured by acupuncture treatment.

But in the other treatment method, asthma is said to be caused only by the lungs. So, they treat the lungs and cannot cure asthma.

Sometimes, an asthma attack can be created due to the energy problem in the heart.

Sleep

The sleeping position of the kidney-affected people will be very different and they can only lie down on their stomachs. They can sleep comfortably only on their stomachs. One must continuously rub the calf muscles, legs and thighs or else someone must press their legs by standing on them. The patient will feel comfortable with more weight and pressure on their legs.

Patients with the faulty kidney energy can sleep only after such vigorous pressing or massages for about half an hour to one hour. These patients suffer by not being able to fall asleep. Some may ask the children to stand and press the part of their bodies from their heels to the hips. The reason is the initiating place of the kidney channel is the heel and it travels to the hips.

If the children do not have enough energy in their kidneys, they will urinate in their beds, even up to the age of thirteen or fourteen years.

After the age of fourteen, if the sperm is discharged spontaneously during sleep, it is normal.

But if this discharge occurs often or daily, then it indicates the weakness of the kidney. The reason is the tiredness of the kidney. This will lead to fatigue in the body. Some of these patients will start talking in their sleep. Some will go on chewing using their teeth, while some will start walking in their sleep.

Some may get epileptic seizures while they sleep. All these are due to the weakness of the kidneys.

Dreams

Persons having problems with the kidney's energy will have excessive fear and an inferiority complex. Their dreams will make them fearful. In general, they get dreams, such as being caught alone in a higher place, feeling scared to look down, becoming desperate to get down, always being chased by animals, being pursued by enemies or getting trapped by animals. They will feel very scared and it will affect their sleep.

The fearful or anxiety-ridden dreams related to examinations, like attending examinations without preparing themselves properly, not being able to write the examination and feeling scared and helpless etc., are also related to weakness of the kidneys.

Excessive sex-related dreams, dreams in which animals, worms and birds get created in the sperm and excessive spontaneous discharge of the sperm are also related to the weakness of the kidneys.

Pericardium:7 pm to 9 pm

The pericardium is the outer sack of the heart. According to allopath treatment, it has no greater significance but in acupuncture, it is one of the major organs. This protects the heart like a fort. Any heart-related problem can affect the heart only by travelling through the pericardium. Hence, it is very important to protect the pericardium to avoid heart disease.

Acupuncture has a large and separate unit to explain the importance of the pericardium, the role of the pericardium, the diseases caused by its malfunction and how to overcome it.

The symptoms such as heaviness in the chest or a blocked feeling while eating, chest burning after eating, bloating of the stomach and a feeling such as piercing in the chest due to gastric problems exist. It travels from the pericardium to the heart. This causes heart failure later in life.

Sleep

Though there is enough time to sleep, the patients cannot fall asleep with a malfunctioning pericardium. They try their level best to fall asleep and go on tossing and turning in bed. They finally get up feeling irritated and not being able to sleep. But when they want to do an important job with full consciousness, they will fall asleep or feel sleepy automatically when they are involved in an important job.

Dreams

They feel heaviness in their chests, feel as if their hearts are going to burst, or feel as if someone is pressing very hard on their chest, etc., while they are in deep sleep.

Due to this, their sleep will get disturbed and they may have palpitations.

Triple warmer:9 pm–11 pm

The malfunction of this organ creates an imbalance in the body temperature and the patient will feel the heat in some parts and cold in other parts of the body. Some of these types of patients will feel more heat in the palms and feet than the other parts of the body, whereas some may feel more chilliness in the palms and feet than other parts of the body. They may sweat profusely on their palms and feet.

Sleep

Patients with a problem in the triple warmer cannot sleep without a blanket covering them. Even if a room's temperature is high, they will clad themselves like a millipede and sleep. They cannot sleep in absolute darkness. Hence, they will have a mild lamplight on and go to sleep.

Dreams

Such patients do not have many dreams. Once they are warmly clad and covered with a blanket, they go into a deep sleep stage and nothing can wake them up. If dreams occur, they will be related to anxiety and suspicion.

Gall bladder:11 pm–1 am

A gallbladder works completely only during these two hours. Persons who eat excessive spices and flavoured food may experience blocks in the energy channels of the gall bladder.

Because of this, they succumb to indigestion. This indigested food creates heat in the body and spreads throughout the body. Because of this, the patients may have swellings or pain in certain parts of the body.

Sleep

Since heat will be created under the skin, muscles and bones, these patients may experience shifting pain and swellings in various places of the body. A patient cannot lie down in any way they like. They must lie down keeping the body's pain in mind. Even a mild change of position will create pain and disturb sleep.

These patients should take care to avoid injury and lie down. Even the blowing wind can cause pain. They cannot get up and walk immediately after getting up.

These patients experience a burning sensation along with the pain. The burning sensation will become very high—as if they were rubbed with raw chilli powder and then the pain will subside. If the pain increases, then the burning will reduce. Like this, the pain and burning occur alternatively and will affect sleep. Though the patient will feel sleepy, it will be disturbed by this pain and burning sensation.

Some of them fear wearing clothes. They wear items that are loose because of a burning sensation and pain. Some hang their legs and hands outside the bed, because the bed may give them pain and a burning feeling. Some will have a fan, especially blowing on the parts of their bodies which burn.

Dreams

Related to forests.

Liver:1 am–3 am

The last organ, to which the food that we eat reaches is the liver. This separates the toxins from the blood and cleans it. The patients with liver problems will get up from deep sleep at 1 am and sleep again at 3 am. All other disciplines except acupuncture do not consider this sort of waking up and sleeping as a disorder.

Only acupuncture can cure this state of disturbed sleep, and it helps a person sleep well and wake up with energy.

Sleep

When the liver is not able to work properly, it cannot separate the toxins and eliminates them from the body. Hence, the skin will get inflammation. In the state of sleep, the patient may scratch his skin excessively and due to this, the inflammation becomes excessive.

Dreams

Usually related to anger, dreams related to homicidal acts and disturbed sleep due to indigestion.

Lungs: 3 am to 5 am

These two hours are like hell for asthma patients. They will be in deep sleep when exactly at 3 am, mild wheezing, nose blockage or a mild cough will start. At 4 am, the symptoms will be very severe and by 5 am, all the observed symptoms will start to subside. This is because some of the energies which must be from the skin by the lungs are blocked. Since the lungs are not able to get enough energy to work at the maximum level during that time, the fluids in the lungs such as phlegm and mucus increase and create asthma.

Sleep

Patients with lung disorders cannot sleep in a normal posture. They cannot sleep if they lie down. They experience suffocation and a blocked chest. They sleep either by sitting or in a slanted posture. Some may lie down on their stomachs with their hands spread widely.

Patients with lung disorders will sweat excessively only when they are sleeping. Generally, the sweat will be excessive around the neck, underarms, thighs, etc. Once the sweat is produced in excess, the allergy, phlegm, etc., will also become excessive.

By using acupuncture treatment, these lung patients can be cured at any point in time.

Dream

Dreams related to weeping, forests and mountains.

Cannot sleep between 3 am and 5 am.

NOTE

(Like the timing chart of acupuncture, Professor Dr. Aathi Jothi Babu has invented a new timing chart based on the six tastes.)

Though all the organs are working for about twenty-four hours per day, the functioning of the organs differs based on taste. This was discovered by Professor Dr. Aathi Jothi Babu. For example, spicy small: 6 am–7 am, bitter small: 7 am–8am, astringent: 8 am–9am, again astringent big: 9 am–10am, bitter big: 10 am–11am, spicy: 11 am–12 noon.

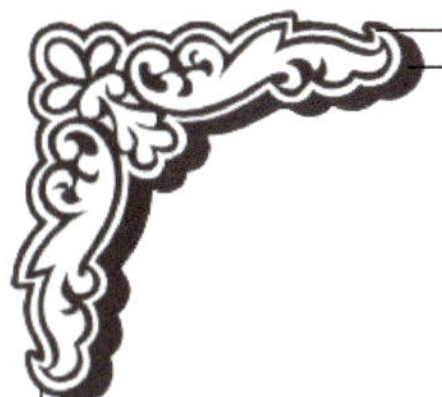
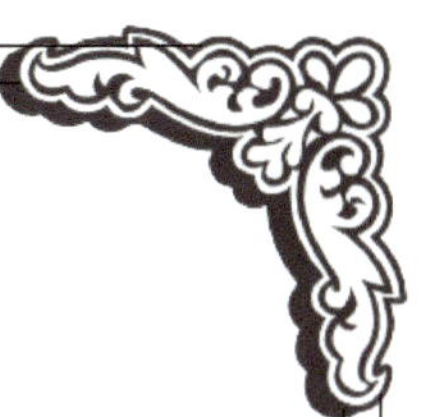

Part Two

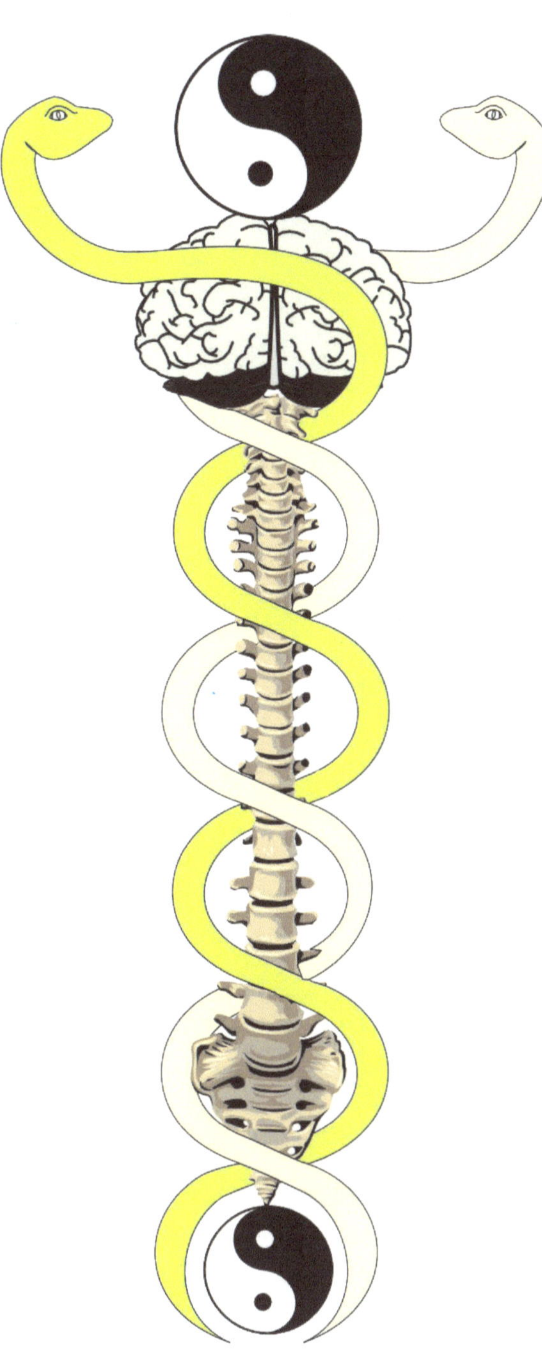

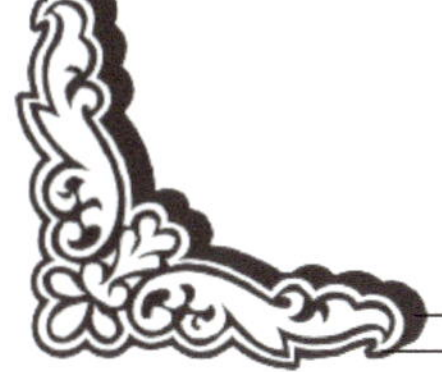

2.1. Large Intestine channel (L.I) six element points method

2.2. Small Intestine channel (S.I.) six element points method

2.3. Triple Warmer (T. W.) six element points method

2.1. Large Intestine Meridian—(L.I.)

Based on the Six Elements

This starts from the index finger's outer side's edge, travels between the first and the second bones of the hand, upwards through the outer side of the elbow's fold, reaches the seventh inner bone of the neck and runs on the front side of it to reach the Clavicle (collarbone). It then goes through the pit on top of it to reach the large intestine by passing through the diaphragm. The branch of this goes up through the outer side of the neck, crosses the cheeks as well as the lips and travels in the front side of the nose to join the stomach.

The time of maximum energy flow is—5am–7am.

The element of L.I. - Metal.

Parallel channel - Lung.

Type of energy - ***Yang***.

The number of points in this meridian - Twenty.

Diseases are cured by puncturing the important points in this meridian.	pain in the large intestine, Breathing related diseases, allergies and constipation.

(From page 62) Diagram 2.1. Large intestine channel (*Yang*).

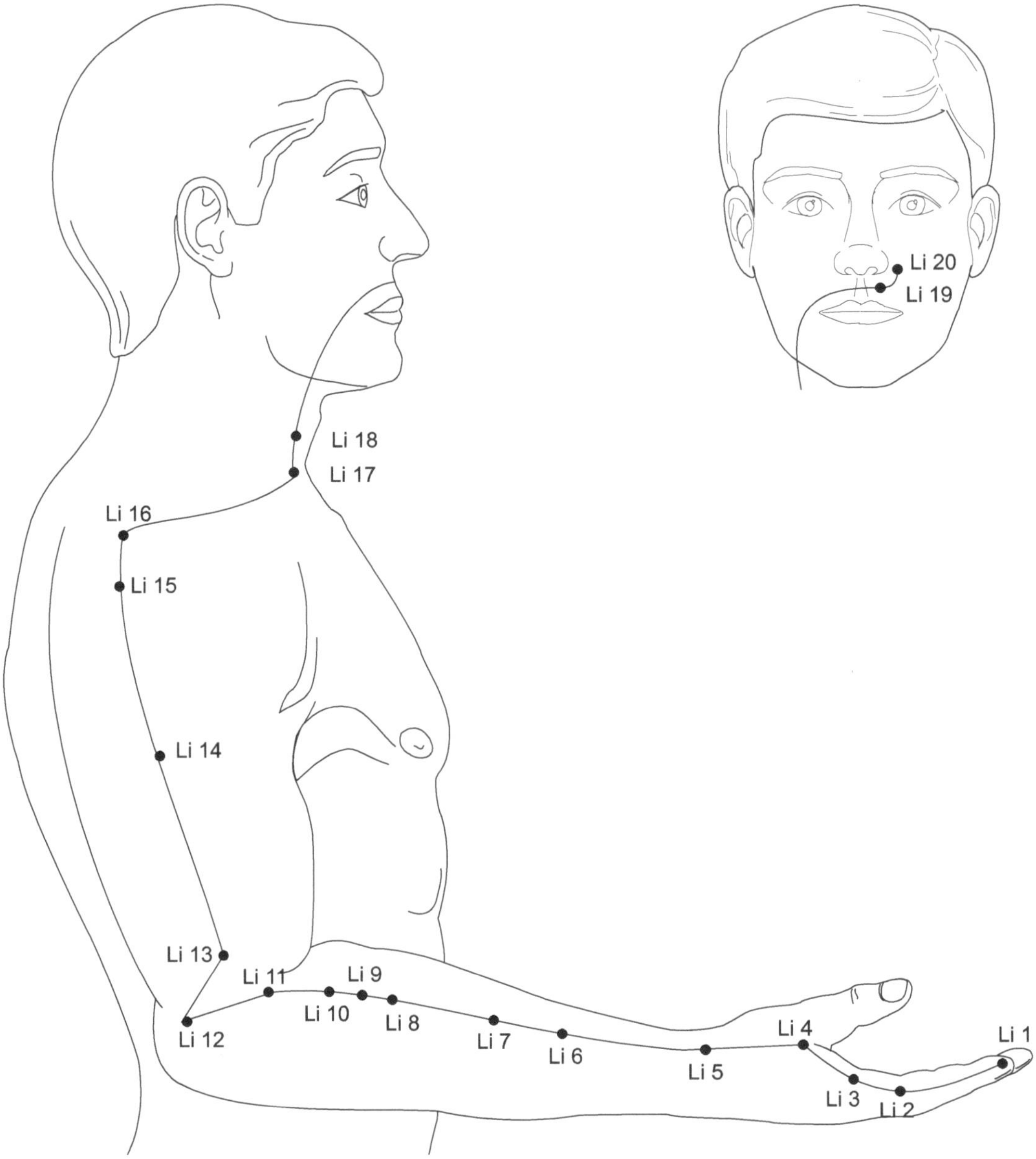

The Lang Intestine (yang) channel of Hand

20 Points

Six Elements Points

Li 1 ⟶ Metal point ⟶ (\ )

Li 2 ⟶ Water point ⟶ (—)

Li 3 ⟶ Wood point ⟶ (I)

Li 4 ⟶ II Fire point ⟶ (II✓)

Li 5 ⟶ I Fire point ⟶ (I ✓)

Li 11 ⟶ Earth point ⟶ (/)

Diseases Which Can Be Cured by Touching the Six Element Points on the Large Intestine.

L.I.—1:Metal point.

Cough, swelling of lips, sudden or acute fever, hearing impairment, dryness of the mouth, swelling of the gums, swelling of the neck, a choked throat, toothache, diarrhoea and jaundice.

L.I.—2: Water point.

Toothache, shoulder pain, facial paralysis or facial palsy tremors, fatigue in the tongue, intestinal pain, diarrhoea and jaundice.

L.I.—3: Wood point.

Numbness in the throat, a choked throat, pain in the eyes, swelling of the tongue, blistered lips, swelling of the nose, a blocked nose, toothache and twisting pain in the body.

L.I.— 4: Second fire point.

Tonsillitis, body pain, headaches, excess phlegm, constipation, hip pain or waist pain, back pain, indigestion, vomiting, lower abdomen pain, wrist pain and diseases of the lungs and large intestine.

L.I.—5: Fire point.

Headaches, tonsillitis, slurring, cough with phlegm, deafness, heat in the ear, ear pain and nerve pain from shoulder to hand.

L.I.— 6: Junction point.

Eye and sight-related disorders, fever, dryness of the throat, tonsillitis, constipation, toothache and mind-related problems.

L.I.— 7:Liquid point: Second fire, Wood.

Toothache, constipation, headache, indigestion and dry tongue.

L.I.— 8: Solid point: Second fire, Earth.

Indigestion, lower abdomen pain, dryness of the lips, headaches and vomiting due to hernia.

L.I.—9: Gaseous point: Metal, Wood.

Knee pain, urinary bladder problem, brain fatigue, headaches, headaches due to chilly wind.

L.I.—10: Junction point.

Toothache, swelling of the neck, tonsillitis, indigestion, stomach ache, less sense in the front hand and swelling of the elbow.

L.I.—11: Earth point.

Red eyes, ear pain, throat pain while swallowing saliva, constipation, fever, blood pressure, skin diseases, elbow-related problems and paralysis.

L.I.—12: Junction point.

Numbness in the wrist, shoulder pain and one cannot lift hands.

L.I.—13: Liquid point—Second fire, Water.

Pain in the lower left chest, pain in the lower heart, vision problems and excessive sleep.

L.I.—14: Solid point—First Fire, Earth.

Neck spasms, contraction or stiffness in the neck, not being able to lift one's hand, headaches, fevers, tremors and nerve pain spreading from shoulder to hand.

L.I.—15: Gaseous point— Metal, Wood

High blood pressure, dryness of the skin, infertile semen (less quantity of semen),fever and nervous pain spreading from shoulder to hand.

L.I.—16: Junction point.

Fits amongst children. Tooth aches, pain in nerves or Neuralgia, spreading from shoulder to hand.

L.I.—17:—Liquid point—Second Fire, Water.

Dumb from birth, (congenital aphasia), choked throat with pain, tonsillitis and pain in the back of the throat.

L.I.—18: Solid point—First Fire, Earth.

Cough, difficulty in inhaling, acute dumbness or acute difficulty in speaking, excessive saliva, hip pain, swelling of shoulder bone and itching in the throat.

L.I.—19: Gaseous point—metal, wood.

Polyp of the nose, stiffness of the nose muscles, facial palsy, bleeding in the nose, blocked nose, toothache, nose without sense or loss of smell (Anosmia).

L.I.—20: Junction point: *Yang.*

Dryness of mouth, less sense in the face, blocked nose, bleeding nose, difficulty in breathing, facial seizures and swelling of gums.

2.2 Small Intestine Meridian (S.I.)

Based on Six Element Points.

This starts from the tip of the small finger, travels upwards through the palm and the side of the ulna bone, reaches the wrists, travels through the back of the forehand, the joint of the elbow, the arms, as well as the circles the shoulder and goes through the meridian, 14. From there, it reaches the upper point of the clavicle, links with the heart meridian and travels through the sides of the food pipe downwards. After crossing the diaphragm, it enters through the stomach to reach the small intestine.

The second branch of this meridian starts from the upper convex of the clavicle bone, goes further up through the sides of the neck and ends at the cheek. Another branch acts as the organ for the cheek and travels at the side of the nose and gets linked with the urinary bladder meridian at the outer side of the eye socket. Another branch goes to the S.I. through the H 39.

The time of maximum energy flow is - 1pm–3 pm

The element - Fire

Parallel channel - Heart

Type of energy - ***Yang***

Number of points in this meridian - 19

Diseases cured by puncturing the important points in this meridian	Myopathy, diseases related to the neurology department. Paralysis, foot drop, joint pain diseases related to the small intestine, deafness, dizziness, eye diseases, spasms of the neck, diseases related to the heart and lungs and psychiatric disorders.

Diagram 2.2 Small Intestine Meridian (S.I.)—Yang

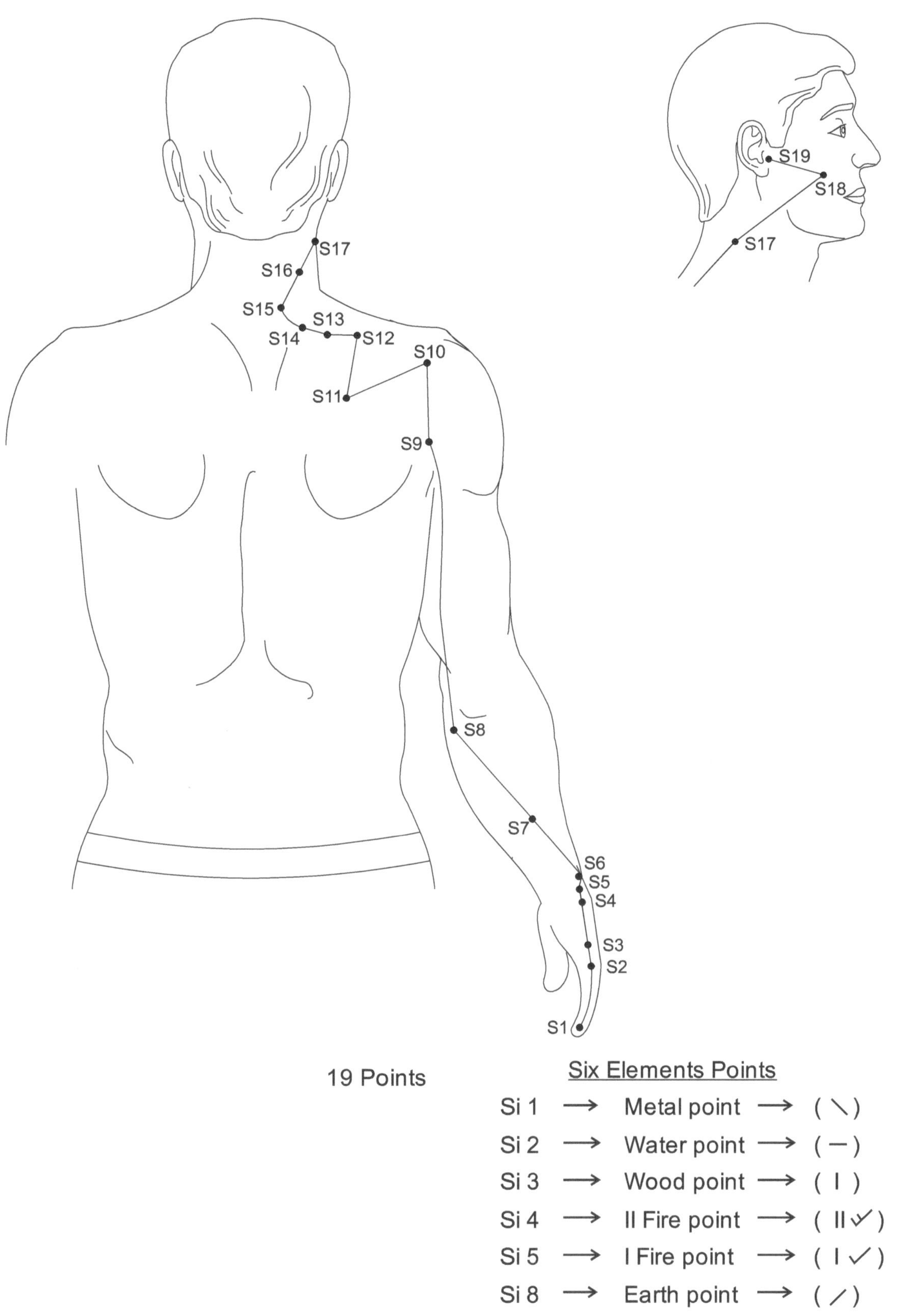

Six Elements Points

The Diseases Which Can Be Cured by Touching the Six Element Points in this Small Intestine Meridian.

S.I.1: Metal point.

* Cough, headaches, tonsillitis, heart pain, diarrhoea, chest pain and difficulty in breathing.

S.I. 2: Water point.

* Fever, Cough, Tonsillitis, Reddish swollen throat and cheeks, blocked nose, epilepsy, cannot lift hands and vision impairment.

S.I. 3: Wood point.

* Mind disorders, epilepsy, not being able to talk, red eyes with pain, tonsillitis, stiffness in the neck, sweating at night, indigestion, cramps or contraction of neck muscles and pain in the backside of the neck.

S.I. 4: Second Fire.

* Paralysis of the muscles in the fingers with pain, cannot fold fingers, headaches, bleeding nose, burning sensation in the stomach and constipation.

S.I. 5: First Fire point.

* Dizziness, bleeding nose, stomach aches, fear, weakness, epilepsy, thickened tongue and painful piles.

S.I.6: Junction point.

* Sudden or acute diseases, vision impairment, paralysis, a cramped neck, wrist pain and a bony feeling in the neck area.

S.I. 7: Liquid point. (Second fire, Water.)

* Cannot fold hands, pain in the hand, cannot hold anything with hand, spinning head, swollen throat, headache, fever and boils on the eyelids.

S.I. 8: Earth point.

*Mind disorders, tremors, lower abdomen pain, fluid retention with the swelling of the heart and indigestion of food in the small intestine.

S.I. 9 Gaseous point: (Metal, Wood).

* Bleeding in the nose, state of dumbness, headache, arthritis numbness, cannot lift a hand, fever, shoulder pain, cramps in the shoulder and joint pain.

S.I. 10: Junction point (*Yang/Yin.*)

Muscle pain, numbness of muscles, arthritis, fatigue, shoulder pain and cannot lift a hand.

S.I. 11: Junction point (Yin).

* Muscle pain, swelling in the lower jaw, cannot lift a hand, headaches, bleeding nose, burning stomach and constipation.

S.I.12: Liquid point (II Fire, Water).

* Numbness, cannot lift a hand, shoulder pain, lung problems, allergies and pneumonia.

S.I. 13:Solidpoint. [First fire (I Fire,) Earth]

* Nervous weakness, numbness, shoulder and elbow pain, heat in the shoulder and cannot hold anything with hands.

S.I. 14: Gaseous point. (Metal (M,), Wood (Wo)

* Dysfunction of the muscles, muscle pain, nervous weakness of the shoulder and front hand, paralysis of the neck muscles and pneumonia.

S.I. 15: Junction point.

* Shallow breath, allergic condition of lungs, vision impaired.

S.I. 16: Liquid point (II Fire, Water).

* Trouble in one half of the body, impaired speech, laziness, cannot turn the neck, swollen lower jaw, state of dumbness, bleeding nose and diseases of the anus.

S.I. 17: Solid point (I Fire, Earth).

* Cannot stand erect, swollen neck, cannot turn the neck, bleeding nose, swollen tongue, nausea, vomiting, state of dumbness, facial palsy and deafness.

S.I. 18: Gaseous point (Metal, Wood).

* Diseases related to the facial nerves, voluntary blinking, voluntary continuous movement of the eye, toothache, numbness, deafness and facial palsy.

S.I. 19: Junction point *Yang.*

* Bleeding nose, state of dumbness, problems of the ears, problems of the outer ear, no sound produced while talking, pain in the ear and noise in the ear.

2.3. Triple Warmer (T.W.)

Points Based on Six Elements

This meridian begins at the outer side of the ring finger, travels up between the fourth and the fifth bone of the hand till the back of the wrist and further travels up the central path of the back side of the hand till the back joint of the elbow. This further travels up through the outer side of the upper arm and reaches the shoulder to cross the gall bladder meridian and reaches the upper curve of the collar bone or the clavicle. One branch goes into the chest, joins with the pericardium as well as travels through the diaphragm to the stomach and joins with the upper and lower organs. Another branch goes up from the heart through the upper curve of the collarbone and the neck and turns at the back of the ear. It reaches the eye pit through the cheeks. The ear path starts from the back of the ear, travels inside the ear, comes out through the outer ear and crosses the previously-mentioned branch track at the cheek area. It joins with the gall bladder. Still, another branch starts from the k–39 point which travels through the stomach and reaches the upper and lower organs of the upper side of the stomach.

The time of maximum energy flow is - 9pm–11 pm

The element - Fire small

Parallel channel - Pericardium

Type of energy - ***Yang***

No of points in this meridian - Twenty-three

Diseases cured by puncturing the important points in this meridian.	Inner ear diseases, constipation, diarrhoea, eye-related diseases, shoulder and back pain, diseases related to the heart and spleen, chest, stomach and lower abdomen-related diseases, as well as pericardium-related diseases.

Diagram 2.3 Triple Warmer Meridian—*Yang*

Based on Six Element Points

The Diseases Which Can be Cured by Touching the Six Element Points in this Triple Warmer Meridian.

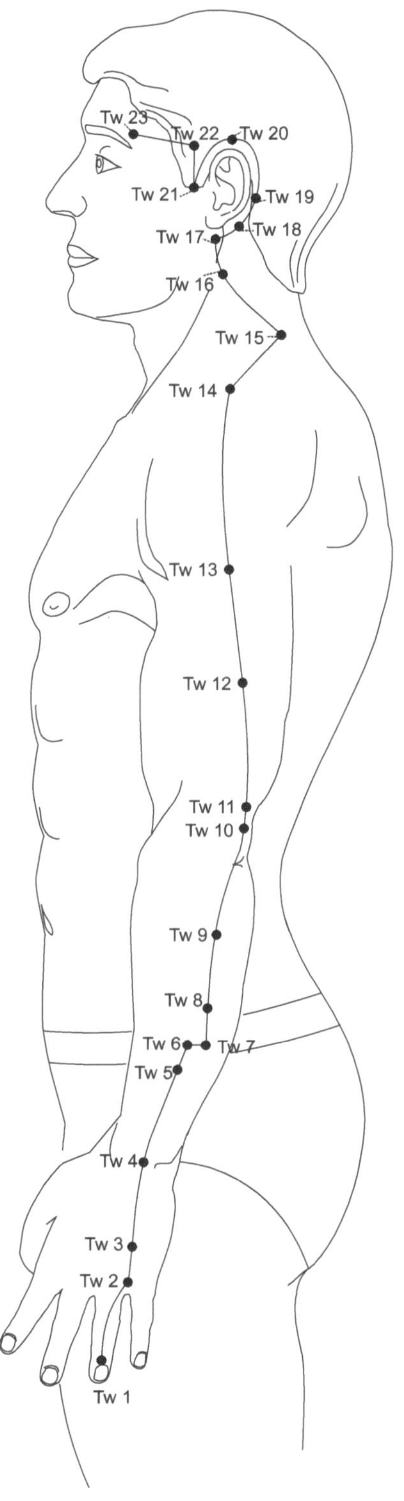

23 Points

<u>Six Elements Points</u>

Tw 1	⟶	Metal point	⟶	(＼)
Tw 2	⟶	Water point	⟶	(—)
Tw 3	⟶	Wood point	⟶	(I)
Tw 5	⟶	II Fire point	⟶	(II✓)
Tw 6	⟶	I Fire point	⟶	(I ✓)
Tw 10	⟶	Earth point	⟶	(／)

TW—1: Metal point.

Headaches, numbness in the throat, dryness of the mouth, summer disease, malaria and shoulder pain.

TW—2: Water point.

Shoulder, hand pain, swelling, pain in the fingers—as if the nerve is pulled, mild deafness, headache, pain in the eye with redness, toothache and malaria.

TW—3: Wood point.

Asthma, allergy condition of the lungs, headaches, sinusitis, elbow pain, not being able to hold anything with the fingers, malaria, fever, dizziness, mild deafness, constipation, gall bladder diseases and numbness of the hand.

TW—4: Junction point. *Yin*

Sinusitis with phlegm, constipation because of gall bladder problem, wrist pain, swelling inflammation of the wrist with swelling and redness, headache, facial palsy, diabetics, dryness of mouth, fever and tremors.

TW—5: Second Fire.

Arthritis, thyroid, parathyroid problems, pain in the fingers, mild deafness, toothache, hyper mental tension, headaches, cough, fever, summer diseases, ulceration of the intestine, cramps in the neck and paralysis.

TW—6: First Fire point.

Fever without sweating, arthritis, pain in the cage, vomiting, deafness, psoriasis, heart diseases and constipation.

TW—7: Liquid point (II Fire, Water)

Epilepsy, tremors caused by nervous problems, mild deafness, as well as pain in the skin and muscles.

TW—8: Solid point (First Fire, Earth)

Elbows, shoulder pain, insomnia, deafness, impaired vision, toothache, pain in the (vertebra) spine.

TW—9: Gaseous point (Metal, wood).

Elbow and shoulder pain, deafness, toothache, pain in the back of the throat and noise in the ears.

TW—10:Earth point

Shoulder, elbow pain, not able to hold anything with fingers, block in the throat, swollen gums with pain, eyes becoming red with pain, mild deafness, cough, lung-related allergic conditions.

TW—11: Liquid point (II Fire, Water).

Elbow pain, shoulder pain, cannot lift a hand because of the pain in the underarm, headaches, noises in the ear, yellowish eyes and pain in the ribs.

TW—12: Solid point (First fire, Earth).

Pain in the hands, swelling, cramped neck, headaches and dizziness.

TW—13:Gaseous point(Metal, wood).

Shoulder pain, cannot lift hands, back pain and swelling of the neck.

TW—14: Junction point (*Yang/yin*); Gaseous point (Metal, Wood).

Neck pain, shoulder pain, hand pain, joint pain, cannot lift hand and skin diseases.

TW—15: Junction point *Yin*—solid point (I Fire, Earth)

Arthritis, thyroid, parathyroid problems, stiffness of the neck, cannot turn the neck, acute deafness, headache due to being in the open air, swelling of the face and pain in the eye.

TW—17: Liquid point (II Fire, Water)

Noises in the ear, deafness, ear pain, itching in the ear, swelling in the jaw and facial palsy.

TW—18: Solid point (I fire, Earth)

Headaches, noises in the ears, partial deafness, high fever in children accompanied by fits, fits or epilepsy ,fear, vomiting and diarrhoea.

TW—19: Gas point (Metal, wood); junction point—*yang*.

The excessive heat of the body, heaviness in the head, fever with fits in children, vomiting in children, noise in the ears, partial deafness, emesis with phlegm or mucus, excessive saliva and not being able to turn the body.

TW—20: Junction point *Yang/Yin*; solid point (I Fire, Earth).

Reddish ear with pain, not being able to chew, swollen gums, eye problems and blisters on the lips.

TW—21: Junction point—Yin; Liquid point (II Fire, Water).

Partial deafness, noises in the ears, pain in the inner ear, ulceration of ears, and toothaches.

TW— 22: Solid point (I Fire, Earth)

Headaches, facial palsy, paralysis of the facial muscles, noises in the ears, swollen neck, swollen jaw, polyps in the nose and diseases of the eyes.

TW—23: Gaseous point (Metal, Wood.)

Headaches due to sinusitis, headaches, redness of the eye with pain, inverted eyes, allergic condition of the eye, vomiting and mind disorders.

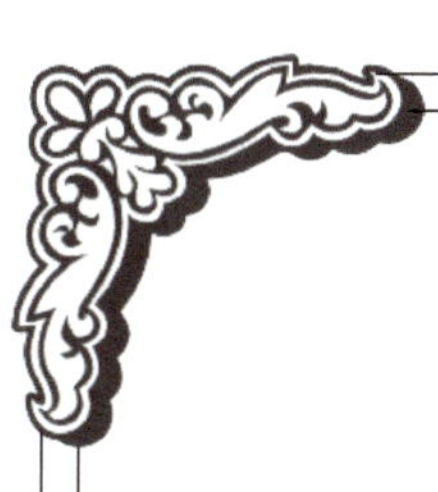

Part Three

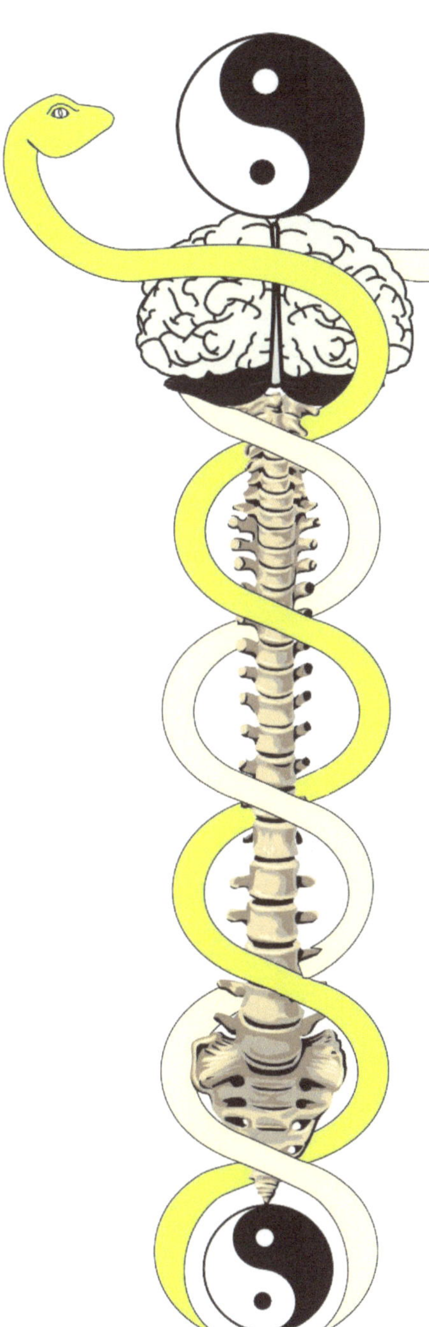

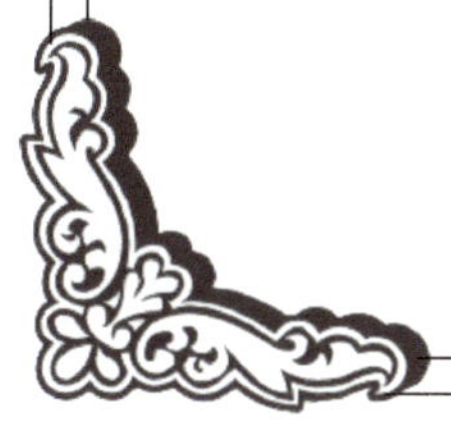

3.1 Lung Meridian (LU) Based on Six Element Points Method

3.2 Heart Meridian (H) Based on Six Element Points Method

3.3 Pericardium Meridian (P) Based on Six Element Points Method

3.1 Lung Meridian (Lu)

Based on Six Elements Points

Based on the six elements points, this meridian starts from the centre of the rib cage, travels down and joins the large intestine. Then, it reaches its organ via the diaphragm and travels upwards across the front side chest and goes down to the front of the elbow through the inner upper arm. Then it travels through the edge of the clavicle bone radius on the right side and crosses the wrist and ends at the inner tip of the thumb.

The time of maximum energy flow is	- 3 am–5am
The element	- Metal
Parallel channel	- Large intestine meridian
Type of energy	- ***Yin***
No of points in this meridian	- 11+1=12

Diseases cured by puncturing the Important points in this meridian	Diseases of the lungs and the skin and diseases related to the large intestine.

Diagram

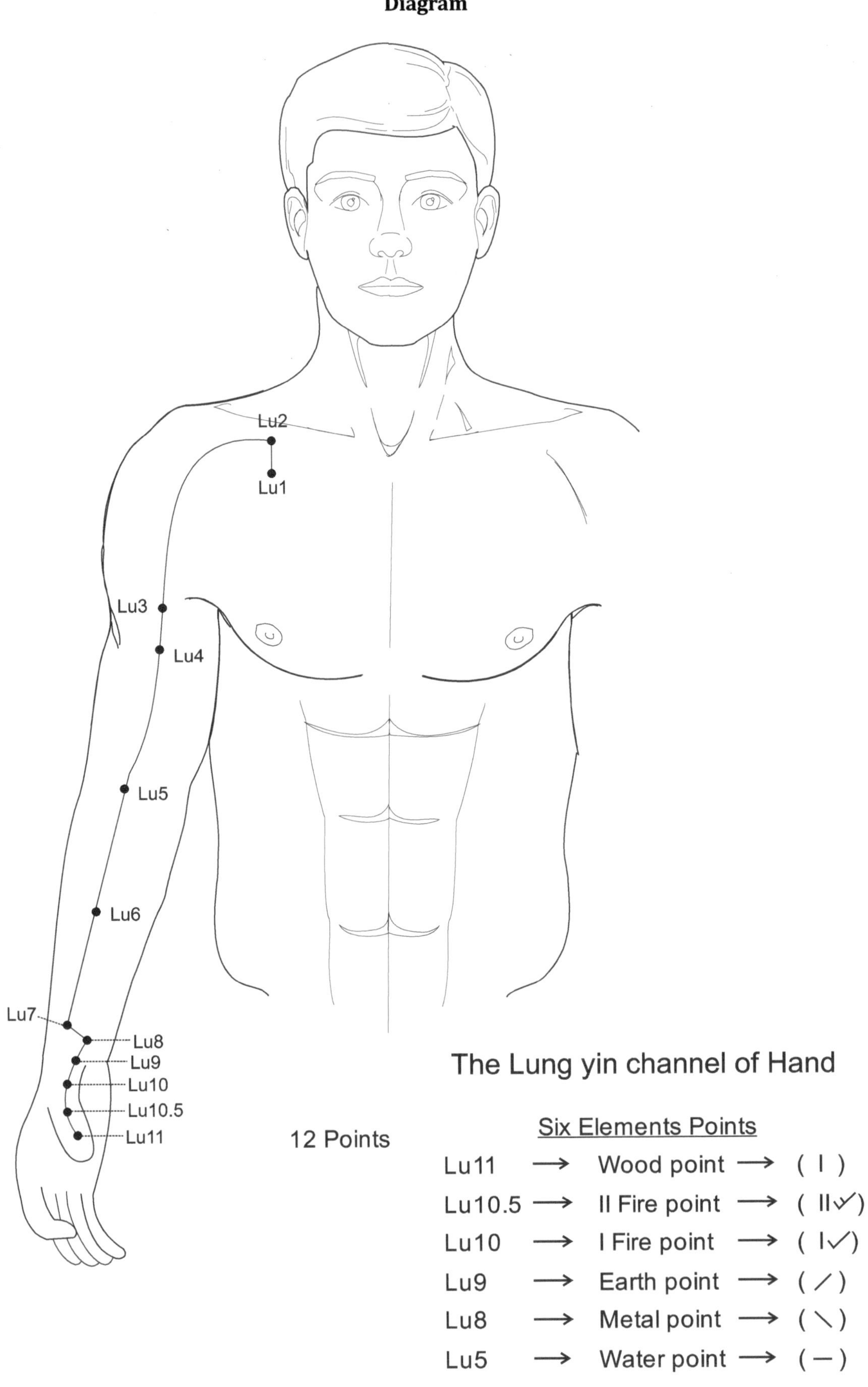

Figure 3.1 Six Element Points on the Lung Meridian

The Diseases Which Can be Cured by Touching the Six Element Points in this Lung Meridian.

L I—1, Junction point: *Yin/Yang*.

The alarm point of the lungs also works as the danger point. This point collaborates with the two states of the air energy which is, in turn, related to the lungs.

Blocked breath, difficulty in breathing, problems in inhaling and/or exhaling, neck pain, shoulder pain, cough, asthma, swelling of the face, rheumatism in the face, neck and chest regions, tonsillitis, pain on the skin, anaemia, redness of the eyes, a foul odour in the urine and congestion with phlegm.

LU—2 Gaseous point (Metal, Wood)

Difficulty in breathing, chest pain, asthma, not being able to lift hands and shoulder, cramps in the muscles of the neck with swelling, heart diseases—in particular—problems in the air going to the heart along the junction point, problems in blood flow from the heart to the lungs, anger and weeping occurring alternatively.

LU—3 Solid point (I Fire, Earth).

Dizziness, contraction and stiffness of the neck muscles, thirst, dryness of the tongue, food gets choked in the throat, getting a common cold after eating sweets, sweating after eating hot or warm food, fever due to food allergy, sad because of a bad experience in life.

LU—4 Liquid point (II Fire, Water)

Chest pain, dark skin under the chest, difficulty in breathing due to water retention, fear, suspicion and hatred.

LU—5 Liquid point.

Lung diseases, rheumatism, pain, throat pain, neck pain, tonsillitis, ulcer in the throat, dry cough, affected often with a common cold, elbow pain, difficulty in breathing, forearm and elbow muscles affected with contraction due to gas, stiffness of the same muscles, sneezing, anger with stubbornness, crying, swelling of the elbow joint and skin diseases.

LU—6 Solid point.

Headache immediately after eating and after the hunger becomes excessive. Piles with blood discharge, shoulder pain, fever, throat ulcer or infection, lung diseases, swelling of the throat, cough, asthma and acute diseases.

LU—6.5. Gaseous point (Metal, Wood)

Gas-related problems after eating, bloating, excessive gas formation, suffocation, belching, excess gas inside an empty stomach and not being able to eat because of excess gas.

LU—7 Liquid point.

Asthma, difficulties in breathing, tremor in hands, teeth sensitivity, cough, phlegm, fear, confusion, hatred, swelling in the wrist, excess sweat in the palms, epileptic, cold palm, facial palsy, back side headache, cramp in neck muscles and lung diseases.

LU—8. Metal point.

Excessive cough in the night, fever and stomach ache, tightening pain in the chest, fast breathing due to anger, swollen wrist, blood-related disease.

LU—9. Earth point.

Body temperature becomes hot and cold alternatively, yellow urine, burning while urinating, chest burning, thirst, dryness in the whole mouth, stressed and tensed mind, difficulty in breathing, burning sensation in the heart, facial palsy, headache ,yellow coloured tongue and white deposit on the tongue.

LU—10. I Fire point.

Throat dryness, thirst cough ,heat in the throat, pain, swelling, redness in the tongue, headache, yellow deposit on tongue and numbness of the tongue.

LU—10. II Fire point. (II)

Chills/fever (fever with shivering), dry cough, astringent taste in the tongue, pale tongue, heavy head.

LU—11. Wood point.

Swelling of the throat, numbness in the palm and the wrist, swelling of the chest, numbness of the tongue and it becomes thick, throat problems, body pain, drilling pain, heart attack, epilepsy, asthma, nervous weakness, feeling helpless mentally.

3.2 Heart Meridian (H)

Based on the Six Element Points

This meridian starts from the heart and one of the branches goes down and gets linked with the S.I. meridian. Another branch goes up through the side of the food pipe and joins the eyes and the brain. The major track of this meridian runs across and reaches the lungs. Then, it goes up through the front side of the underarm, crosses the back side of the upper hand and travels downwards to the palm. It reaches the inner tip of the little finger and joins the S.I.'s path.

The time of maximum energy flow is	- 11 am to 1pm
The element	- First Fire/Fire Big/I Fire
Parallel channel	- Small intestine meridian
Type of energy	- ***Yin***
No of points in this meridian	- 9+1=10

Diseases cured by puncturing the important points in this meridian.	Diseases related to the brain, speech impairment, insomnia, fear, daydreaming, fever with fits, epilepsy, dizziness, hyperactivity, mind-related problems and heart diseases.

Diagram

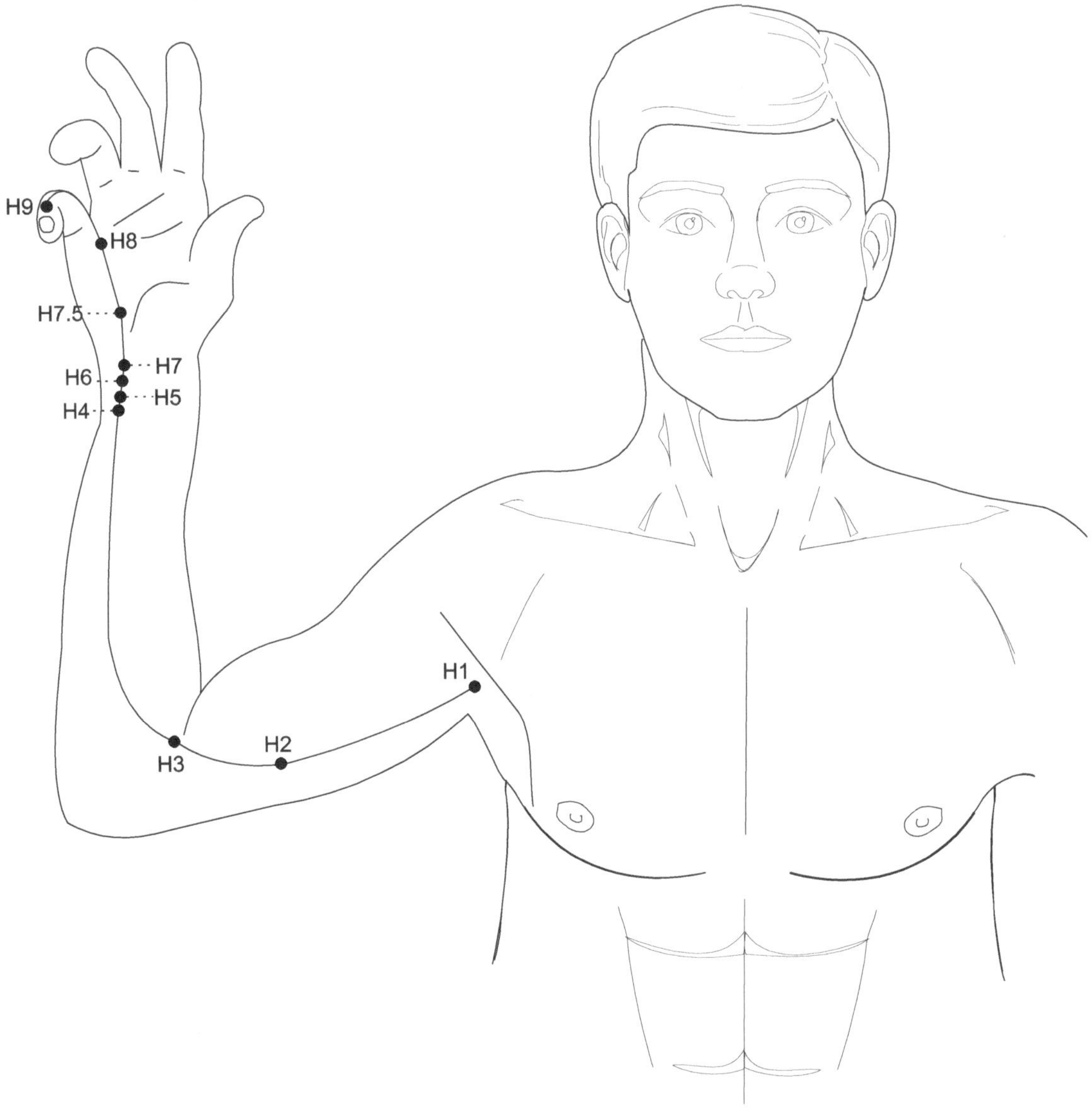

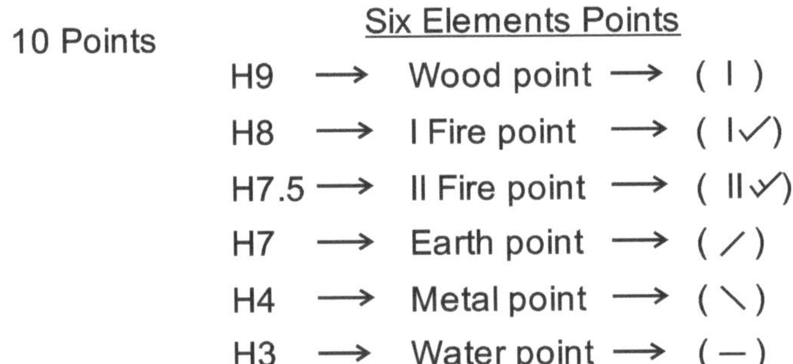

10 Points

<u>Six Elements Points</u>

H9	⟶	Wood point	⟶	(I)
H8	⟶	I Fire point	⟶	(I✓)
H7.5	⟶	II Fire point	⟶	(II✓)
H7	⟶	Earth point	⟶	(/)
H4	⟶	Metal point	⟶	(\ )
H3	⟶	Water point	⟶	(–)

Figure 3.2 Six Elements Points on the Heart Meridian

The Diseases Which Can be Cured by Touching the Six Element Points in this Heart Meridian

H1—Junction Point, Gaseous Point (Metal, Wood)

Heart diseases, dry throat, pain in the heart, excessive thirst, heaviness in the chest, nausea, myopathy of the chest muscles, psychiatry disorders, not being able to fold the tongue, numbness in the tongue, fatigue and chillness in the elbow.

H 2—Solid point (I Fire, Earth)

Cannot tolerate cold, fever, tremors, headaches on the front side of the head, general headaches, shoulder pain and paralysis of the shoulder muscle.

H 3—Water point—Liquid point (II Fire, Water).

Epilepsy, psychiatry disorders, toothache, dizziness, facial palsy, shoulder pain, paralysis of the shoulder muscles, headaches, headaches due to heat or cold, tremors in the hand, stress and depression, chest pain, anxiety, swollen elbows, stiffness and heart pain.

H 4—Metal point—Gaseous point (Metal, Wood)

Arthritis in the elbows and wrists, heart pain, psychiatry problems, the tongue getting pulled (dystonia), a state of dumbness, nausea and a feeling of severe chillness in the bone.

H 5—Solid point (I Fire, Earth)

Headaches, dizziness, tonsillitis, an acute state of dumbness, paralysis of the throat muscles and shoulder muscles, psychiatric problems, uncontrolled urine, without sweat flushed hot face, yawning, vomiting, constipation, swelling of the lower abdomen, hoarse voice and slurring.

H 6—Liquid point (II Fire, Water)

Blocked nose, dizziness, headaches, anxiety, tonsillitis, psychiatric problems, shortness of breath, heaviness of chest, tremors, sweating at night, acute dumb state, acute diarrhoea, cannot fold elbows and chest pain.

H 7—Earth point

Psychiatric problems, heart diseases due to other ailments, enlargement of the heart, pain and heat around the heart, suffocation, palpitation, allergic nose, blocked nose, tremors, unconscious state, constipation, headaches, insomnia, nervous weakness and epilepsy.

H 7.5—II Fire point

Heart disease due to kidney problems, palpitation, anxiety, less warmth in blood and feeling dull-headed.

H 8—I Fire point

Numbness of the hands, difficulty in urination, prostate enlargement, palpitation of the heart and chest, psychiatric disorders, fear and tremors.

H 9—Wood point (Wo)

Heart diseases, palpitation, a weak heart, impaired vision, dryness of throat, fever, fatigue due to fever, white discharge, dizziness and heart pain.

3.3 Pericardium Meridian (P)

Based on the Six Element Points

This starts from the heart, reaches its organ—the pericardium, travels through the diaphragm, descends to the stomach and joins the triple warmer. One of the branches starts from the chest, travels through the rib bone up to 3 *zun* measurement, from the front folds of the underarm, travels upwards, descends through the inside of the upper arm, travels between the lungs and heart meridians till the elbow fold, travels further along the ulna bone side and reaches the tip of the central finger through the palm. Another branch reaches the ring finger, starting from the palm where the triple warmer meridian joints are located.

The time of maximum energy flow is	- 7 pm to 9 pm
The element	- Second Fire/Fire small/II Fire
Parallel channel	- Triple warmer meridian
Type of energy	- ***Yin***
No of points in this meridian	- 9+1=10

Diseases cured by puncturing the important points in this meridian are:	Diseases related to the wrists area, glands-related diseases, heart-related diseases, psychiatric disorders, insomnia, fear, intestinal ulcer, hiccups and triple warmer-related diseases.

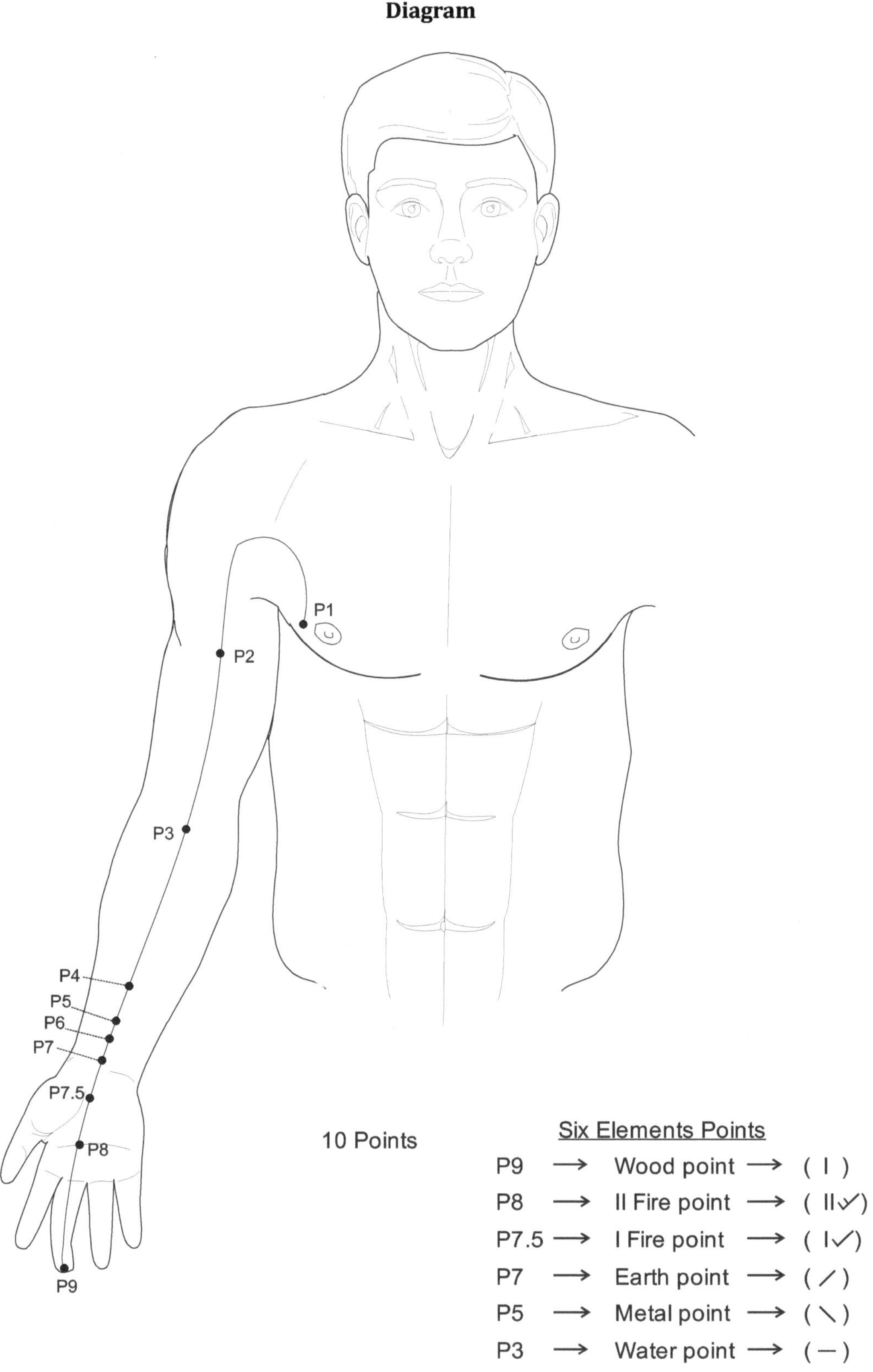

Figure3.3 Six Elements Points on the Pericardium Meridian

The Diseases Which Can be Cured by Touching the Six Element Points in this Heart Meridian

P 1—Gaseous point (Metal, Wood)

Stomach ache, headaches, fever, swelling in the underarm, chest pain and smoky vision.

P 2—Solid point (I Fire, E)

Chest pain, palpitation due to fear, pain in the whole chest, cough, allergic condition of lungs, swelling of the chest and the whole of the back, pain in the entire underarm, impaired vision and the fear of getting exposed to the chilly wind.

P 3—Water point, Liquid point (II Fire, Water)

Stomach pain, vomiting, diarrhoea, tremors in hands, pain, sweat on the face and the neck, infertile men/ women, diseases related to cardiac muscles, chest pain, palpitation of the heart and skin diseases.

P 4—Liquid point (II Fire, Water)

Diseases related to the cardiac muscles, chest pain, nausea, weakness and memory loss.

P 5—Metal point—Solid point (I Fire, E).

Heart pain, heart diseases, nausea, gastric problems, swollen underarm, menstrual problems, fear of getting exposed to cold wind and the fear of ghosts.

P 6—Gaseous point (M, W.)

High blood pressure, pituitary gland diseases, headache, anaemia, palpitation of the heart, epilepsy, psychiatric diseases, swollen underarm, heart pain, nausea, stomach pain, gastric problems, lower abdomen swelling, diarrhoea, cough, rheumatism of the feet, jaundice, summer diseases, depression, asthma, insomnia and shoulder pain.

P 7—Earth point.

High blood pressure, body heat, chest rib pain, fever, chills and sweat, choked throat, ulcer in the chest, swollen underarm, pain, sadness, being in a state without happiness, intestinal ulcer, painful red eye, nervous weakness and wrist problems.

P 8—First Fire point.

Anger, laughing or sadness, shoulder pain, indigestion, blood in urine, haemorrhoids around the anus, jaundice, thirst and excessive sweat.

P 8.5.—Second Fire point.

An alternate feeling of heat and cold, swelling in the pericardium due to water retention, palpitation of the heart, clotting of blood, very slow heartbeat, feels chilliness in the heart, fear, feels suspiciousness.

P 9—Wood point(Wo)

Asthma, allergic content of lungs, dizziness, unconscious state, less memory, shoulder pain, nausea, vomiting, diarrhoea, hypo/hyper depression.

Part Four

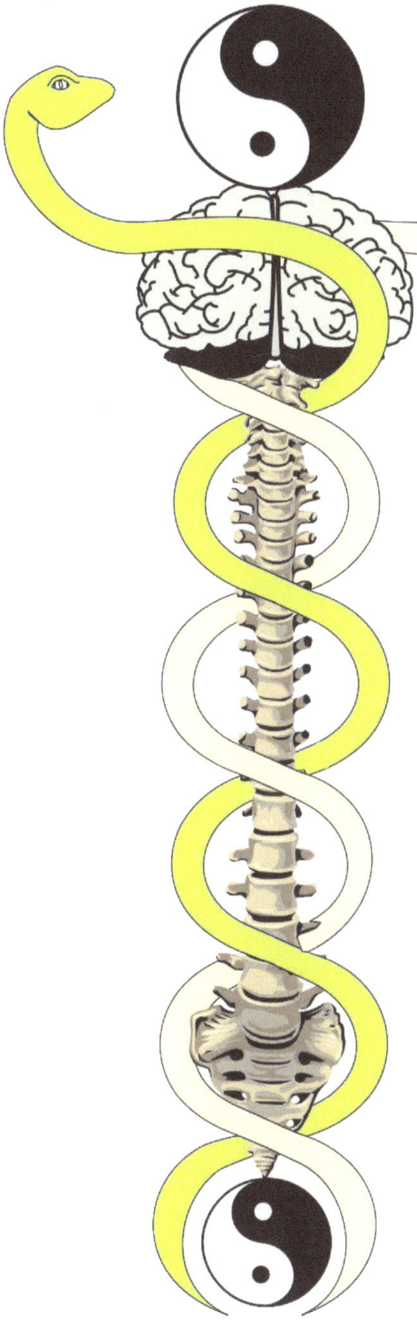

4.1. Gall bladder meridian (GB) based on six element points method

4.2. Stomach meridian (ST) based on six element points method

4.3. Urinary bladder meridian (UB) based on six element points method

4.1 Gall Bladder Meridian (GB)

Based on Six Elements Points

This meridian starts from the outer area of the eye socket, goes up to the front of the forehead, travels through the back of the ear lobe towards the side of the neck and reaches the front of the TW meridian on the shoulders. It then goes to the backside of the TW meridian and ends at the upper curve of the collarbone. The gall bladder meridian branch of the ear begins at the back of the ear, enters the ear and comes out from the front ear to reach the back of the eye socket.

The branch from the outer side of the eye socket goes down toST.5, crosses the TW point situated at the lower side of the eye socket and joins with its mother meridian by crossing the neck side and the upper curve of the collarbone. Then again, through the diaphragm, it goes to the chest region and gets linked with the LIV meridian. It enters its organ, the gallbladder.

Diagram

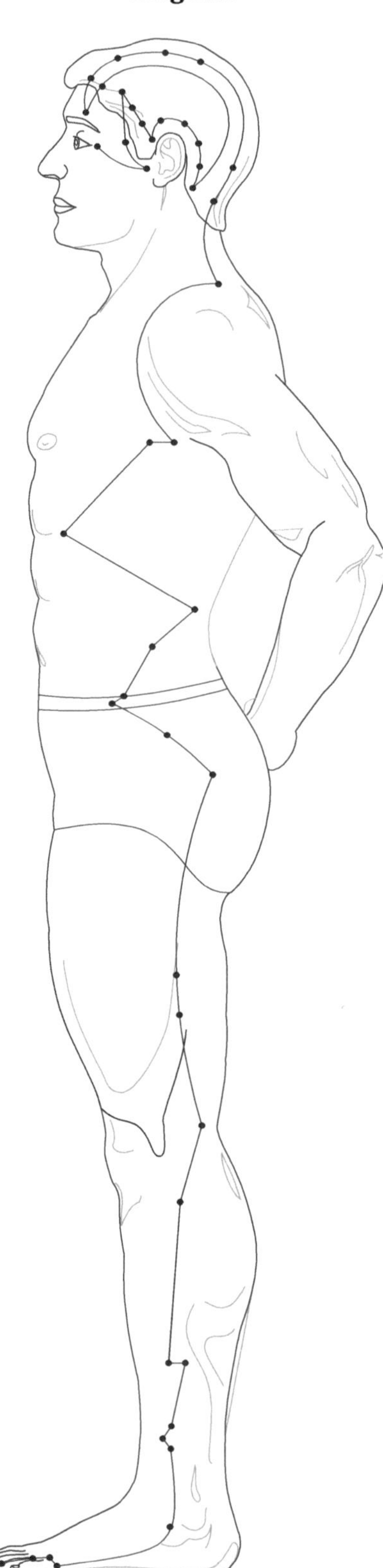

Figure 4.1 Gall bladder meridian—*Yang*

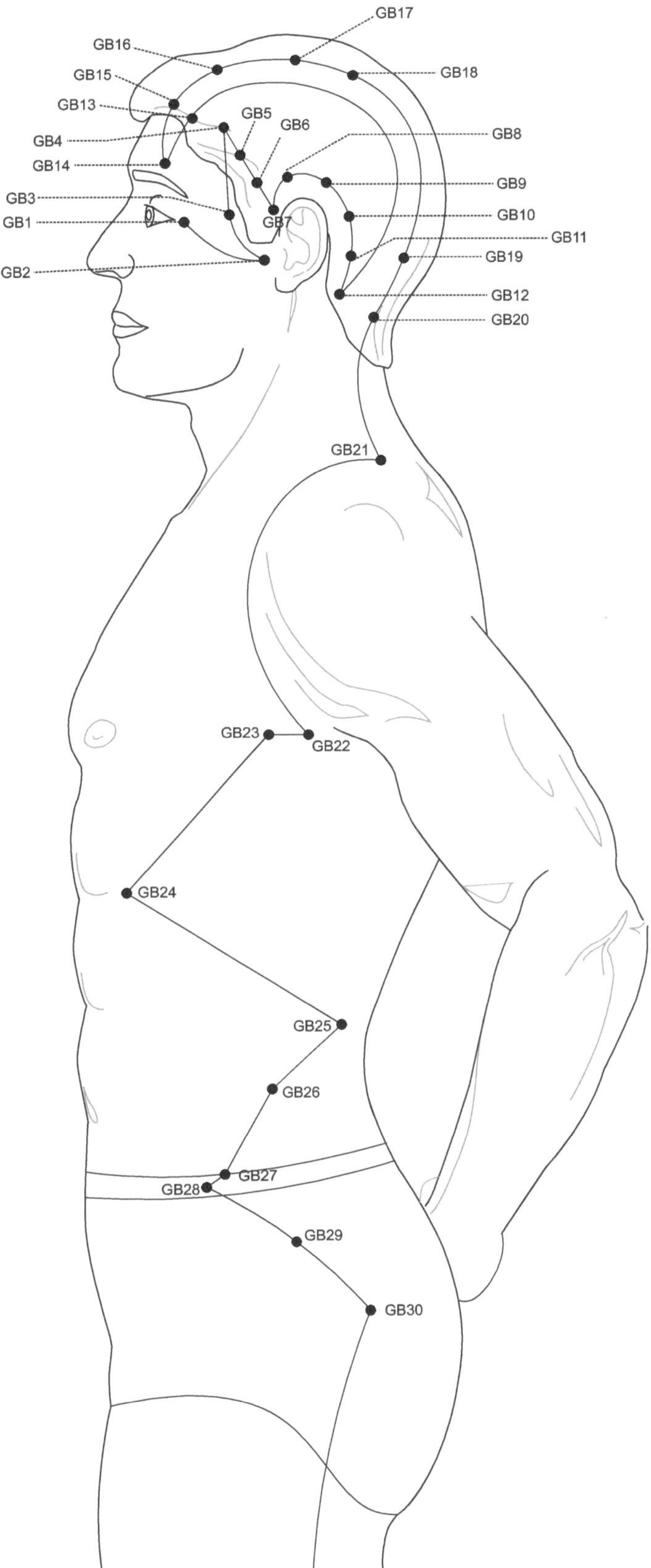

Figure 4.2 Gall bladder meridian—*Yang*

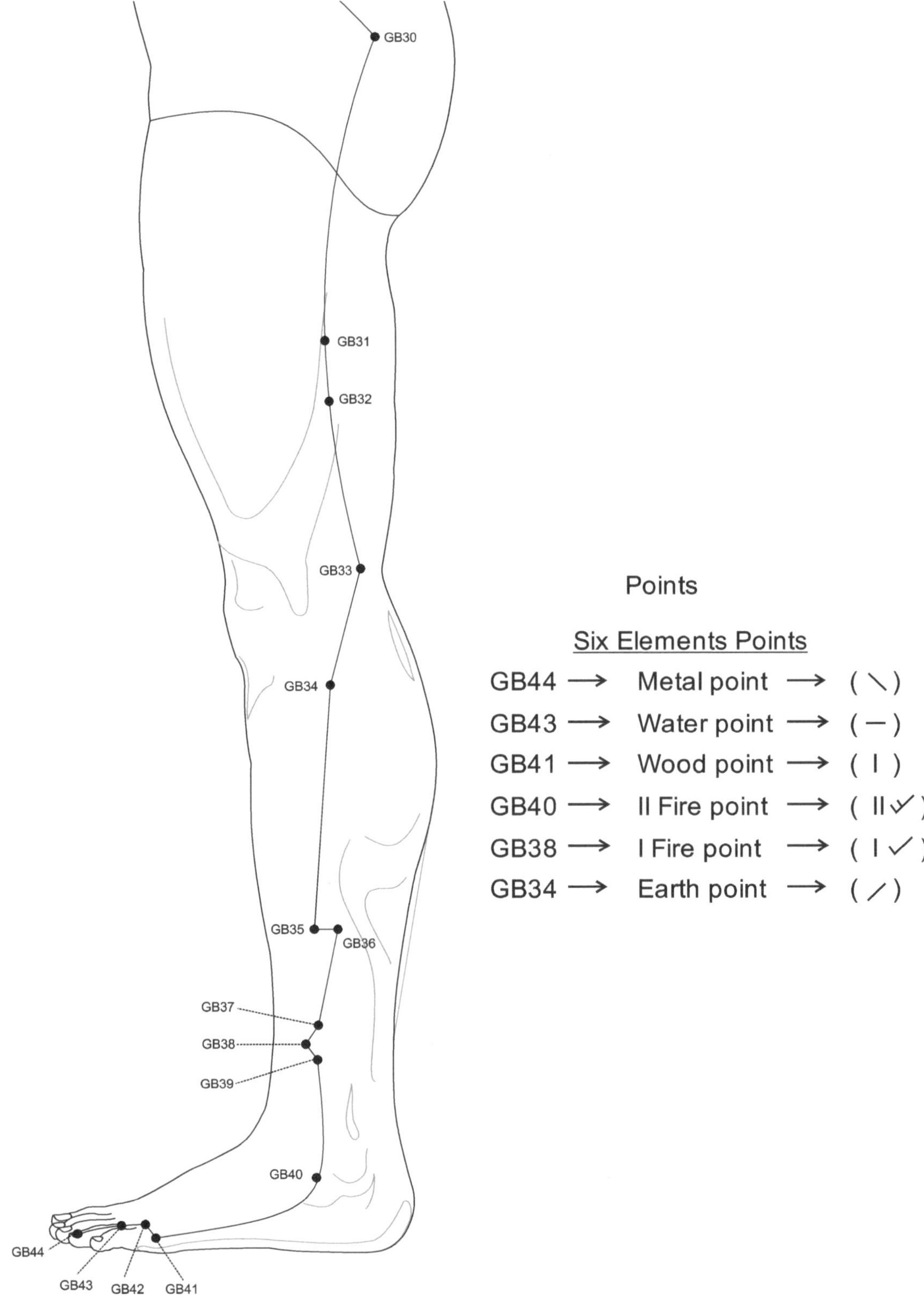

Figure 4.3 Gall bladder meridian—*Yang*

The time of maximum energy flow is -11 pm–1 am

The element -Wood

Parallel channel -Liver meridian

Type of energy -***Yang***

Number of points in this meridian - 44

Diseases cured by puncturing the important points in this meridian:	Facial palsy, nerve pain on one side of the cheeks and diseases related to an allergy to milk.

Glands, diseases related to liver and gall bladder, headaches, diseases related to liver and gall bladder, headaches, anger, indigestion and diseases related to the ears and the eyes.

The Diseases Which Can be Cured by Touching the Six Element Points in this Gall Bladder Meridian.

Gall Bladder1: Junction point—*Yang.*

Headaches, colour blindness, eye diseases and trigeminal neuralgia.

Gall Bladder 2: Water point(II Fire, Water)

Deafness, noises in the ear, ear pain, pain in the lower jaw, Pain after consuming cold food, do not like to drink water, sadness and facial palsy.

Gall Bladder 3: Solid point (I Fire, Earth)

Does not like to go out in the cold windy weather, has dizziness, migraines, toothache, does not like to look at a bright light and Glaucoma.

Gall Bladder 4: Gaseous point (Metal, Wood)

Migraines, noises in the ear, deafness, dizziness, toothache, sneezing, fits in children, epilepsy, neck pain and rheumatic arthritis.

Gall Bladder 5: Gaseous point (Metal, Wood)

Migraines, toothaches, reddened face with pain, heat in the body and no sweat.

Gall Bladder 6:Fever without sweat, migraines, trigeminal neuralgia, swollen red face with pain and heart disease.

Gall Bladder 7: Liquid point (II Fire, Water)

Swelling of the jaw and cheeks, pain, contraction of neck muscles with pain, migraines, headaches and eye-related diseases.

Gall Bladder 8: Junction point: *Yang/Yin.*

Headaches, pain in the centre of the head, headaches due to exposure to the air, vomiting, eye diseases, continuous headaches and ear disease.

Gall Bladder 9: Gaseous point (M, Wo)

Headaches, toothaches, swollen gums and pain.

Gall Bladder 10: Solid point (I Fire, Earth)

Numbness of the throat, cough, noises in the ears, deafness, toothache, swollen neck, pain, tonsillitis and shoulder pain.

Gall Bladder 11: Liquid point (II Fire, Water)

Headaches, neck and jaw pain, bitterness with pain in the mouth, stiffness of the tongue, noises in the ears, dizziness, eye pain, an hidrosis or hypohidrosis (no sweat).

Gall Bladder 12:Gaseous point (M, Wo)

Headaches, headaches if exposed to the wind, swollen face and head, facial palsy, neck pain, deafness, yellow or red urine, anaemia and weak legs.

Gall Bladder 13: Water point (II Fire, Water)

Unconsciousness, dizziness, sudden dark vision, stiff neck with pain, cannot turn the neck, epilepsy, spitting of saliva, fear, psychiatric disorders.

Gall Bladder 14: Solid point (I Fire, Earth)

Eyes become swollen, painful and reddened, squinted eyes, does not like to see the light, headaches, facial palsy, trigeminal neuralgia and nausea.

Gall bladder 15:Liquid point (II Fire, Water)

Pain in the outer side of the eyes, watery eyes, blocked nose, fear to get exposed to the cold wind and stiffness in the spine.

Gall bladder 16: Gas point (metal, wood)

Colour blindness, eyes becoming red with pain, swollen face and eyes, impaired vision, headaches, dizziness, giddiness and fever without a sweat.

Gall Bladder 17: Solid point (I Fire, Earth)

Head and neck pain, tooth pain, swollen lips, vomiting, giddiness, cannot listen, vision impaired.

Gall Bladder 18: Liquid point (II Fire, Water)

One has headaches, does not like to go out in the chilly wind, blocked nose and bleeding nose.

Gall Bladder 19: Gaseous point (Metal, Wood)

Headaches, dizziness, headaches to the extent that one cannot open one's eyes, excessive heat in the body, physical weakness, cramped neck and cannot turn.

Gall Bladder 20: Solid point (I Fire, E)

Body becoming hot and cold recurrently, summer diseases, headaches, nervous weakness, boils in the spinal cord, drowsy eyes, excessive water discharge in the eyes, weakness of the eye, night blindness, bleeding nose, blocked nose, headache at the back of the head, cramped neck and common cold.

Gall Bladder 21: Liquid point (II Fire, Water) Junction point.

Arthritis, cramped neck, cannot turn neck, shoulder and back pain, cannot lift a hand, dizziness, abscess in the chest, tremor in hands, gall bladder diseases, rheumatism and dumbness.

Gall Bladder 22: Junction point: *Yang.*

Chest pain, weakness of chest, cannot lift a hand.

Gall Bladder 23:Gaseouspoint (Metal, Wood)

Cannot sleep because of heaviness in the chest, asthma, wheezing, sleeplessness because of lung diseases, vomiting and heat in the lower abdomen.

Gall Bladder 24: Solid point (I Fire, Earth).

Pain in the chest ribs, heart problems due to problems in the kidneys pain while swallowing, excessive saliva, cough, difficulty in speaking and heat in the lower abdomen.

Gall Bladder 25: Liquid point (II Fire, Water)

Pain in the spine, cannot bend, hip pain, hip muscle and bone pain, cannot stand for a long time, diarrhoea, asthma, difficulty in excreting urine and yellow-coloured urine.

Gall Bladder 26: Junction point: *Yin*

Lower abdominal pain, intermittent menstruation, white discharge, myopathy of the lower abdomen, as well as no menstruation or amenorrhea.

Gall Bladder 27: Junction point: *Yang.*

Spinal cord pain, myopathy of the kidney, constipation, white discharge, cysts in the intestine, as well as the allergic condition of the testis.

Gall Bladder 28:Gaseous point (Metal, Wood)

Hip pain, leg pain, spinal pain, swelling, vomiting, infections in the intestine, difficulty in urination and infection in the testis.

Gall Bladder 29:Solid point (I Fire, Earth)

Paralysis, lower back pain, amenorrhea or absence of menstrual periods, irregular periods, white discharge, a difference during urination, allergy in testis, as well as shoulder pain.

Gall Bladder 30: Liquid point (II Fire, Water)

Half of the body does not cooperate, paralysis, epilepsy, hip pain, thigh pain, numbness and pain in the legs, inability to twist the body, rheumatism and joint pain.

Gall Bladder 31: Gaseous point (Metal, Wood)

Paralysis, hands and legs not working amongst children, weak legs, pain and numbness in one's legs.

Gall Bladder 32: Solid point (I Fire, Earth).

Half of the body does not cooperate, numbness and pain in the legs, weakness in the legs and myopathy of the leg muscles.

Gall Bladder33: Liquid point (II Fire, Water)

Swollen inflamed reddish joints, cannot bend or stretch the wrist joints, no sense in the joints.

Gall Bladder 34: Gaseous point (Metal, Wood) Earth point.

Half of one's body does not cooperate properly, chilliness, especially a shivering sensation in one's legs and because of less blood circulation leg becomes numb and hurts. It becomes red, swollen and painful, the face becomes swollen, psychiatric disease, constipation and itching in the skin.

Gall Bladder 35: Solid point (I Fire, Earth)

Numbness in the throat, oedema of the face, pain with numbness in legs, fatigue, weak legs and cold feet.

Gall Bladder 36: Leg point(II Fire, Water)

Paralysis, hip muscles do not function, neck pain, swollen neck, pain, allergic to cold wind and psychiatric problems.

Gall Bladder 37: Gaseous point (Metal, Wood)

Pain in the leg muscles, cannot stand for long, paralysis, fever without sweat and acute psychiatric problems.

Gall Bladder 38: Solid point (I Fire, Earth)

Paralysis, myopathy, boils or cysts, chest pain, joint pain, numbness and pain in legs, pain in eyes, numbness of the throat and bleeding nose.

Gall Bladder 39: Liquid point (II Fire, Water)

Hands and legs do not cooperate, swelling of the stomach and lower abdomen, loss of appetite, diarrhoea, rheumatism, choked throat, bleeding nose, psychiatric problems, fear, contracted neck and pressure in the chest.

Gall Bladder 40:II Fire

Pain in the chest and ribs, difficulty in breathing, swelling of the underarm, paralysis, lower hip pain, numbness and pain in the legs, reddened, swollen feet with pain, vomiting, burping with a sour taste, atrophy of the muscles and chills/fever.

Gall Bladder 41:Wood point

Rheumatism, oedema of legs, pain, pain in the ribs, irregular menstruation, dizziness, fever, excessive sweat, fever with shivering, and pain due to sagging breasts.

Gall Bladder 42: Solid point (I Fire, Earth)

Pedal oedema with reddishness, wound in the chest, eyes red in colour with pain.

Gall Bladder 43: Water point, Liquid point (II Fire, Water)

Pedal oedema and red, myopathy of the muscles in the feet joints, swollen jaws, deafness, dizziness and fever without any sweat.

Gall Bladder 44: Metal point—Junction point

Headaches, dreams of ghosts, heart diseases, pain in the eyes, difficulty in breathing, cough, excessive sleep, anaemia, heat in the feet and palms, stiffness of the tongue, dryness of mouth, deafness, chest pain and drowsiness.

4.2 Stomach Meridian (St)

Based on Six Elements Points

This path starts from the outer walls of the nose (Stomach 20), goes up through the sides of the nose and reaches the related path at the beginning point of the kidney near the nostrils. Then it goes down leftwards via the upper lip and reaches the gum area. Then it goes around the lips, descends and reaches the lower jaw. It joins the parallel path of its kind at the curve under the lower lips.

Then it goes out through the tip of the jaw, crosses the gall bladder track at the front of the ear and reaches the forehead through the edge of the skull along the hairline.

The lower track starts from stomach 5, descends through the throat and neck and reaches the upper curve of the collarbone. From there, straight away, it reaches its organ—the diaphragm. This is in connection with the spleen's track.

Another important branch descends from the upper curve of the collarbone through the centre line on the breast's ripple, goes up to the outer side of the umbilicus and reaches the stomach.

The stomach branch goes to the lower side of the stomach, and the feet and descends through the outer side of the thigh bone, knee and leg bone and ends at the second finger of the upper foot.

Diagram

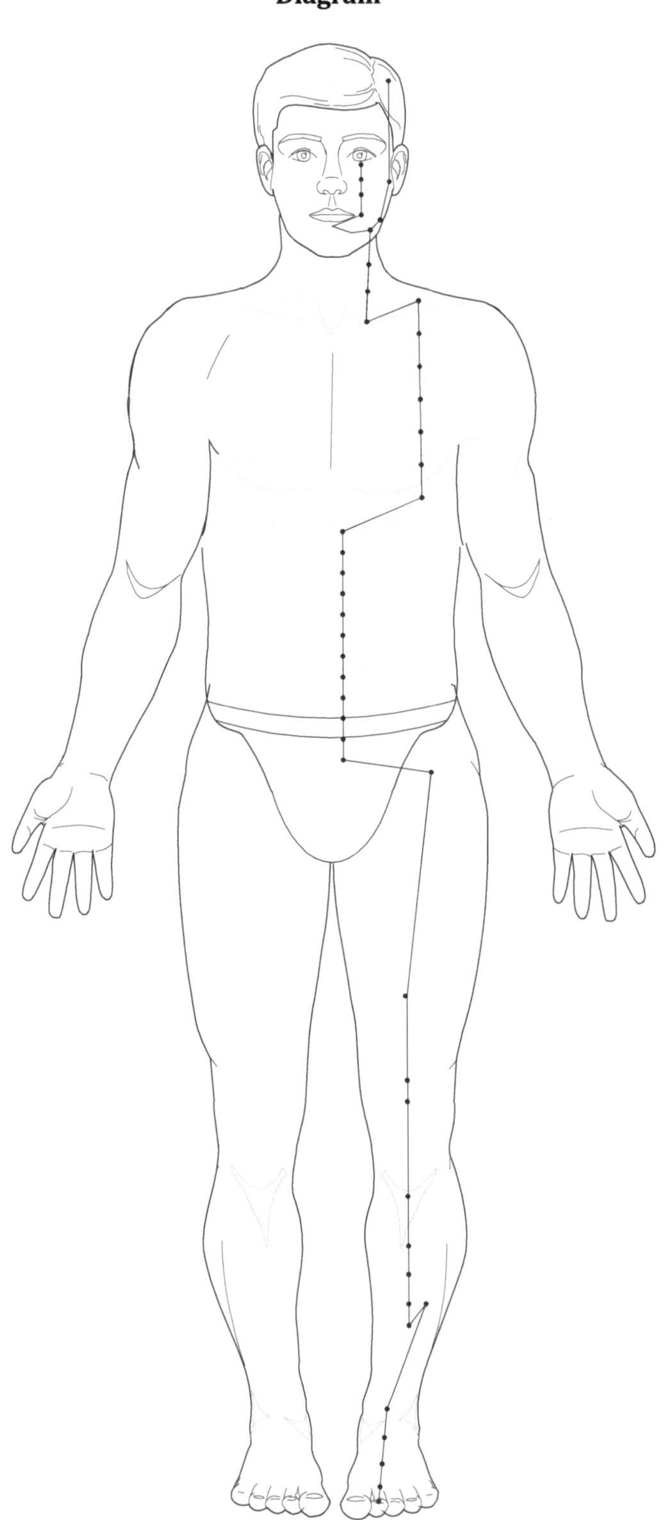

Figure 4.4 Stomach Meridian—*Yang*

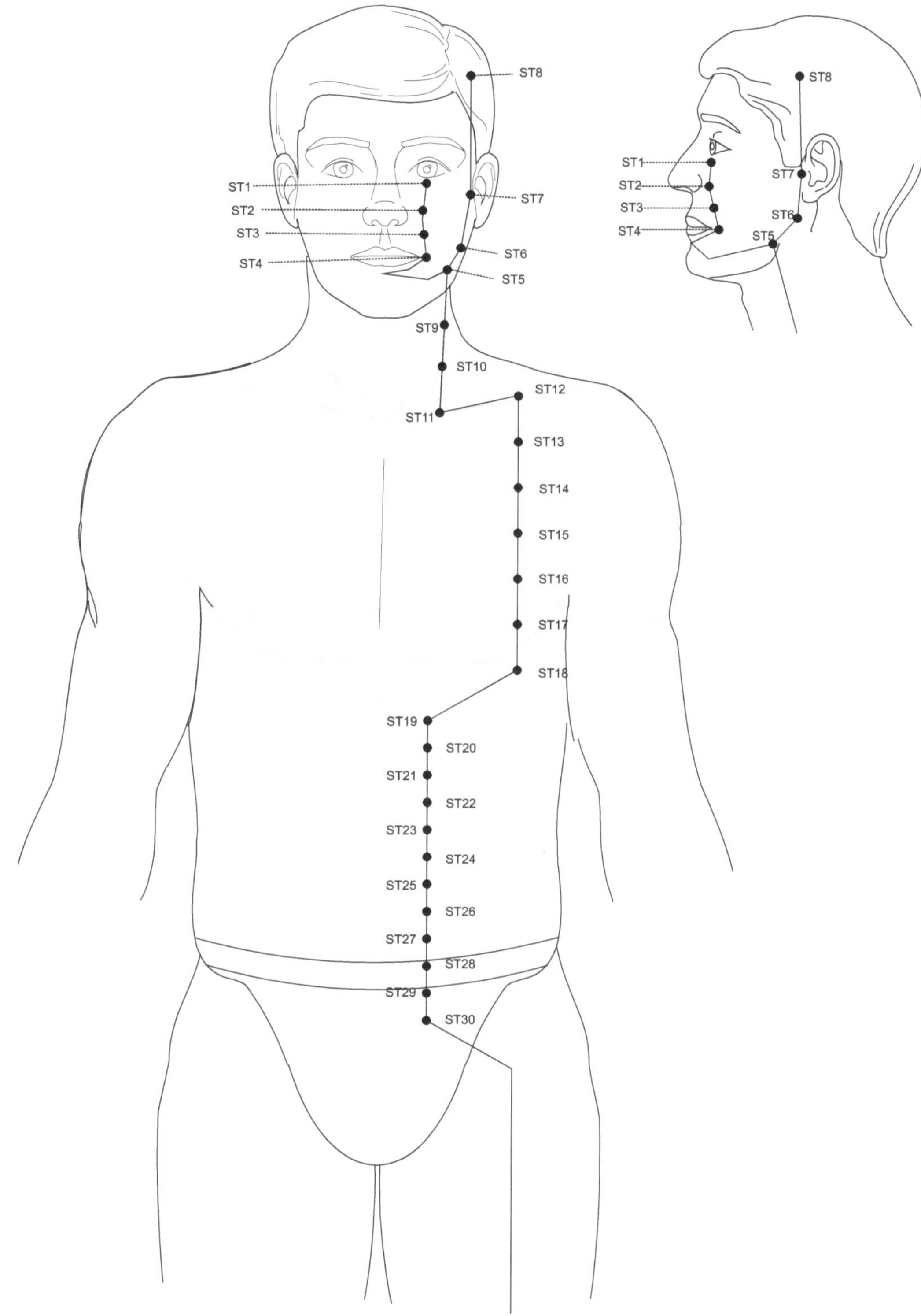

Figure 4.5 Stomach meridian—*Yang*

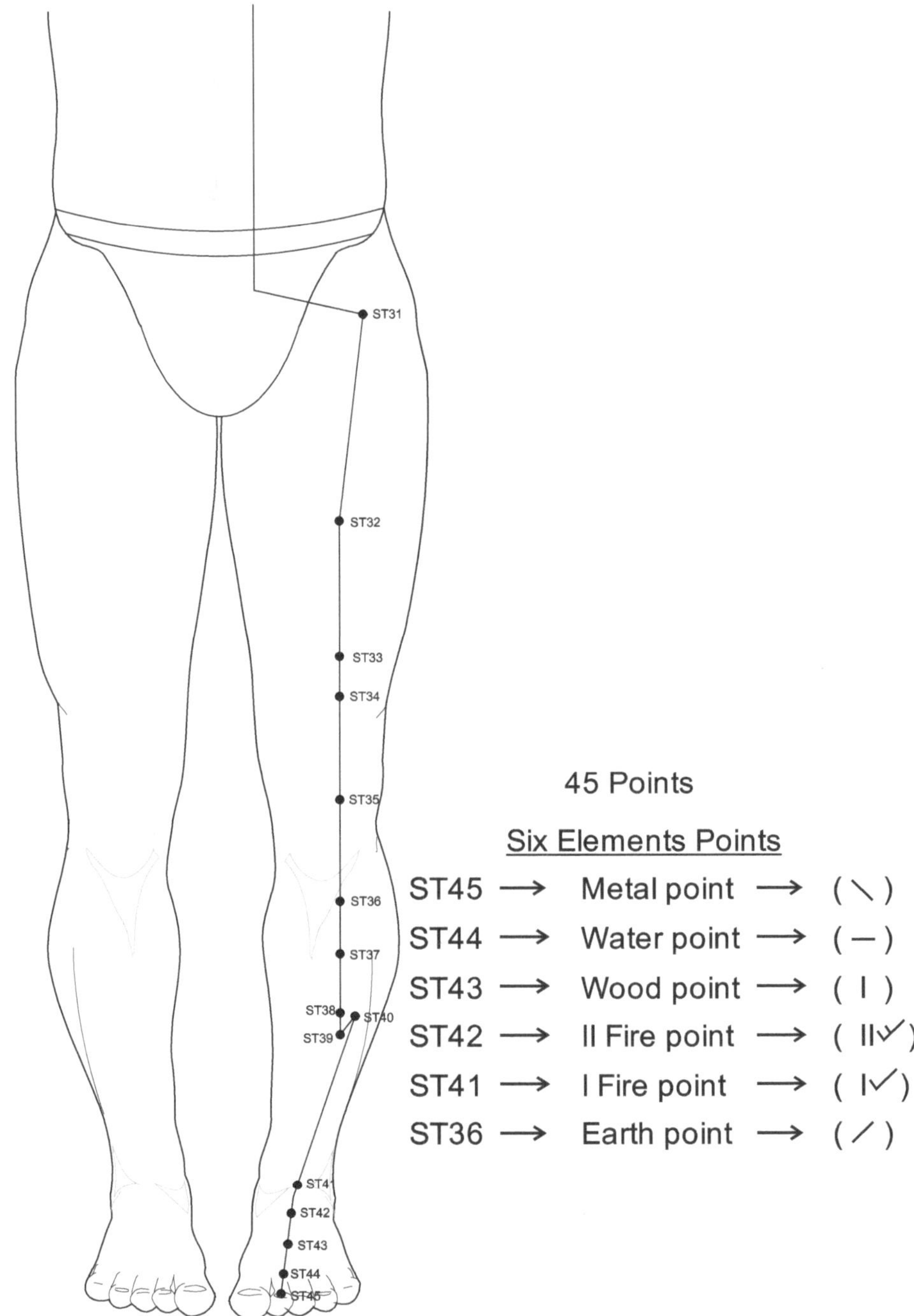

Figure 4.6 Stomach Meridian—*Yang*

The time of maximum energy flow is	- 7 am–9 am
The element	- Earth
Parallel channel	- Spleen meridian
Type of energy	- ***Yang***
Number of points in this meridian	- 45

Diseases are cured by puncturing the important points in this meridian.	Toothache, headache, paralysis of the cheeks ,polio, stomach diseases, ulceration of the intestine, rheumatism, menstruation-related disease, spleen-related diseases.

The Diseases Which Can be Cured by Touching the Six Element Points in This Stomach Meridian

ST—1—Junction point.

Vision impaired, right impaired, facial palsy, contraction of the facial muscles, myopathy of the facial muscles, tiredness, continuous watery discharge in one's eyes, tiredness in the eyes, deafness, cannot see bright lights, green colour around the eye muscles and noisy ears.

ST: 2 Gaseous point. (Metal, Wood)

Headaches, eye dystonia, continuous or involuntary blinking of the eyes, watery eyes, contraction of the facial muscles, high blood pressure, thyroid and parathyroid problems and nervous weakness.

ST: 3 Solid point. (I Fire, Earth)

Nose block due to moisture in the air, nose block due to common cold, cyst in the nose, long-sightedness vision impaired, nervous of the teeth becomes weak, swollen gums, swollen lips, pedal oedema, facial palsy and toothache.

ST: 4: Liquid point. (II Fire, Water)

Acute deafness or sudden deafness, a state in which one cannot speak, impaired blinking or cannot blink, oedema of legs, cheek pain, facial palsy, excessive saliva and swollen lips.

ST: 5—Liquid point. (II Fire, Water)

Neck pain, stiffness of the tongue, cannot talk, epileptic, blindness, fever with chills and shivering.

ST: 6 Solid point. (First fire, Earth)

Swelling in the gums, cannot talk, black spots in the eye, facial palsy, pimples on the face, toothache.

ST: 7: Gaseous point. (Metal, wood)

Bleeding nose, deafness, smoky vision, red eyes with pain, headache, dizziness, yawning, drowsiness, facial palsy and teeth becoming loose.

ST: 8—Junction point—*Yang.*

Headache, headache as if the head is going to burst, facial palsy, less sense in the face, eye pain, feels like the eyes are coming out, watery eyes, cannot see the sunlight, pain in the eyebrow, migraine and headache.

ST: 9 Junction point—Yin.

The heaviness of the chest, swollen reddish throat with pain, tonsillitis, vomiting, tension and high blood pressure.

ST: 10—Gas point. (metal, wood)

Tonsillitis, cold, laceration at the back throat and infection of the lungs.

ST: 11—Solid point. (First fire, Earth)

Numbness of the throat, swollen neck, pain, swollen glands in the neck, pain in the back of the throat, along with a swollen thyroid gland.

ST: 12—Liquid point. (II Fire, Water)

Numbness of throat, one side of the chest feels hot and swollen, cough, pain around the neck and pedal oedema due to water stagnation.

ST: 13—Gaseous point. (Metal, Wood)

The heaviness of the rib cage and joints, cannot sense the taste nor smell anything, no appetite and sweat in the foot.

ST: 14—Liquid point. (Second Fire, Water)

The heaviness of the rib cage and joints in the stomach area, phlegm along with bloody discharge, lung-related allergies, as well as body and mind affected by shock.

ST:15 Solid point. (First Fire, Earth)

The heaviness of rib cage and joints, swollen stomach, itching of the body, asthma, cyst in the chest, as well as pain due to compressed nerves.

ST: 16 Liquid point. (Second Fire, Water)

Large breast, ulceration of chest, short breath, common cold due to chilly weather, fever, swollen lips, diarrhoea, bitter taste in mouth and sensation of chest burning.

ST: 17 Solid point. (First Fire, Earth)

Breast/nipple-related diseases, indigestion, heart diseases, pericardium diseases, lung diseases.

ST: 18 Gaseous point. (Metal, Wood)

Chest pain, cough, prolonged menstruation, continuous cough, heart diseases, pericardium diseases, lung diseases.

ST 19: Gas point. (Metal, Wood)

Chest pain, cough, pain in the ribs, eye diseases, heart pain.

ST 20: Solid point. (First Fire, Earth)

Diarrhoea with noisy intestine(growling stomach) cannot swallow either liquid or food/jaundice.

ST 21:Liquid point. (Second Fire, Water)

Diarrhoea due to intestinal infections, gastric problems, burning stomach, ulcer, vomiting and nausea.

ST22: Liquid point. (Second Fire, Water)

Swollen lower abdomen, gastric problems, swelling because of water retention, diarrhoea, diarrhoea with a growling stomach.

ST 23: Solid point. (First Fire, Earth)

Psychiatric problems, palpitation of heat, indigestion, phlegm, talks when alone.

ST 24:Gaseous point (Metal, Wood)

Psychiatric problems, vomiting, thickened tongue, indigestion, pain under the tongue.

ST 25: Gaseous point.(Metal, Wood)

Pain around the naval, enlargement of the lower abdomen, menstrual problems, oedema due to water return, retention of urine, diarrhoea, dysentery, ulcer and stomach diseases.

ST 26: Solid point. (I Fire, Earth)

Pain around the naval, enlarged lower abdomen, oedema due to water retention, atrophy of the muscles in the colon.

ST 27: Liquid point. (II Fire, Water)

Hernia, lower abdomen swelling, quick ejaculation, weakness of bone joints, constipation, insomnia.

ST 28: Liquid point. (II Fire, Water)

Body heat, the mild reaction of urine, disease related to the ovary and genitals and pain in the female genitals.

ST29: Solid point. (I Fire, Earth)

Pain in the male genitals, diseases of genitals, atrophy of testis, allergic condition of the testis, amenorrhea, white discharge, swollen testis, menstruation problems.

ST30: Gaseous point. (Metal, Wood)

Lower abdomen pain, swelling in the genitals(in the male), feeling the heat in the stomach, hernia, contraction of the renal muscles, cannot walk, amenorrhea.

ST31: Junction point. (*Yang*)

Knee pain, numbness in the joints, pain travelling from the lower abdomen to the throat, swelling of the hip joint bone.

ST32:Gaseous point. (Metal, Wood)

Thigh/leg pain, the recurrent feeling of cold and heat in the knees, heaviness of the head, varicose vein, oedema in the leg with water stagnation, asthma at night.

ST33: Solid point. (First Fire, Earth)

Pain due to hernia, lower abdomen pain, contraction and pulling feeling of the pedal muscles, thirst, tremors of the fingers, fatigue.

ST 34: Liquid point. (II Fire, Water)

Knee and pedal pain, stomach ache, swollen breast/chest with pain, diarrhoea, Stomach diseases.

ST 35: Junction point.

Knee pain, cannot fold knees, crippled feet, pedal oedema due to water retention.

ST 36: Earth point.

Psychiatry problems, gastritis, growling stomach, pain in the lower abdomen, constipation, fatigue, eye diseases ,bleeding nose, body pain, tonsillitis, dizziness, state of dumbness ,nausea, diarrhoea and appendicitis.

ST37: Joint point (*Yang)*

Ribs and joints swelling, arthritis of the knee, cannot lift hand and leg, empty feeling in the stomach, gastritis, intestinal pain, chillness in the bone.

ST 38:Gaseous point. (Metal, Wood)

Weakness in the leg, no sense of urinating, tonsillitis, gastritis, pain in the intestine, diarrhoea, shoulder joint contraction.

ST39: Solid point. (I Fire, Earth)

Diarrhoea, lower abdomen pain, leg pain, psychiatry problem, tonsillitis, dryness of lips, no sweat, loss of hair.

ST40: Liquid point. (II Fire, Water)

Blocked throat, state of dumbness, headache, swollen face, asthma, cough, constipation, diabetes ,liver diseases, phlegm, epilepsy.

ST 41: Fire point.(I Fire)

Headache, swollen face, psychiatric problems, dizziness, heat in the shoulder, burning of eyes, indigestion, numbness of muscles, slurring, oedema in the ankle, tiredness in the fingers, ulceration of the heel.

ST 42: Second fire.(II Fire)

Periodical psychiatric problems occur every month, toothaches, vomiting, yawning and continuous walking.

ST43: Wood point.

Heaviness in the rib bones and joints, swollen face, fever with thirst, stomach problem, excessive belching with swollen lower abdomen and fever.

ST 44: Water point.

Pain around the umbilicus, fear and tremor because of pain, blood and mucus with stools, fever, diarrhoea, skin disease, toothache, headache and body pain.

ST 45: Metal point

Constipation, sinusitis, giddiness, numbness in the throat, tonsillitis, psychiatric disorders, excessive dreams, swollen face, toothache.

4.3 Urinary Bladder Meridian

Based on Six Elements Points

This meridian starts from the inner tip of the eye socket, ascends parallel to the centre line through the forehead and front side of the fontanelle and descends by the back of the head. From the fontanelle, a small branch goes towards the temporal bone. The straight track of this meridian connects with a part of the brain. Then it descends from the back of the skull and divides itself into two branches at the front of the neck, each of which descends at the inner side of the shoulder bone and parallel to the spinal cord. It reaches the hip and enters the body. It connects to the kidney and joins with its paired organ, the urinary bladder.

The branch from the joint of the pelvis descends through the buttocks and reaches the back fold of the knee. The branch from the upper part of the neck descends by the side of the shoulder bone, goes through the buttocks via the backside of the thigh and joins with the branch coming from the pelvic area and joins along with it at the back of the knee fold. From there, it becomes a single track and goes down through the calf muscles and the outer lower joint area of the backside of the leg. It reaches the outer tip of the small finger of the foot. There, it joins with the kidney meridian.

The time of maximum energy flow is - 3 pm –5 pm

The element - Water

Parallel channel - Kidney meridian

Type of energy - ***Yang***

Number of points in this meridian - 67

Diseases cured by puncturing the important points in this meridian:	Hemiplegia, headache nerve pain in the cheeks, disease related to the neck, cramps, joint pain, some related diseases, pain around the hip, kidney-related diseases, venereal diseases, urinary related diseases.

Diagram

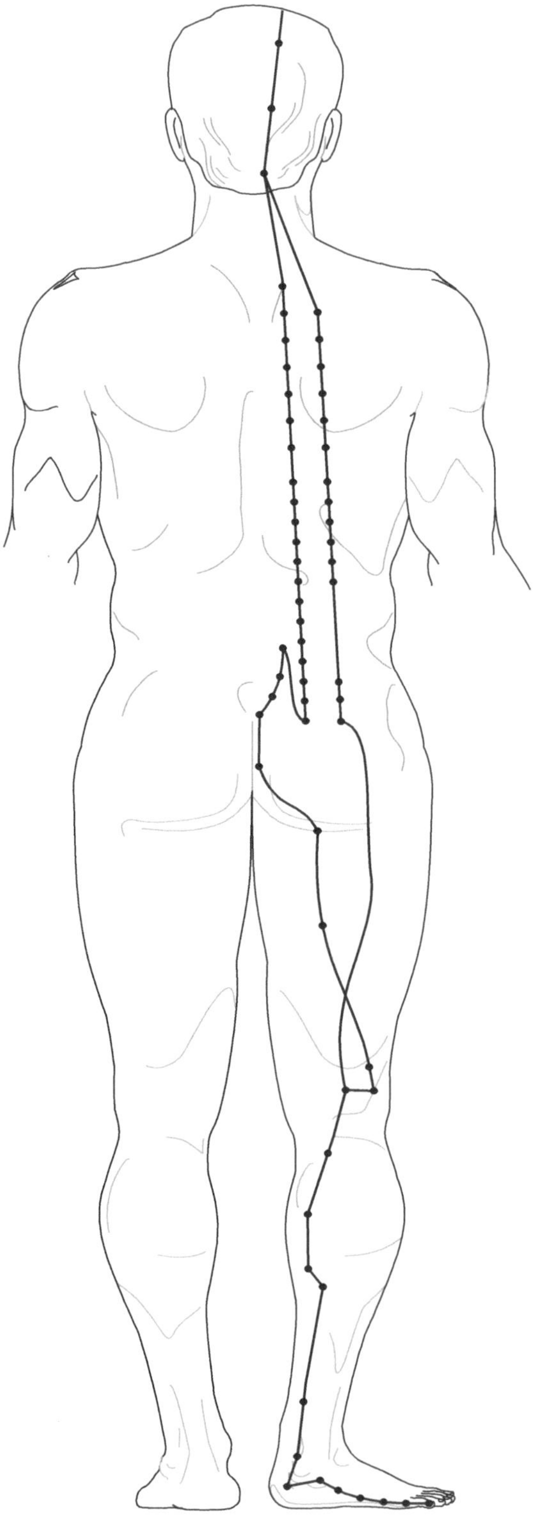

Figure 4.7 Urinary Bladder *Yang*

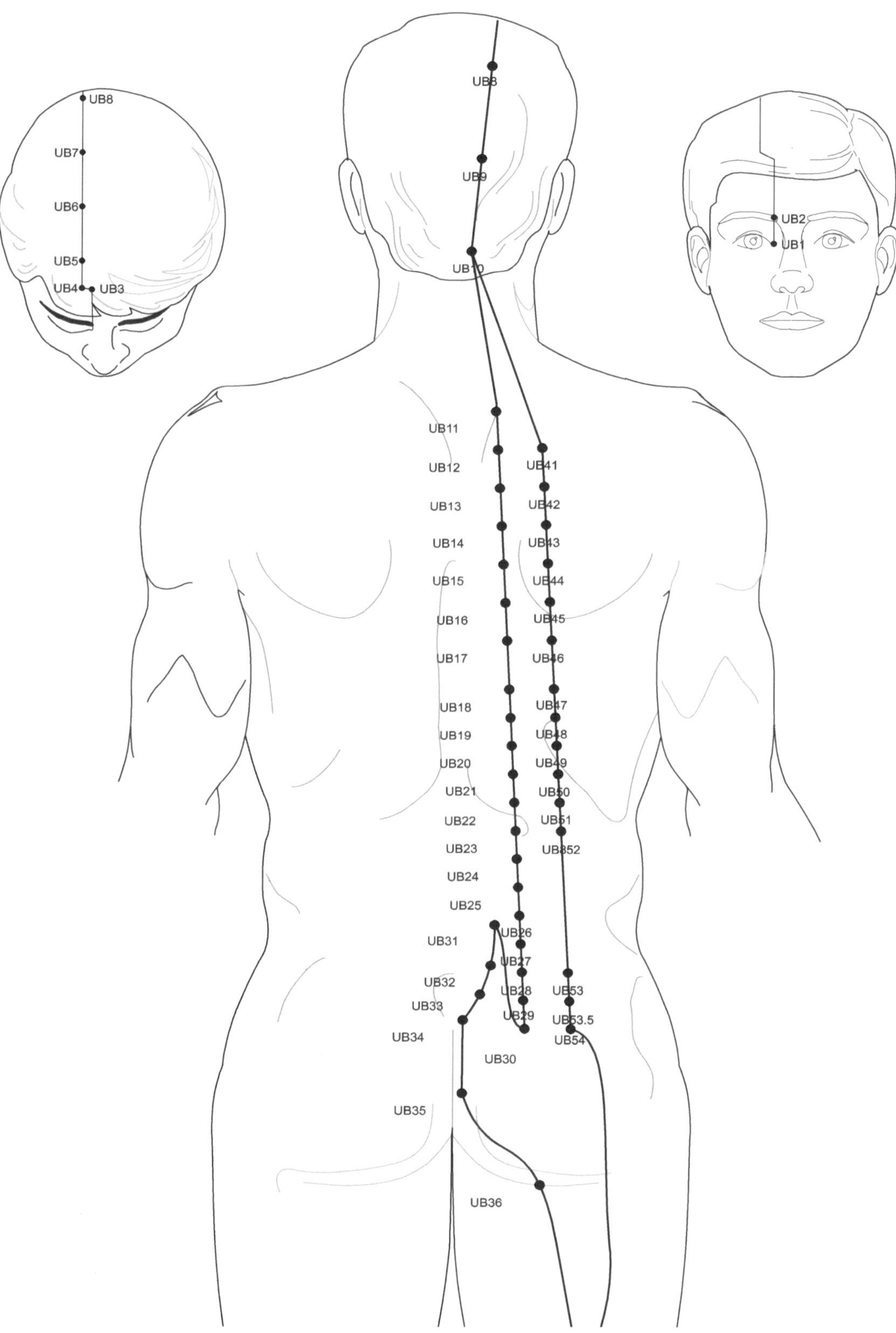

Figure 4.8 Urinary Bladder *Yang*

Six Elements Points

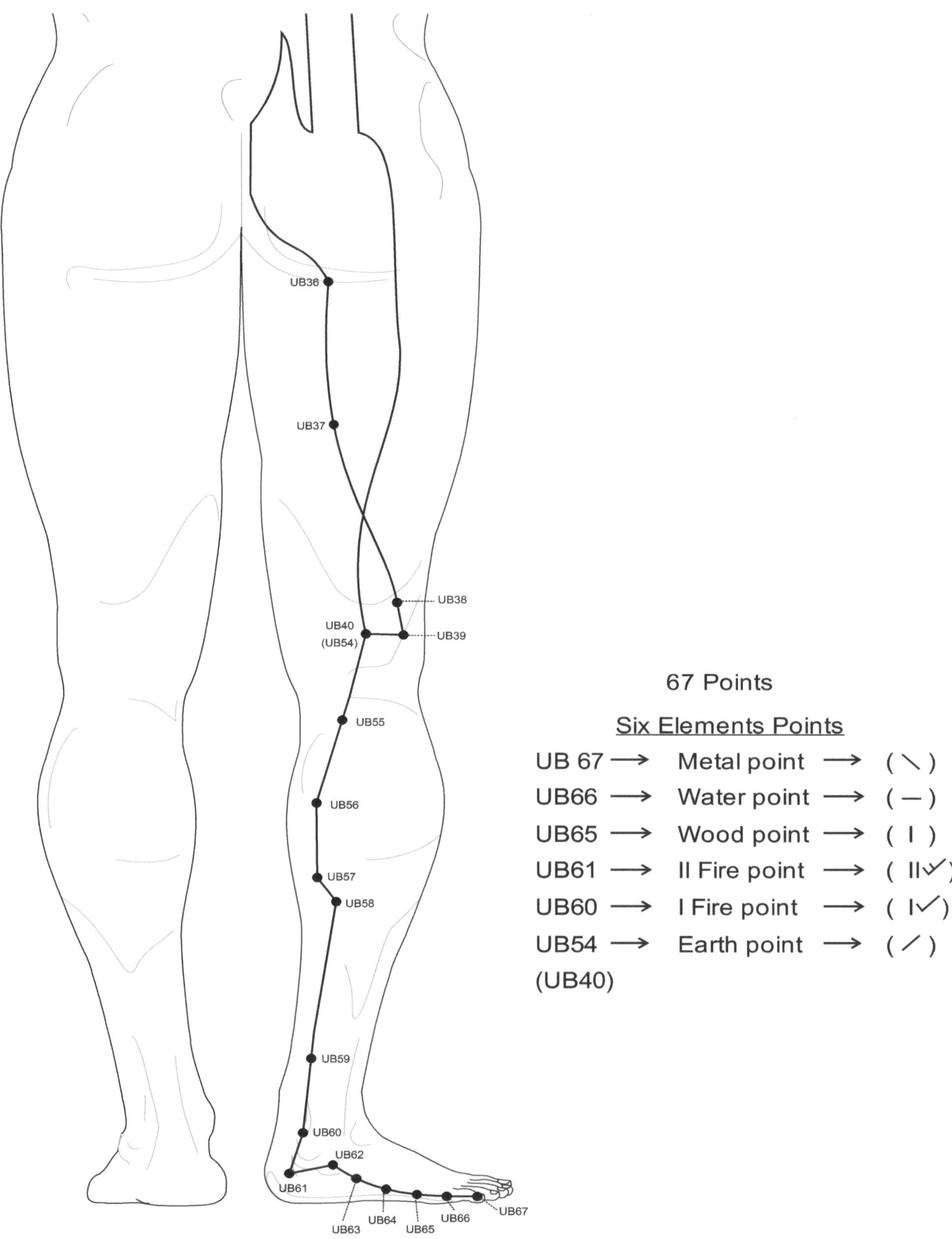

Figure 4.9. —Urinary Bladder *Yang*

The Diseases Which Can be Cured by Touching the Six Element Points in this Urinary Bladder Meridian

Urinary Bladder—1 Liquid point. (II Fire, Water)

Eye diseases, all sorts of diseases related to the eyes, vision is impaired, swelling of eyes, dizziness, night blindness and headaches.

Urinary Bladder—2 Solid point. (I Fire, Earth)

Brain fatigue, contraction of neck muscles, psychiatric diseases, redness of the eye, pain and redness of the eyes, excessive blinking, smoky feeling in the eyes, excessive fever, sneezing, sneezing if exposed to wind, sinusitis, nausea, vomiting.

Urinary Bladder—3 Gaseous point. (Metal, Wood)

Headaches, drowsiness, epilepsy, blocked nose, cataract formation, cannot sense any smell, complete sinusitis.

Urinary Bladder—4 Junction point—*Yang*

Headaches, facial nerve pain, burning heat in the head, contraction of the neck muscles, enlargement of the nose with skin diseases, blocked nose, ulcer or laceration.

Urinary Bladder—5 Water point. (II Fire, Water)

Headache, unconscious state, less memory, pain in the spine, heartburn.

Urinary Bladder—6 Solid point. (I Fire, Earth)

Fever without sweat, vomiting, dizziness, palpitation white colour around the eyes, vision impaired, nose block, heart diseases, pain in the shoulder muscles.

Urinary Bladder—7 Gaseous point. (Metal, Wood)

Headaches, heaviness in the head, blocked nose, swollen face, dryness in the mouth, allergic condition of the lungs, dizziness thirst and impaired vision.

Urinary Bladder—8 Gaseous point.(Metal, Wood)

Epilepsy, psychiatric diseases, impaired vision, swollen lower abdomen, as well as pain in the neck and shoulders.

Urinary Bladder—9 Solid point.(I Fire, Earth)

Pain in the eye, blocked nose, head and shoulder pain, dizziness, as well as neither being able to look down nor lift the head.

Urinary Bladder—10 Liquid point.(II Fire, Water)

The heaviness of the head, myopathy of the neck muscles, paralysis of the legs, swollen throat, state of dumbness, blocked nose, no sense of smell, phlegm, headaches, back of the head pain, sprain or contraction in the neck.

Urinary bladder—11 Junction point.

Fever sweat, fever, rheumatism, headaches, dizziness, epilepsy, drowsiness, heaviness in the chest, myopathy of the backside muscles, joint pain, blocked nose, skin diseases, asthma and shoulder bone diseases.

Urinary Bladder—12 Gaseous point.(Metal, Wood)

Paralysis or myopathy of the neck muscles, headache, cough, asthma, cannot sit, vomiting, sneezing, cyst in the back and shoulders.

Urinary Bladder—13 Solid point.(I Fire, Earth)

Cough, asthma, allergic condition of the lungs, sweat, vomiting, dryness of the mouth and tongue, feeling sad and blocked nose.

Urinary Bladder—14 Liquid point. (II Fire, Water)

Depression, cough, heart pain/chest pain, enlargement of the heart, vomiting, problems in the nervous system of the dentures, sudden stroke .Cannot go to the hill stations, cannot go to places at higher altitudes.

Urinary Bladder—15 Liquid point. (II Fire, Water)

Cannot stop talking, epilepsy, brain diseases, nervous weakness, palpitation with wheezing and cannot lie down and sleep, heart pain, feeling sad, vomiting, psychiatric problems, reddened face and infertility.

Urinary Bladder—16 Solid point.(I Fire, Earth)

Heart pain, pain in the intestines, cough, pain in the lower abdomen, shivering due to a fever with chillness, nervous breakdown.

Urinary Bladder—17 Gaseous point. (Metal, Wood)

Heart pain, numbness in the throat, tiredness of the body, fatigue or weakness, vomiting after eating, indigestion, wheezing, difficulty in breathing, hiccups and loss of appetite.

Urinary Bladder—18Gaseous point. (Metal, Wood)

Enlarged liver, black circle under the eyes, bitterness in the mouth, jaundice, ulcer, asthma, lung allergy, liver diseases.

Urinary Bladder—19 Solid point. (I Fire, Earth)

Fever, shivering/tremors, dryness of mouth, bitter taste in the mouth, pain in the ribs, vomiting after eating, high blood pressure, haemorrhage in the eyes and diseases of the urinary bladder.

Urinary Bladder—20 Liquid point. (II Fire, Water)

Heart pain, swollen lower abdomen, spleen-related point and spleen alarm point, abdominal pain, indigestion, thin physique despite eating well (not able to put on weight). Urinary bladder diseases and swollen intestines.

Urinary Bladder—21 Liquid point. (II Fire, Water)

Hip pain, acidity, indigestion, stomach ache, vomiting, diarrhoea, lower abdomen swelling, gastric problems, diarrhoea in children with green-coloured stools, liver and kidney related point and stomach diseases.

Urinary Bladder—22 Solid point.(I Fire, Earth)

Indigestion, cannot control urine, acidity, contraction of the shoulder, neck and muscles, hair loss, problems in the genital organs, urinary bladder diseases, ear diseases and diseases related to the bones.

Urinary Bladder—23 Gaseous point.(Metal, Wood)

Deafness, kidney diseases, prior indication point of the kidney problem, leg rheumatism or related problems, asthma, thyroid-related problems, pain in the spine, hair loss, ear diseases and venereal diseases.

Urinary Bladder—24Junction point.

Backbone pain, high blood pressure, intestinal muscles not functioning, V.D., haemorrhoids in the anus.

Urinary Bladder—25 Gaseous point. (Metal, Wood)

Pain around the umbilicus, diarrhoea, dryness of the large intestine, pain in the small intestine, chillness in the backbone, weakness in the legs, less urination, constipation and dysentery.

Urinary bladder—26 Solid point.(I Fire, Earth)

Lower abdomen swelling, diarrhoea, numbness and pain in the leg, fertility problems, pain in the hip muscles and bone and urinary tract diseases.

Urinary bladder—27 Liquid point. (II Fire, Water)

Diarrhoea, oedema of the leg, haemorrhoids around the anus, small intestine diseases and genital diseases.

Urinary Bladder—28 Liquid point. (II Fire, Water)

Yellowish urine, hip muscles and bones pain, lower abdomen pain, pain in the foot sole, feeling of chilliness in the head and pain while urinating.

Urinary Bladder—29 Solid point.(I Fire, Earth)

Weakness of the kidneys, hip muscles and bone pain with cramps, numbness and pain in the leg, hernia, lower abdomen pain and blood in the stools.

Urinary Bladder—30 Gaseous point. (Metal, Wood)

Yellow or reddish urine, anus muscles become paralysed, numbness and pain in the legs and from the hip, the pain extends to the whole of the lower body.

Urinary Bladder—31 Junction point *Yang.*

Constipation, uterus not able to function, white discharge, infertility, genital diseases, numbness and pain in the legs and infertility amongst women.

Urinary Bladder—32 Gaseous point. (Metal, Wood)

Backbone and muscles are constrained, knee swelling and pain, red-coloured urine, diarrhoea, white discharge, diseases of the testis, irregular menstruation and venereal diseases of both genders.

Urinary Bladder—33 Solid point.(I Fire, Earth)

Constipation, vomiting, swollen lower abdomen, diarrhoea, white discharge, hip pain, VD in both genders and infertility.

Urinary Bladder—34 Liquid point. (II Fire, Water)

Blood in stool, diarrhoea, constipation, pain and numbness in the thigh with the feeling of chillness, venereal diseases (VD) in both genders and cannot urinate.

Urinary Bladder—35 junction point: *Yin.*

Diarrhoea, pain in the anus, bloody stools, fluid discharge from the anus, numbness and pain in the legs, VD., and haemorrhoids in the anus.

Urinary Bladder—36 Gaseous point. (Metal, Wood)

Myopathy of the shoulder muscles, stiffness and pain in the neck, allergic to wind and chillness, allergic condition of the lungs.

Urinary Bladder—37 Solid point.(I Fire, Earth)

Feel emptiness in the lungs, lung allergy, vomiting and shoulder pain.

Urinary Bladder—38 Liquid point. (II Fire, Water)

Weakness, vomiting, sweating at night, psychiatric problems, less memory, slurring and bloody discharge while coughing.

Urinary Bladder—39 junction point. (*Yin/Yang*)

Asthma, heart diseases, tremors and atrophy of the kidneys.

Urinary Bladder—40 Earth point.

Calf muscles cramps, paralysis of the testicles, asthma, fever without sweat, headaches, pericardium diseases, difficulty in breathing, dizziness, vision is impaired, backbone pain and vomiting.

Urinary Bladder—41 Gaseous point. (Metal, Wood)

Bloody discharge from the intestines, vomiting, burping, cannot swallow water and food, excessive secretion of saliva, nausea and yellow urine.

Urinary Bladder—42 Solid point.(I Fire, Earth)

Cannot swallow water and food, indigestion, yellow or red urine, paralysis.

Urinary Bladder—43 Liquid point. (II Fire, Water)

Diarrhoea, water-borne diseases, red or yellow urine, body heat, yellowish eyes, rheumatism.

Urinary Bladder—44 Liquid point. (II Fire, Water)

Diarrhoea, rheumatoid, continuous vomiting, yellow eyes, yellow urine, fear of getting chills, excessive thirst.

Urinary Bladder—45 Solid point.(I Fire, Earth)

Cannot swallow food and water, is vomiting and has back pain with swelling.

Urinary Bladder—46 Gaseous point. (Metal, Wood)

Infection in the chest, lower heart pain, paralysis of the stomach muscles and constipation.

Urinary Bladder—47 Gaseous point. (Metal, Wood)

Pain in the penis, swelling, VD, difficulty in urination, weakness of the kidneys, vomiting, swelling of the lower abdomen and pain in the back of the kidney.

Urinary Bladder—48 Solid point.(I Fire, Earth)

Lower abdomen pain, constipation, retention of urine, difficulty in urination, VD, haemorrhoids around the anus and uterus-related diseases.

Urinary Bladder 49—Liquid point. (II Fire, Water)

Numbness and pain in the legs, swelling in the genital organs, diseases after undergoing pregnancy, difficulty in urination and haemorrhoids around the anus.

Urinary Bladder 50—Liquid point.(II Fire, Water)

Haemorrhoids around the anus, constipation, backbone pain, hip pain, numbness and pain in the legs, penis pain, diseases related to pregnancy and diseases related to sperm.

Urinary Bladder—51 Solid point.(I Fire, Earth)

Hip bone and muscle pain, numbness with pain in the legs, one cannot move the legs, paralysis of the legs, haemorrhoids around the anus and thigh problems.

Urinary Bladder—52 Gaseous point. (Metal, Wood)

Cannot fold the knee, paralysis of thigh muscles and calf muscles, heat in the lower abdomen, constipation and vomiting.

Urinary Bladder—53 Liquid point. (II Fire, Water)

Pain in the backbone and the neck, arthritis of the knees, pedal oedema, sweat at night due to weakness, psychiatric problems, nervous weakness, lower abdomen pain with swelling, tremors, loss of hair, loss of eyebrows, skin diseases and back pain.

Urinary Bladder—53.5 Solid point.(I Fire, Earth)

Stomach disorders, hip pain, hip cramps, nerve pain (as if pulling a nerve).

Urinary Bladder—54 Gaseous point. (Metal, Wood)

Hernia, rheumatoid, psychiatric problems, fits in children, paralysis of the lower abdomen muscles, knees, calves, and female genital organs, pedal oedema.

Urinary Bladder—55 Junction point *Yang*.

Hernia, psychiatric problems, hip pain, paralysis of the lower abdomen, muscle failure of the female genital organs.

Urinary Bladder—56 Gaseous point. (Metal, Wood)

Pedal oedema, the nerves in the calf area get stretched, haemorrhoids around the anus and constipation.

Urinary Bladder—57 Solid point.(I Fire, Earth)

Heat in the head, epilepsy, lower abdomen pain, bleeding haemorrhoids around the anus, VD(both sexes), pain in the heels, calf cramps and diseases of the reproductive organs.

Urinary Bladder—58 Liquid point.(II Fire, Water)

Epilepsy, weakness of the legs, backbone pain, numbness and pain in the legs, constipation and haemorrhoids around the anus.

Urinary Bladder—59 Junction point *Yin*.

Arthritis in the knees, painful stretched nerves, cannot fold the knees because of the pain, heaviness in the head, pain, cannot lift hands, swelling of the thigh and rheumatoid in the knees.

Urinary Bladder—60 Fire point.

Delirium in small children, backbone pain, thigh pain, numbness and pain in the legs, rheumatoid of the foot, pedal oedema, headaches, dizziness, haemorrhoids around the anus and ankle pain.

Urinary Bladder—61 Second Fire. (II Fire, Water)

Foot arthritis, weakness of the foot, backbone pain, nerve pain in the calf, psychiatric diseases, fear of ghosts, dizziness and genital diseases in both sexes.

Urinary Bladder—62 Gaseous point. (Metal, Wood)

Psychiatric diseases, epilepsy, electrical units' emission through the skin, knee pain, reddish swollen face, numbness and pain in the foot, backbone pain, headache and brain diseases.

Urinary Bladder—63 Solid point.(I Fire, Earth)

Headaches, paediatric delirium, knee pain, lower abdomen pain, vomiting and leg pain.

Urinary Bladder—64 Liquid point.(II Fire, Water)

Backbone pain, numbness and pain in the legs, stiffness of the neck, headaches, epilepsy, psychiatric diseases, heart diseases, impaired vision and cannot eat food and drink water.

Urinary Bladder—65 Wood point.

Diarrhoea, fever, one does not like air and chilliness, psychiatric problems, dizziness, deaf, cramp in the neck, numbness and pain in the leg, all sorts of abscesses and all sorts of haemorrhoids around the anus.

Urinary Bladder—66 Water point.

Headaches, dizziness, constrain in the neck, impaired vision, indigestion, intestinal diseases and allergic to changes in food and water.

Urinary Bladder—67 Metal point.

Heaviness in the head, blocked nose, pain in the eye, fever, difficulty in urination and venereal diseases in both sexes.

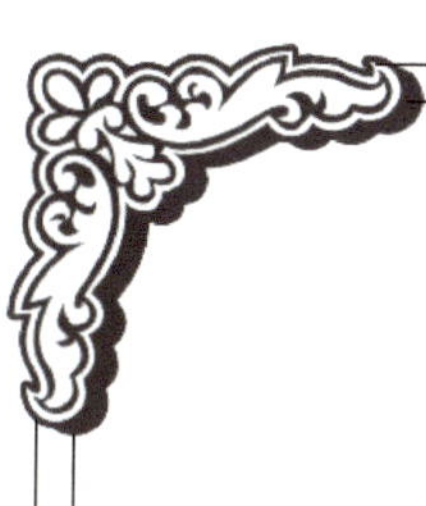

Part Five

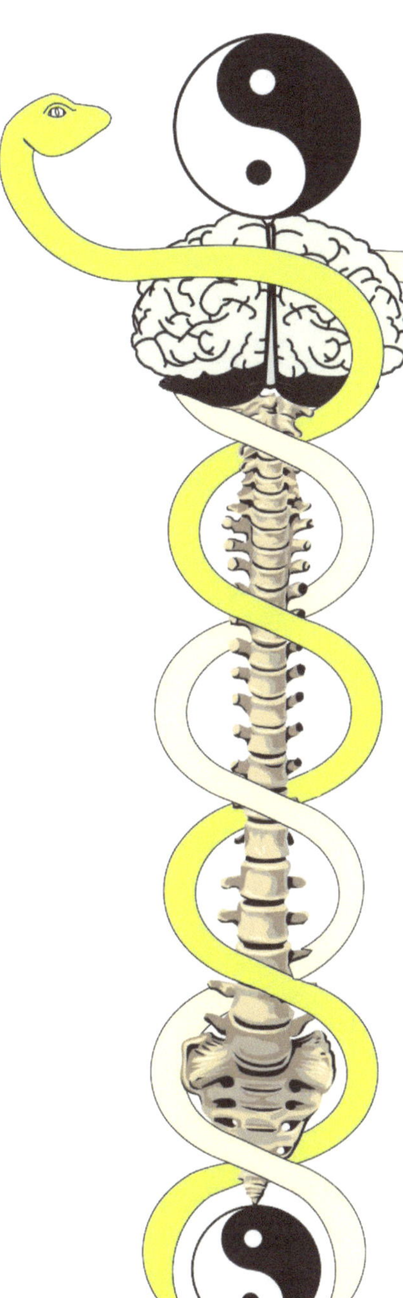

5.1.Liver Meridian (LIV) Based on Six Element Points Method

5.2.Spleen Meridian (SP) Based on Six Element Points Method

5.3.Kidney Meridian (K) Based on Six Element Points Method

5.1 Liver Meridian (LIV)

Based on Six Elements Points

This meridian starts from the top of the toe and travels on the top of the foot up to 1 cm distance and reaches the lower side of the front bone of the leg. From there, it goes up through the inner side up to an8 cm distance and crosses the spleen meridian. Again, it travels down the inner side through the knees and thighs and reaches the front of the pelvic area. It goes around the reproductive organs and enters the lower side of the stomach.

From there, it goes up to circle the stomach area. Then, it enters its organ to link with the gall bladder.

Again, from there, it goes up through the diaphragm and reaches the upper part of the chest. Again, it goes through the back of the throat, the air passage, joins with the eyes and goes to the meridian situated at the centre of the skull through the front side of the head. One branch from the eye goes down through the cheeks and reaches the inner side of the lips. Then the branch starts from the liver, goes through the diaphragm and reaches the lungs. There it gets connected with the lung meridian.

The time of maximum energy flow - Up to 3 am.

The element - Wood.

Parallel channel - Gall bladder.

Type of energy -***Yin***

Number of points in this meridian - 14 + 1 = 15

Diseases cured by puncturing the important points in this meridian.	Eye-related diseases, Spleen, liver diseases, epilepsy, headache, indigestion, gall bladder-related diseases.

Diagram

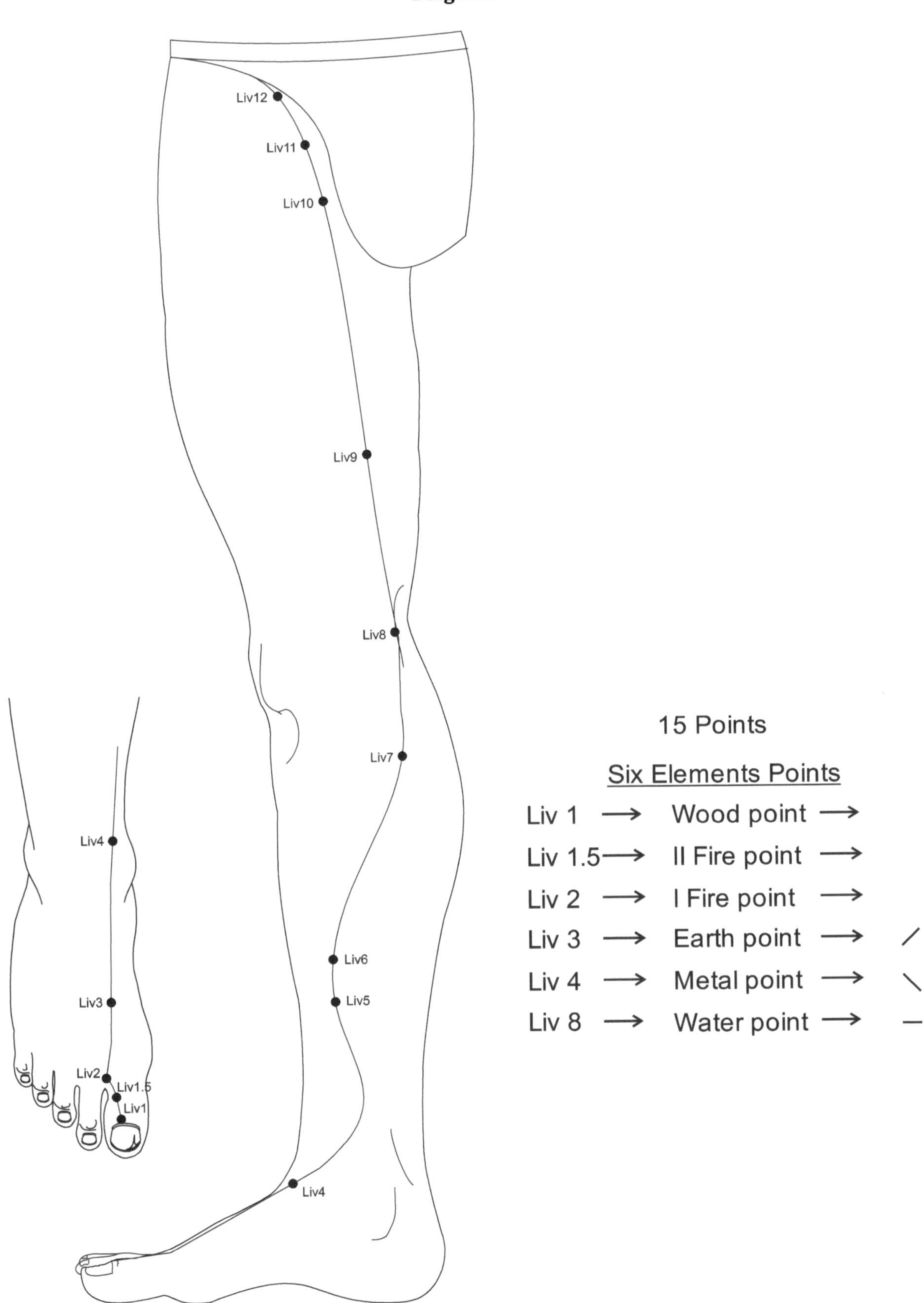

Figure 5.1 Liver meridian—*Yin.*

The Diseases Which Can be Cured by Touching the Six Element Points in this Liver Meridian.

Liver—1 Wood point.

Continuous headache, one of the testicles becomes enlarged, pain in the penis, bleeding nose, uterus problems, lower abdomen pain, stomach pain, unconscious state, drowsy, likes to sleep, excessive sweat and backbone pain.

Liver—1.5. Second Fire: (II Fire)

Indigestion, winter diseases, kidney problems, palpitation of the heart, wheezing, less breathing or shortness of breath and the whole body becomes numb.

Liver—2 Fire point. (I Fire)

Headache, anaemia, excessive anger, dryness of throat, irritation, cough, swelling of the lower abdomen, urine retention, knee pain, swelling of the lower abdomen, urine retention, knee pain, swelling, cannot fold knee because of pain, psychiatric diseases, epilepsy, delirium in children abscesses in the breasts and ulcer in the breast.

Liver—3 Earth point.

Headache, anaemia, getting angry, swollen red eye, dryness and burning sensation in the throat, rib pain, cough, pain due to gastric problems, swollen body, lower abdomen swelling, retention of urine, hip muscles and bone pain, knee pain, cannot fold knee, psychiatric diseases, epilepsy, abscesses in the breasts, eye diseases and low blood pressure.

Liver—4 Metal point.

Swollen lower abdomen, yellowish eyes, fever, jaundice, fever after eating, pain around the umbilical area, the chilliness of hands and legs, shrinking of muscles or atrophy of muscles and pain in the vagina.

Liver—5 Liquid point. (II Fire, Water)

Severe lower abdomen pain, swelling in the lower abdomen, retention of urine, swelling in the testicles, pain, irregular menstruation, burping, blocked or choked throat, anxiety, cannot bend the body backwards, depression or stress, cannot fold knees, as well as liver diseases related to kidney and urinary bladder.

Liver—6 Solid point. (I Fire, Earth)

Lower abdomen pain, diarrhoea, knee pain and numbness of skin due to chilliness, liver and gall bladder diseases and liver diseases related to the digestive organs.

Liver—7 Gaseous point. (Metal, Wood)

Arthritis, throat pain, knee pain, cannot fold knee, liver diseases related to the lungs, large intestine and gaseous state-related organs.

Liver—8 Water point.

Abscesses, swelling of the lower abdomen, menstrual problems, pain in the penis, difficulty in urination, retention of urine, knee pain, bleeding nose and psychiatric problems.

Liver—9 Liquid point.(II Fire, Water)

Hip muscles and bone pain, lower abdomen pain, hip muscles fail to function, difficulty in urination, heaviness in the chest, urinary bladder-related liver diseases.

Liver—10 Solid point. (I Fire, Earth)

Heaviness in the lower abdomen, retention of urine, testicles swell, itching, no sweat, insomnia, irregular periods, white discharge, intestine-related liver diseases.

Liver—11 Gaseous point. (Metal, Wood)

Pain in the penis, pain in the thighs, pain in the whole of the lower hip, irregular periods; Lungs and intestine–related liver diseases.

Liver—12 Liquid point.(II Fire, Water)

Penis pain, thigh pain, pain in the lower hip ,kidney and urinary bladder-related liver diseases.

Liver—13 Solid point.(I Fire, Earth)

Spleen diseases-related alarm point, lower abdomen swelling, indigestion, diarrhoea stomach pain, dryness of mouth, excessive eating, high blood pressure, loss of body weight, Intestinal-related liver diseases.

Liver—14 Gaseous point.(Metal, Wood)

Alarm points of liver diseases, cough, burping, vomiting with a sour taste(fermented) dryness of mouth, excessive thirst, body pain on both sides, pain in the wrist, diseases of the chest, Lung-related liver diseases.

5.2 Spleen Meridian (SP)

Based on Six Elements Points

This meridian starts from the inner tip of the toe, travels outside to the foot and reaches the bottom of the upper leg's bone. It then travels inside the calf muscles and crosses the liver meridian. Then, it travels upward through the inner side of the thighs, reaches the stomach region and enters its organ, the spleen. Then, it gets connected to the stomach from which it travels through the diaphragm towards the direction that runs up—at the sides of the food pipe and reaches the tongue. Another branch joins the heart meridian by travelling through the diaphragm and the heart.

The time of maximum energy flow is - 9 am to 11 am

The element - Earth.

Parallel channel - Stomach.

Type of energy -***Yin***

Number of points in this meridian - 21 + 1 = 22

Diseases cured by puncturing the important points in this meridian:	The stomach, the spleen, liver diseases, allergies, problems in blood formation and swelling of the intestines, intestinal problems, Elephantiasis, diseases related to urine ,fertility issues.

Diagram

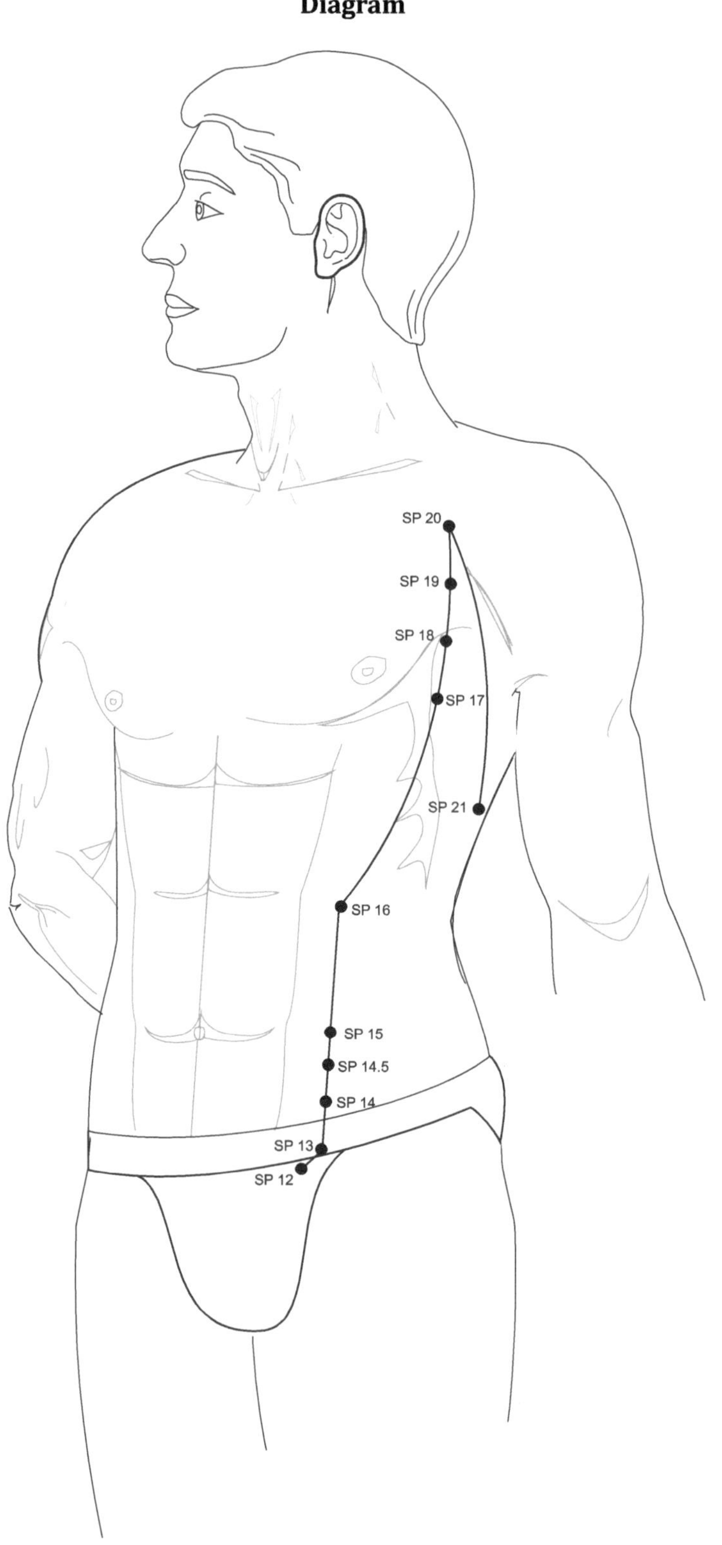

Figure 5.2.—Spleen *Yin*

Figure 5.3.—Spleen *Yin*

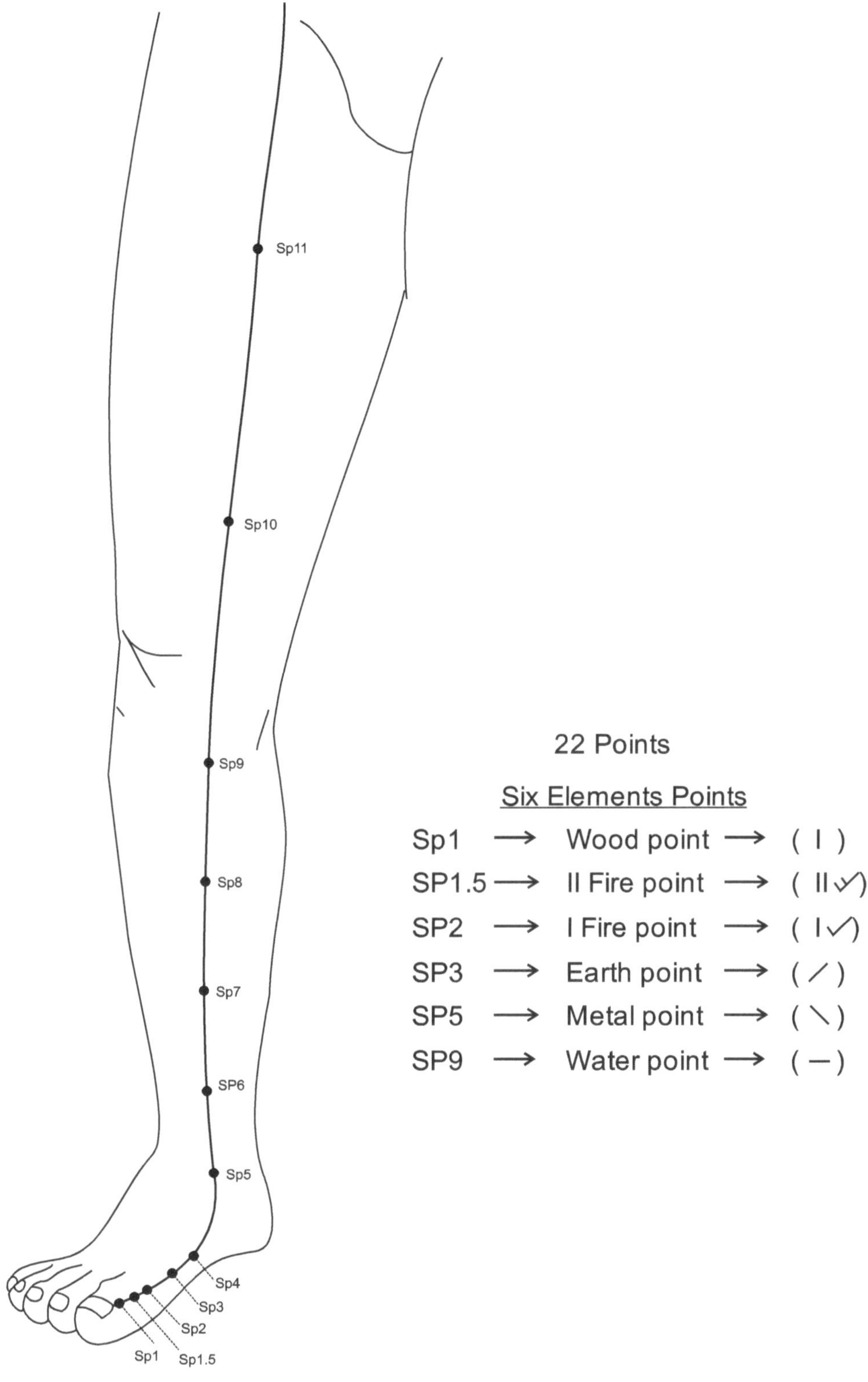

Figure5.4.—Spleen *Yin*

The Diseases Which Can be Cured by Touching the Six Element Points in this Spleen Meridian.

SP 1—Wood point.

Asthma, swelling of the lower abdomen, excessive vomiting, thirst, paralysis due to the chilliness of the foot and psychiatric problems.

SP 2—Second Fire. (II Fire)

Asthma, excessive phlegm during winter, cannot breathe, allergic to chilly air, often fever with chilliness, all the eaten food converts into phlegm.

SP 3—Earth point.

Fever, swelling of the lower abdomen, severe pain with intestinal sounds, diarrhoea, constipation, heaviness of the body, psychiatric problems, pain in the heart and chilliness of the foot.

SP 4—Junction point. *Yang.*

Swelling of the intestine, severe pain in the intestine, swelling of the lower abdomen, heart pain, vomiting all the food eaten, fever, jaundice, swelling of face, excessive thirst and non-healing ulcer.

SP 5—Metal point. (M)

Vomiting, whatever is eaten is vomited, headache, swollen face, one feels as though the spleen is empty, indigestion, pain in the thigh, hernia ,pain in the lower abdomen, dreams of ghosts, jaundice, non-healing ulcer, ankle pain and menstruation problems.

SP 6—Liquid point. (II Fire, Water)

All diseases related to both genders' genital organs, pain in the genitals, swollen lower abdomen, asthma, diabetes, indigestion, acidity, skin diseases and fertility problems.

SP 7—Solid point.(I Fire, Earth)

Swelling of the lower abdomen, indigestion, cannot gain weight despite excessive eating, numbness, cannot walk, psychiatric problems, pain in the foot and the ankle, swelling and ejaculation in one's sleep.

SP 8—Gaseous point. (Metal, Wood)

Lower abdomen swelling, irregular periods, less urination, fever and nocturnal emission (wet dreams).

SP 9—Water point.

Oedema around the naval with water retention, nocturnal emissions, knee pain, heaviness of the chest, fever, weakness of the legs, oedema of the intestines, swollen blood arteries/veins and blocked urine.

SP 10—Solid point. (I Fire, Earth)

Menstruation with lower abdomen pain, indigestion, skin diseases, eczema, itching due to indigestion, menstrual problems and allergies.

SP 11—Gaseous point. (Metal, Wood)

Less urine, cannot control urine, spontaneous urine discharge and urination if one coughs.

SP 12—Liquid point. (II Fire, Water)

Lower abdomen swelling with pain, indigestion, retention of urine(less quantity), hernia, menstruation with pain in the lower abdomen and abscesses in the breasts.

SP 13—Solid point. (I Fire, Earth)

Hernia, indigestion, lower abdomen pain and pain under the hip.

SP 14—Gaseous point.(Metal, Wood)

Lower abdomen pain, diarrhoea and weakness in legs, cough and heart problems.

SP 14.5—Liquid point.(II Fire, Water)

Lower abdomen swelling with water, urine retention, urination at intervals and excessive urine during the winter season.

SP—15 Solid point.(I Fire, Earth)

Stools with blood, mucus in stool, acidity, pain from around the naval to the lower abdomen, intestinal pain, intestinal paralysis, worms in the intestines and loose motion.

SP—16Gaseous point. (Metal, Wood)

Blood in the stools, dysentery, pain from the naval to the lower abdomen and ulcer of the stomach.

SP—17 Liquid point. (II Fire, Water)

Heaviness in the chest, severe noise in the intestines, fever, spleen fever, paralysis, forgetfulness and difficulty in breathing due to heart problems.

SP—18 Solid point.(I Fire, Earth)

Pain in the centre of the chest, swelling, the breast becomes enlarged due to swelling, less milk secretion, ulcer in the stomach, cough and throat irritation.

SP—19 Gaseous point.(Metal, Wood)

Heaviness in the rib bones and joints, no appetite or hunger, problems in turning, cannot sit and lung problems.

SP—20 junction point: *Yang.*

Cough, bloody discharge with phlegm, swelling, swelling in the eyebrows and swelling in the lower abdomen.

SP—21 Junction point: *Yin.*

Migraine, headaches, pain on one side of the body and shifting pain.

5.3 Kidney Meridian (K)

Based on Six Elements Points

This meridian starts from the bottom of the small finger of the foot, travels in a slanting direction to the back of the lower knot of the front leg bone and enters the heel. Then it goes up by travelling inside the leg. Through the inner fold of the knee, it travels further up by the side of the thigh towards its meridian and enters its organ, the kidneys near the backbone. Then it gets connected to the urinary bladder. One straight track starts from the kidney and travels up via the liver and diaphragm. It goes through the lungs and the sides of the throat till the middle of the tongue and ends there. Another track starts from the lungs, reaches the heart and joins the pericardium by travelling through the ribs.

The time of maximum energy flow is - 5pm to 7 pm

The element - Water.

Parallel channel - Urinary Bladder.

Type of energy -***Yin***

Number of points in this meridian - 27 + 1 = 28

Diseases cured by puncturing this meridian:	Fertility, menstrual problems, important points in impotence in males, loss of hair, ear, bone and heart-related diseases, heel pain and swelling, the small intestine, the kidneys and urinary bladder-related diseases.

Diagram

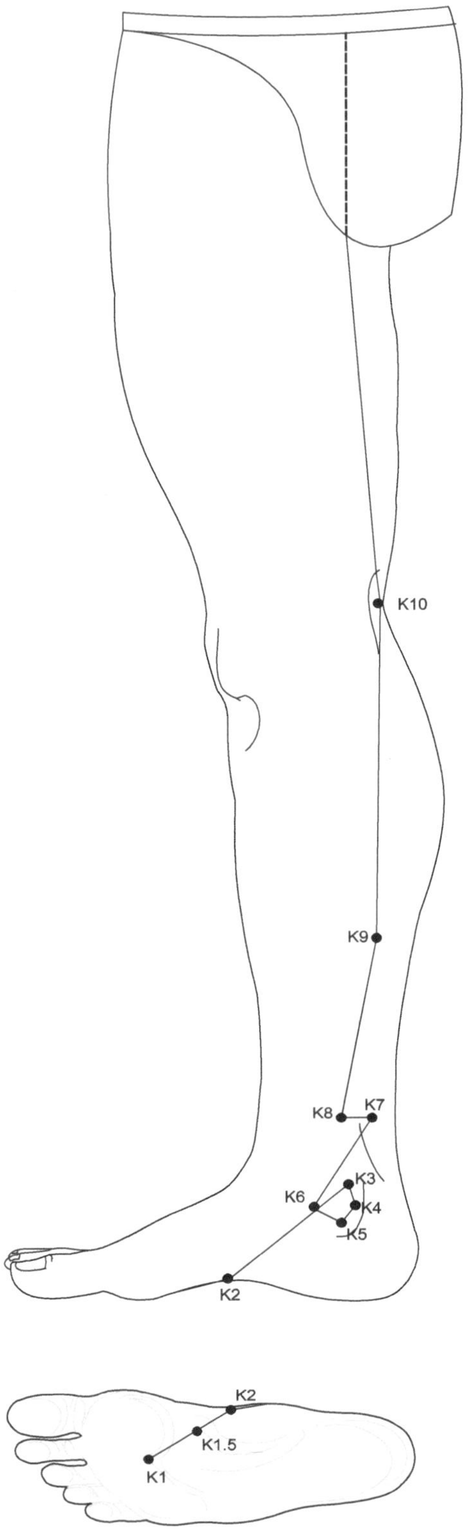

28 Points

Six Elements Points

K 1 → Wood point → (I)

K 1.5 → II Fire point → (II✓)

K 2 → I Fire point → (I✓)

K 3 → Earth point → (/)

K 7 → Metal point → (\ )

K 10 → Water point → (—)

Figure 5.4 Kidney *Yin*

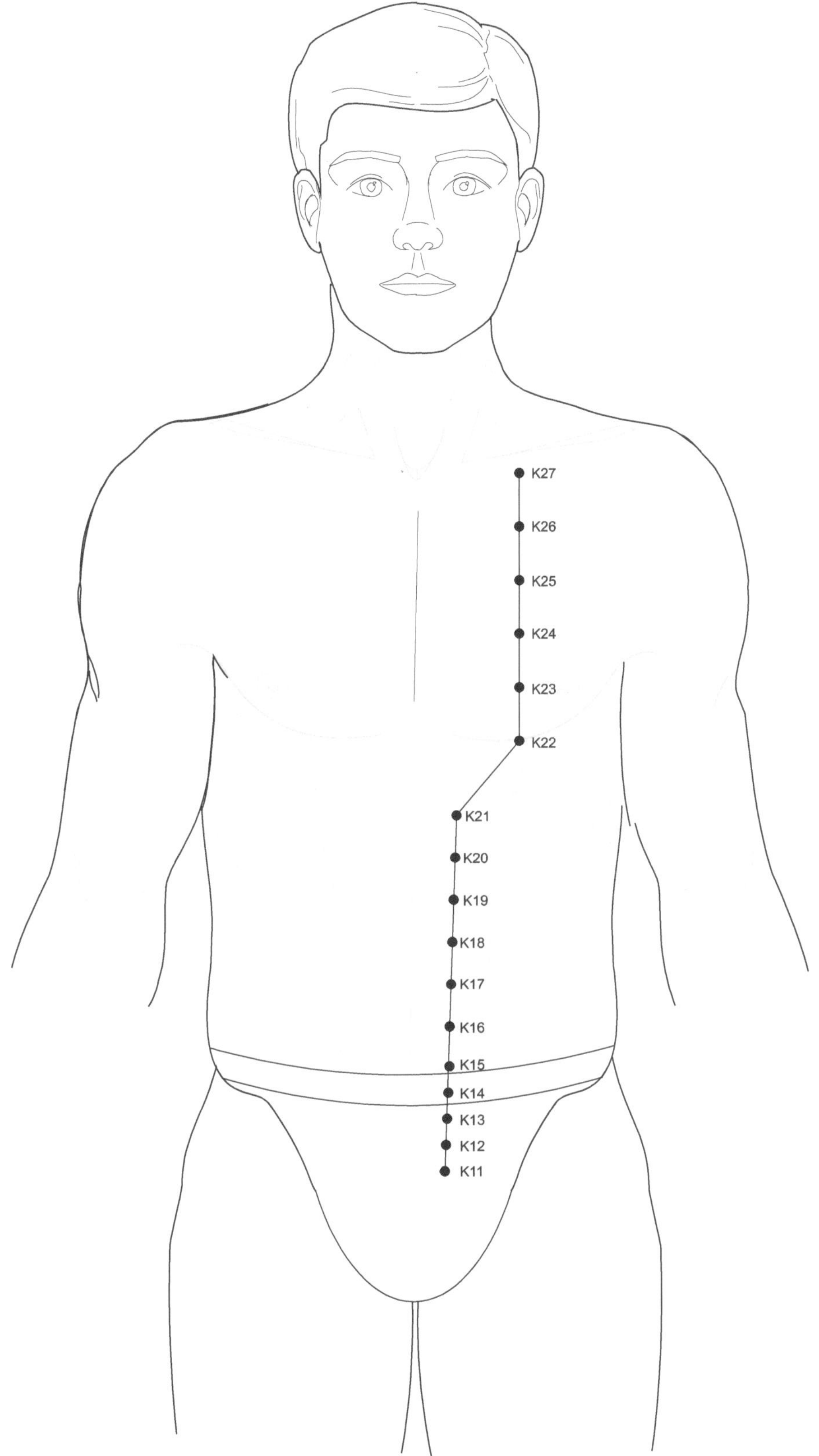

The Diseases Which Can Be Cured by Touching the Six Element Points in this Kidney Meridian.

Figure 5.5 Kidney *Yin*

K—1 Wood point.

Deafness, dizziness, fear, psychiatric diseases, epilepsy, head and neck pain, throat pain and swelling, bleeding from the nose, blockage in the throat, pain in the small intestine, backbone pain, dizziness, constipation, retention of urine, shock and senselessness.

K—1.5. Second Fire.(II Fire)

Low blood pressure, psychiatric problems, hatred, fear, one feels as though he/she would die in the cold weather, scared to sleep at night, excessive chilliness and numbness.

K—2 Fire point.

High blood pressure, asthma, lung allergy, pain and swelling of the throat, blocked throat, diseases of the genitals, infertility, irregular periods and sweating at night.

K—3 Earth point.

Diabetes, pituitary diseases, dryness of the throat, sadness, psychiatric diseases, epilepsy, lower abdomen pain, irregular periods, constipation, asthma, headaches, anaemia, ankle pain, less strength in fertility and hip pain.

K—4 Liquid point.(II Fire, Water)

Stiffness and pain in the whole of the backbone, pedal oedema and pain, constipation, heat in the whole mouth, dryness of the tongue, swelling of the chest, blockage in the throat, cannot swallow, unhappiness, one vomits everything after eating and VD in both sexes.

K—5 Solid point.(I Fire, Earth)

Backbone pain, blocked throat, vomiting, fear, unhappiness, asthma, difficulty in breathing and kidney-related diseases.

K—6 Earth point.

Cough, cough with phlegm, pain like pins and needles in the heart, pinning pain in the heart, yellow urine, fever, throat swelling, irregular menstruation, toothache, pedal pain and sweating, ankle swelling and VD.

K—7 Metal point.

Sweating, continuous sweating, constipation, diarrhoea, diabetes, no sweat, indigestion, venereal diseases in the testicles, haemorrhoids around the anus, vision problems and hair and bone-related diseases.

K -8 Liquid point.(II Fire, Water)

Menstruation problems, white discharge, muscle pain in the thigh and leg areas ,venereal diseases, difficulty in urinating, testis-related diseases, constipation, dysentery with mucus and blood and lower abdomen pain.

K—9 Solid point.(I Fire, Earth)

Weakness, foot pain, swelling in the tongue, failure of the lower abdomen muscles, less milk secretion in women ,immunity point.

K-10—Liquid point.(II Fire, Water)

Thigh pain, knee pain, lower abdomen and the whole genital area pain ,pain around the navel area, itching in the testicles, difficulty in urination, yellow urine and excessive secretion of saliva.

K-11—Gaseous point. (Metal, Wood).

Lower abdomen swelling and pain, difficulty in urination, penis and testis pain swelling, reddish eyes with pain, pain in the kidney area and one cannot stand for a longer period.

K—12 Solid point.(I Fire, Earth)

Swelling in the lower abdomen with pain, venereal diseases, penis pain, infertility in women, retention of urine and backbone pain.

K—13 Liquid point.(II Fire, Water)

Infertility amongst women, irregular menstrual discharge, lower abdomen pain, painful reddish eyes, diarrhoea, infertility, pain in the penis and venereal diseases.

K—14 Gaseous point. (Metal, Wood).

Umbilical hernia, indigestion, stabbing pain around the navel, chilliness with shivering, venereal diseases and eye diseases.

K—15 Liquid point.(II Fire, Water)

Heat in the upper abdomen, constipation, intestinal pain, difference in urination, irregular periods, reddish painful eyes, swelling and pain in the fingers of the hands.

K—16 Solid point.(I Fire, Earth).

Pain in the whole of the lower abdomen and swelling, stabbing pain in the lower abdomen, constipation diarrhoea, failure of stomach muscles, jaundice, reddish painful eyes and failure of the neck muscles.

K—17 Gaseous point. (Metal, Wood)

Lower abdomen pain or stabbing pain, loss of appetite, constipation, diarrhoea, failure of intestinal muscles, sorrowful feelings and a patient does not want to live.

K—18 Junction point *Yin*

Breathing problems due to asthma, cough, empty feeling in spleen and stomach ,allergic to cold beverages, vomiting, retention of impure blood in organs, unbearable lower abdomen pain, constipation, genital diseases or venereal diseases and yellow urine.

K—19 Liquid point.(II Fire, Water)

Sound in the lower abdomen, gastric ulcer, burning of the heart (at the bottom of the heart), vomiting, suffocation due to asthma, reddish eyes with pain and jaundice.

K—20 Solid point.(I Fire, Earth)

Dryness of mouth, deafness, yawning ,pain in the ribs, diarrhoea, chronic gas problems, ulcers in the intestines and cramped neck.

K—21 Gaseous point. (Metal, Wood)

Pain in the whole of the chest, allergy of the lungs, pain while swallowing, upper abdomen swelling, dysentery with blood, ulcer of the intestines, vomiting during pregnancy, abscesses in the breasts and reddened eyes with pain.

K—22 Gaseous point. (Metal, Wood)

The heaviness of the chest, cough, asthma, blocked nose, vomiting, infections of the chest and failure of lower abdomen muscles.

K—23Solid point.(I Fire, Earth).

Cough, the heaviness of the chest, difficulty in breathing, lung allergy, ulcer in the breasts and vomiting.

K—24 Liquid point.(II Fire, Water)

Heaviness in the chest, pain, vomiting, blocked nose, lung allergy and anaemia.

K—25 Liquid point.(II Fire, Water)

Heaviness in the chest, difficulty in breathing, cough, vomiting, anaemia caused by self-neglect due to sorrow, sounds less audible, does not want to live.

K—26 Solid point.(I Fire, Earth)

Cough, a difference in breathing due to asthma, cannot eat, lung allergy, palpitation, heaviness of the chest, the chilliness of the hands and failure of the stomach and intestinal muscles.

K—27 Gaseous point. (Metal, Wood)

Cough, heaviness of the chest, asthma, pain in the tongue, headaches, stomach pain before menstruation, tension and chest pain.

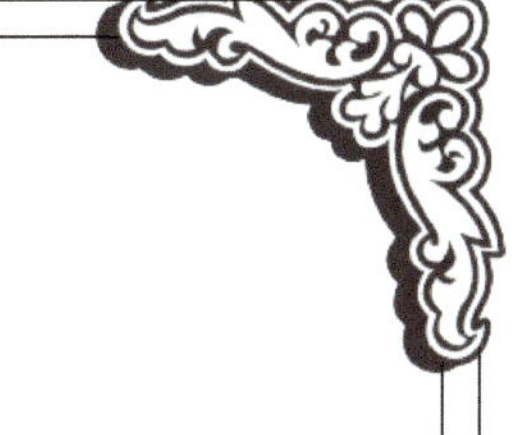

Part Six

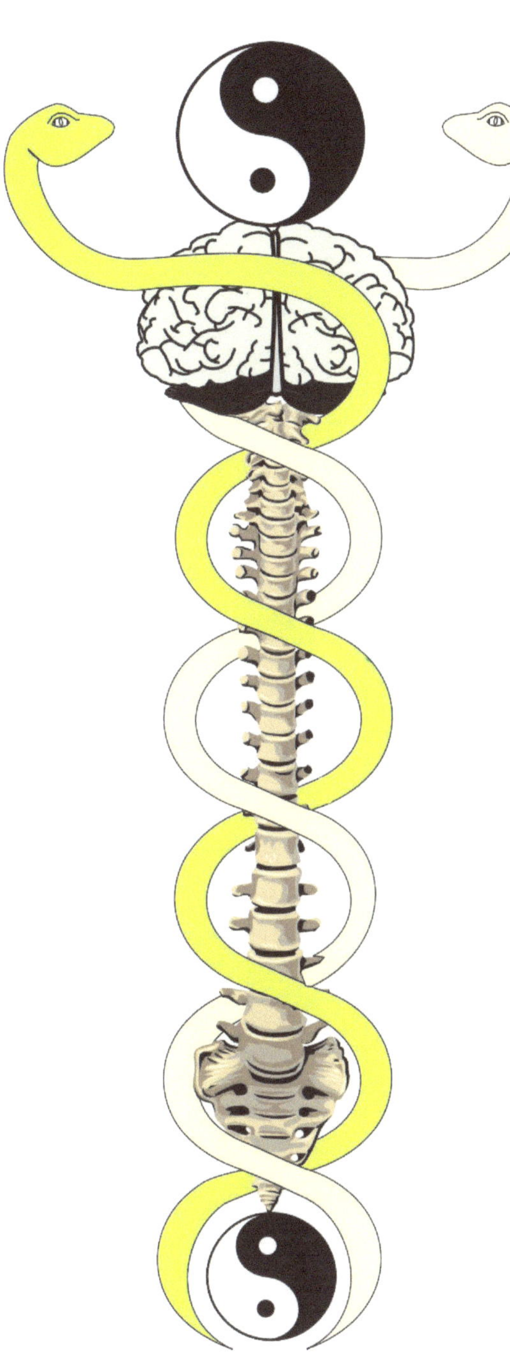

6.1 Governing Vessel Meridian (Gv) Based on Six Element Points Method

6.2 Conception Vessel Meridian (Cv) Based on Six Element Points Method

6.1 Governing Vessel Meridian (GV)

Based on Six Elements Points

This starts from the anus, travels up the backbone, goes through the centre of the neck and skull and descends in the front through the forehead and eyebrows. It reaches the inner membrane in the upper lip, the inner fold via the tip of the nose and the upper lip. All the ***yang*** meridians come under this governing vessel meridian. This meridian is one of the main meridians of the major eight meridians. This is not connected to any organ. This is called a ***single track***. This travels through the backbone and the brain. One can treat the central nervous system through this track.

Nature of the track ***Yin***.

The number of points 28.

Important points of this meridian by which diseases can be cured (by needling):	Epilepsy, psychiatric diseases, facial palsy, insomnia, nervous disorder, cannot speak, backbone pain and neck-related pain.

Diagram

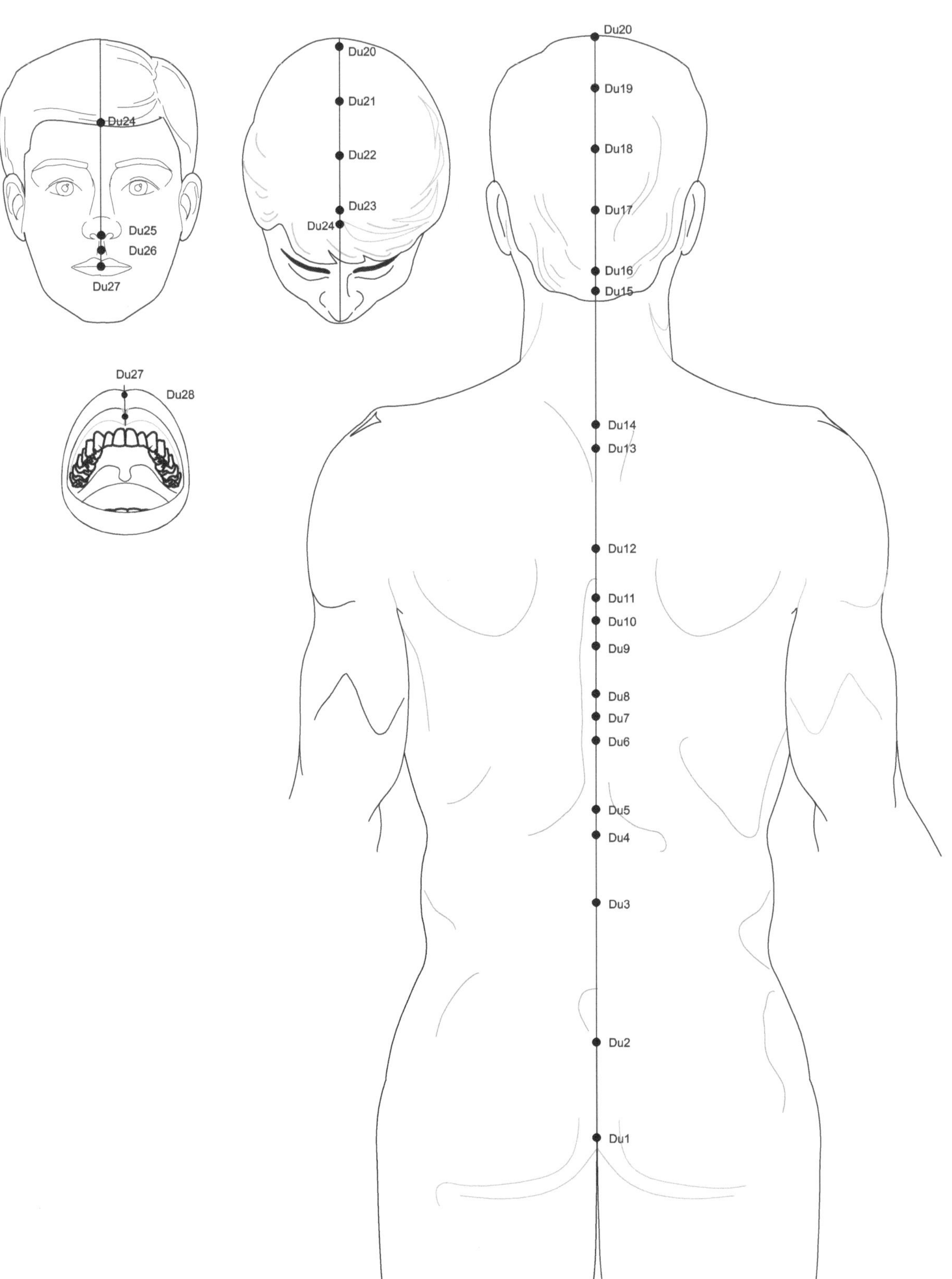

Figure 6.1 Governing Vessel Meridian—*Yin*

The Diseases Which Can be Cured by Touching the Six Element Points in this Governing Vessel Meridian.

Governing vessel—1(GV-1).

Piles, bloody discharge from the anus, pain in the vagina, penis pain, constipation and sweating.

Governing vessel—2 (GV-2).

Swelling of the lower abdomen, pain, retention of urine, discharge from the vagina—either white or red coloured, infertility, swelling of the testis, itching, VD in both genders, hip pain, irregular periods, malaria and haemorrhoids around the anus.

Governing vessel—3(GV-3).

Knee pain, hip bone and muscle pain, not being able to fold the knee, diarrhoea, intestinal pain, and urine-related diseases, one becomes less vigorous.

Governing vessel—4 (GV-4).

Headaches, no sweat, fever, lower abdomen pain, white discharge, anaemia, swelling, haemorrhoid around the anus, bleeding nose, hip pain and is less potent.

Governing vessel—5(GV-5).

Hip bone and muscle pain, as well as indigestion.

Governing vessel—6(GV-6).

Epilepsy, jaundice, stools with blood, diarrhoea and haemorrhoids around the anus.

Governing vessel—7(GV-7).

Lower backbone pain, stomach pain and vision problems.

Governing vessel—8(GV-8).

Epilepsy, psychiatric problems, heart pain, stiffness of the lower backbone and stomach pain.

Governing vessel—9(GV-9).

Lower backbone and muscle pain, chest pain, back pain, dumbness, not being able to speak, jaundice and fever.

Governing vessel—10(GV-10).

Asthma, lung allergy, anaemia, lower back muscle and bone pain.

Governing vessel—11(GV-11).

Heart diseases, fever, headaches, nervous weakness, fits in children, stiffness and pain in the back.

Governing vessel—12(GV-12).

Epilepsy, body heat, coarseness of one's voice, psychiatric diseases and diseases related to rheumatic arthritis.

Governing vessel—13(GV-13).

The heaviness of the head, dizziness, depression, stiffness of the backbone, pain in the shoulder, neck and back, fever with chilliness, fever, with no sweat and brain diseases. **Governing vessel—14(GV-14).**

Headaches, constrain in the neck muscles, not being able to turn the neck, hernia, cough, fever, vomiting, jaundice, summer diseases, asthma, lung allergy and common cold.

Governing vessel—15(GV-15).

Headaches, constrain of the neck, epilepsy, cannot talk, deafness and stammering.

Governing vessel—16(GV-16).

Headaches, dizziness, blocked nose, swelling of the throat with pain, constrain of the neck, phlegm and brain-related disease.

Governing vessel—17(GV-17).

Vision problem, head heaviness and constrained neck with pain.

Governing vessel—18(GV-18).

Severe headache, dizziness, epilepsy, anaemia, depression, constrain of the neck and heart diseases.

Governing vessel—19 (GV-19).

Headaches, fear of exposure to the chilly air, constrained head and neck, dizziness ,epilepsy, psychiatric diseases and anaemia.

Governing vessel—20 (GV-20).

Headaches, dizziness, blocked nose, infertility in females, psychiatric diseases, stiffness of the backbone with pain, heaviness of the head ,loss of memory, loss of hair and insomnia.

Governing vessel—21 (GV-21).

Headaches, dizziness, epilepsy, polyps of the nose and a swollen red face.

Governing vessel—22 (GV-22).

Dizziness, less memory, swollen face and a blocked nose.

Governing vessel—23 (GV-23).

Headaches, eye pain, blocked nose, nose polyps, swollen red face and fever without sweating.

Governing vessel—24 (GV-24).

Severe headache, swollen red eyes, less memory, stiffness of the tongue, thirst and vomiting.

Governing vessel—25 (GV-25).

Blocked nose, polyps of the nose and ulcer in the nose.

Governing vessel—26 (GV-26).

Dizziness, epilepsy, psychiatry diseases, swelling, thirst, summer diseases, hip muscles and bone pain, nervous weakness and facial palsy.

Governing vessel—27 (GV-27).

Drowsiness, epilepsy, dizziness, stiffness of the lips, toothache and dryness of the tongue.

Governing vessel—28 (GV-28).

Itching and reddened eyes, blocked nose, polyps in the nose, heart pain, less talkative and bleeding.

6.2 Conception Vessel Meridian (Cv)

Based on Six Elements Points

This starts from the anus and goes up through the central line of the front of the body and ends in the mouth. This is one of the important eight tracks. This governs all the ***yin*** tracks of the body. This meridian has no connection with the inner organs. This is related to reproduction through this meridian. One can treat all sorts of diseases of any of the organs in the body.

Nature of the track	***Yang***.
The number of points	24.

Important points of this meridian by which diseases can be cured.	Diseases related to fertility, heart and brain diseases, impaired speech, excessive saliva, discharge, facial palsy, oedema of the intestines ,child delivery without labour pain, enlarged stomach and ***yin/yang***-related diseases.

Diagram

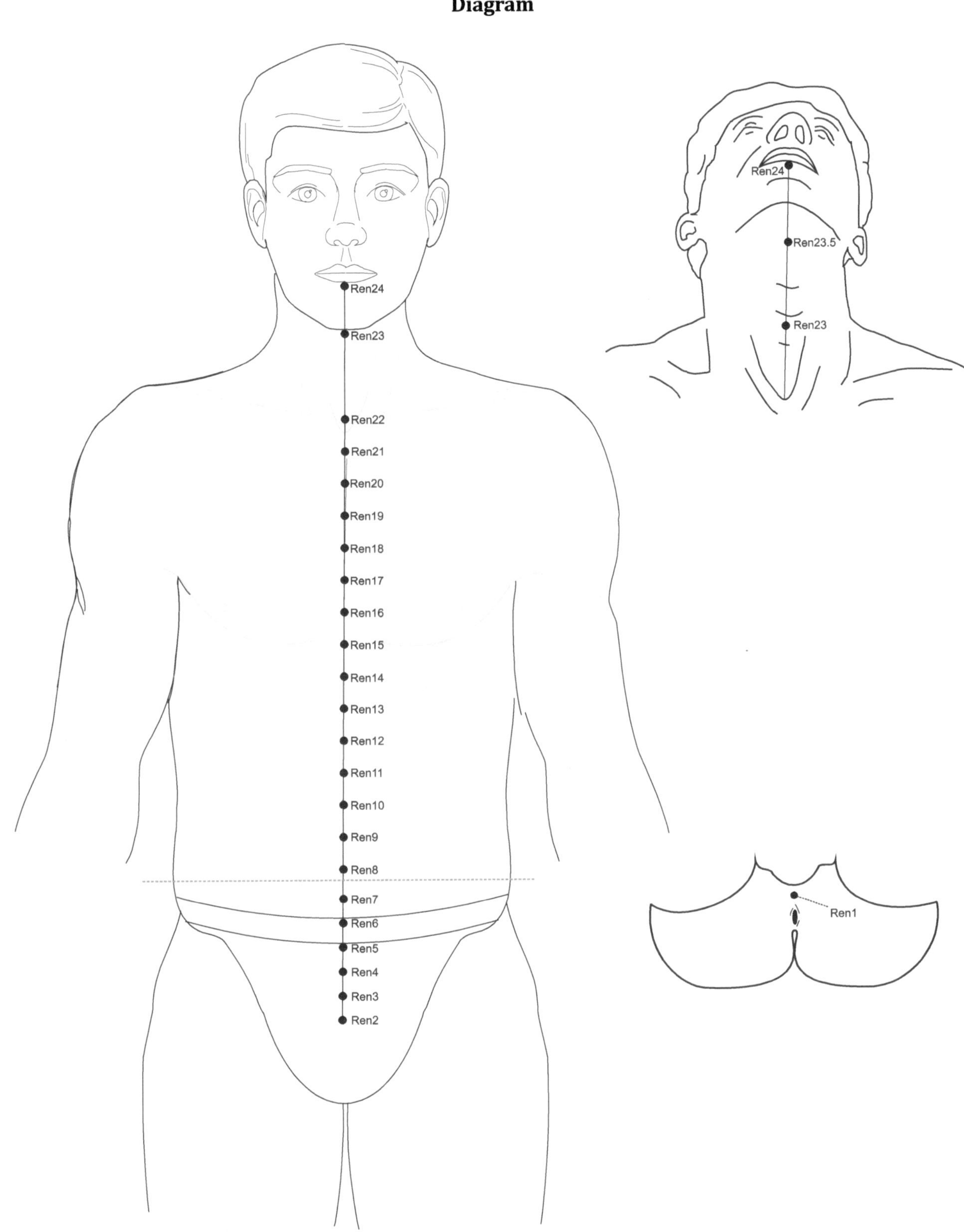

Figure 6.2 Conception Vessel Meridian—*Yang*

The Diseases Which Can be Cured by Touching the Six Element Points in this Governing Vessel Meridian.

Conception vessel 1 (CV-1)—junction point—*yin.*

Vaginal pain, swelling, irregular periods, pain in the penis, chilliness in the testis, constipation, sweat, piles, fistula, fertility and meridian junction point.

Conception vessel—2 (CV-2), Gaseous point. (Metal, Wood)

Lower abdomen swelling, severe stomach pain, retention of urine, white discharge, venereal diseases, uterus not shrinking, infertility, itching in the testis, kidney diseases, reproductive diseases/disorders and the liver junction point of the ***yin*** organs.

Conception vessel—3—(CV-3) Solid point. (I Fire, Earth)

Pain in the bones and the muscles of the thigh, cannot fold the knees, pain in the intestines, diarrhoea, kidney diseases, reproductive disorders and spleen diseases.

Conception vessel—4—(CV-4) Liquid point.(II Fire, Water)

Headaches, body heat, no sweat, irregular fever, epilepsy or seizures, white discharge, infertility, VD of both genders, haemorrhoids around the anus, swelling, anaemia, uncontrolled urine, reproductive diseases and kidney diseases.

Conception vessel—5—(CV-5) Liquid point.(II Fire, Water)

Pain in the hip bone, stiffness, indigestion, headaches, diarrhoea, diseases related to the anus, nervous weakness, swelling in the body and alarm point of the triple warmer.

Conception vessel—6—(CV-6) Solid point.(I Fire, Earth)

Epilepsy, swelling of the lower abdomen, jaundice, haemorrhoids around the anus, stools with blood, anus diseases, nervous weakness, point for all urine-related problems of all the energies and junction point of the triple warmer.

Conception vessel—7—(CV-7) Gaseous point.(Metal, Wood)

Pain in the hip bone and muscles, stomach ache, impaired vision, psychiatric problems, hernia, gastric problems, ulcer in intestines and tonsillitis.

Conception vessel—8—(CV-8) Gaseous point.(Metal, Wood)

Epilepsy, psychiatric diseases, eye diseases, heart pain, stiffness in the hip area, stomach ache and diseases related to the brain.

Conception vessel—9—(CV-9) Solid point.(I Fire, Earth)

Hip pain, chest and back pain, problems in speech, chilliness in the stomach, cannot eat, jaundice, fever and lung junction point.

Conception vessel—10—(CV-10) Liquid point. (II Fire, Water)

Asthma, lung allergy, pneumonia, anaemia, as well as pain in the hip muscles and bones.

Conception vessel—11—(CV-11)Liquid point.(II Fire, Water)

Heart diseases, fever, one is averse to chilliness, headaches, forgetfulness, nervous weakness, psychiatric diseases, epilepsy, as well as pain and stiffness of the backbone.

Conception vessel—12—(CV-12) Solid point.(I Fire, Earth)

Epilepsy, nervous weakness, excessive body heat, hoarseness in the speech, psychiatric problems, pain and stiffness in the hip muscles and bones, rheumatism hernia, intestinal ulcer and the centre point of T.W.

Conception vessel—13—(CV-13)Gaseous point. (Metal, Wood)

Heaviness in the head, dizziness, epilepsy, depression, shoulder pain, back pain, neck pain, fever with chills, no sweat, bone diseases, numbness and the junction point of the gall bladder.

Conception vessel—14—(CV-14) Liquid point. (II Fire, Water)

Headaches, stiffness of the neck, cannot turn the head, rheumatoid arthritis, paralysis, cough, pain in the hip muscle and bones, fever, junction point of all the ***yang*** organs and alarm point of all the heart diseases.

Conception vessel—15—(CV-15) Liquid point. (II Fire, Water)

Headaches, stiffness of the neck, the backbone, epilepsy, immovable tongue, not being able to talk, deafness and the junction of the urinary bladder.

Conception vessel—16—(CV-16), Gaseous point.(Metal, Wood)

Headaches, dizziness, blocked nose, swelling with pain in the throat, deafness, constrained neck, toothache, brain-related diseases, psychiatric diseases, urinary bladder junction point and congestion with phlegm.

Conception vessel—17—(CV-17) Gaseous point. (Metal, Wood)

Pain in the eye, diseases related to the eyes, heaviness in the head, contraction and pain in the neck muscles and joint point of the urinary bladder and ST.

Conception vessel—18—(CV-18)Solid point. (I Fire ,Earth)

Severe headache, dizziness, vomiting, epilepsy or seizures, anaemia, depression, cramp in the neck and heart diseases.

Conception vessel—19—(CV-19)Liquid point.(II Fire, Water)

Headache, muscle spasms of the head and neck, dizziness, psychiatric diseases and anaemia.

Conception vessel—20—(CV-20) Liquid point.(II Fire, Water)

Headache, dizziness, diseases related to the brain, drowsiness, forgetfulness, crying, psychiatric diseases, heart diseases, deafness and joint point of the liver and urinary bladder.

Conception vessel—21—(CV-21) Liquid point.(II Fire, Water)

Headache, dizziness, epilepsy, neuro-diseases, polyps in the nose and flushed face.

Conception vessel—22—(CV-22)Gaseous point. (Metal, Wood)

Dizziness, nervous weakness, oblivion, swelling of the face, blocked nose, paleface, asthma, cough and hiccups.

Conception vessel—23—(CV-23) Liquid point.(II Fire, Water)

Headache, reddish eyes, blocked nose, polyps in the nose, fever, swelling of the face and excessive saliva secretion in the mouth.

Conception vessel—23.5—(CV-23.5) Solid point.

Very severe headaches, eyes-related diseases, dementia, psychiatric diseases, vomiting, thirst, facial palsy and joint point of ST.

Conception vessel—24—(CV-24)Gaseous point.(Metal ,Wood)

Nervous weakness, headache, dizziness, diseases related to the eyes, a blocked nose, facial palsy, vomit and blood in the urine.

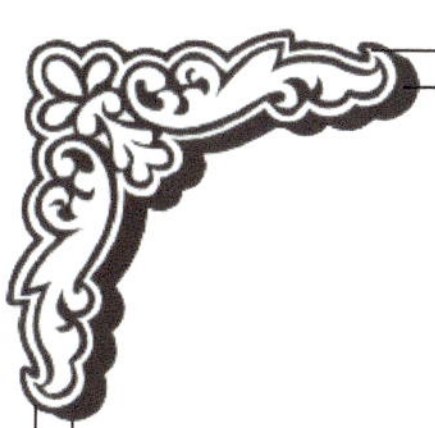

Part Seven

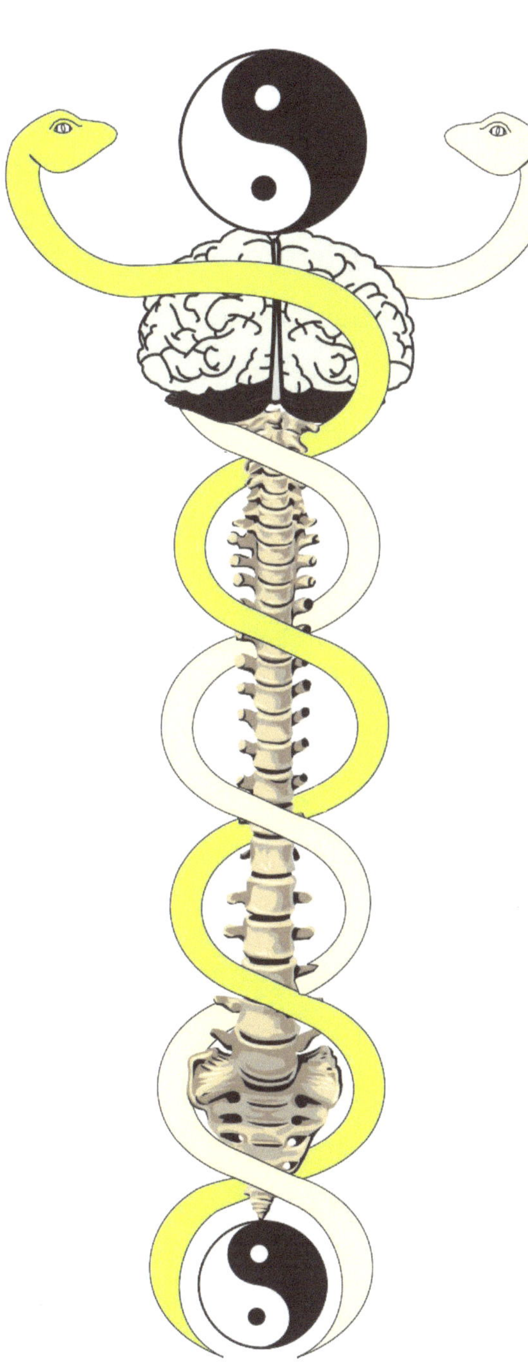

7.1 14 Index of Meridians/Tracks

Tracks	Time	*Panchaboodha* Nature	Related track	Nature of track	No. of points	Disease cured by the points in this track. With needle
Lungs (LU)	3-5 am	Metal	LI	Yin	11	Lung and skin-related diseases, asthma, blocked nose, knee pain.
Large intestine LI	5-7 am	Metal	Lung	Yang	20	Body pain, lung diseases and allergies, LI diseases.
Stomach ST	7-9 am	Earth	Spleen	Yang	45	Body pain, toothache, headache, facial palsy, polio, paralysis, ST-related disease, ulcer in ST, ulcer in the intestines, menstruation problems and rheumatism.
Spleen SP	9-11 am	Earth	ST	Yin	21	Production of blood, reproduction, UB problems, oedema of the intestines, inflammatory bowel diseases (IBD) elephantiasis and delivery without labour pain.

(Contd.)

Heart H	**11-1 pm**	**Fire**	**Small intestine**	**Yin**	**9**	**Brain-related diseases, impaired speech, insomnia, fear, daydreams, tremors, delirium, epilepsy, dizziness, psychological problems and vertigo.**
Small Intestine SI	**1-3 pm**	**Fire**	**Heart**	**Yang**	**19**	**Myopathy, atrophy of muscles, neuro disorders, paralysis wrist drop, arthritis, SI-related diseases, deafness, vertigo, eye diseases, cervical spondylitis, heart and brain-related diseases.**
Urinary Bladder UB	**3-5 pm**	**Water**	**kidney**	**Yang**	**67**	**This track is considered important. Many diseases can be cured by puncturing at many places on this track as this track travels from head to toe.**

						Eye-related diseases, nose-related diseases, headaches, trigeminal neuralgia, neck-related and cervical-related diseases. Pain around the hip reproductive disorders, UB diseases, paralysis, sciatica, cramps, knee pain or joint pain.
Kidney K	**5-7 pm**	**Water**	**UB Urinary bladder**	**Yin**	**27**	**Urinary tract-related diseases impotence and infertility. Menstrual problems, hair fall, ear, bone, lungs, heart, brain, SI, related diseases liver, UB related diseases**
Pericardium P	**7-9 pm**	**Fire**	**Triple warmer TW**	**Yin**	**9**	**Wrist diseases, glands, heat-related diseases, psychiatry problems, insomnia, fear, tremors, stomach ulcer, mainly hiccups, ST-related diseases.**

(*Contd.*)

Triple warmer	**9-11 pm**	**Fire**	**Pericardium**	**Yang**	**23**	**Ear, inner ear diseases, constipation, diarrhoea, eye diseases, shoulder, heart and back-related problems and spleen-related problems.**
Gall bladder GB	**11-1 Night**	**Wood**	**Liver**	**Yang**	**44**	**Facial palsy, neuro problems at one side eye, lacto-glandular diseases, liver, GB-related diseases, nervous constraint, paralysis and polio.**
LIV	**1-3 am**	**Wood**	**Gall bladder**	**Yin**	**14**	**Eye, liver, spleen-related problems, epilepsy, headache, psychological problems.**
Governing Vessel	**The whole of the night**	**A mix of wood, water and earth**	**GV**	**Yin**	**28**	**Neuro related, insomnia, not being able to speak, neck pain, back pain, fatigue, to control fever, for e.g., Governing vessel 14.**

Conception Vessel CV	**The whole of the day**	**A mix of metal, fire Cold Fire**	**CV**	**Yang**	**24**	**Reproduction, urine-related problems, stomach, heart, lungs, diseases, toothache, excess saliva secretion, toothache, facial palsy, oedema of the intestine and enlarged small intestine.**

7.2 Psychiatric Disorders

- **Hysteria**
- **Anxiety neurosis**
- **Neurasthenia**
- **Insomnia**
- **Mental retardation**
- **Schizophrenia**
- **Impotence.**

Hysteria

Occurs because of unpleasant circumstances, mainly caused by failures, disappointment, and not being able to express oneself. G.V. 20,H7,P6,LI 4,k3,ST 40,UB62.

Ear acupuncture: Shenmen

Emergency points GV 26, K-1

When the three energies, namely, wood, fire and cold fire combine with the right side upper energy cycle to form this state.

Impotence

Near points: CV 2, CV 3, CV1.

Far points: K3, SP 6

Ear acupuncture: External genitalia

When cold fire and fire combine with the right side downward energy cycle, this state is created.

Anxiety Neurosis

Anxiety, being excited or fierce are the features of this disorder.

Important points GV 20, X-6.

Other points H7,P-6

Ear acupuncture—Shenmen.

When the fire joins with the upper right cycle and the lower right cycle, this state occurs.

Neurasthenia.

Fatigue, insomnia and hatred are the signs of this disease.

GV 20, H-7,SP 6

When fire and cold fire connect with the upward left energy cycle, this state occurs.

Insomnia.

GV 20, X-6, X-8, X-9,H-7, P-6

Ear acupuncture: Shenmen.

When fire and second fire connect with the upward left energy cycle, this state occurs.

Mental Retardation.

Mental and physical retardation are the natural manifestations of this disease. Some may have cerebral palsy too.

Important point.

GV 20, X-6,ST 8, H-7,P 6, GB-34,ST 36.

Ear acupuncture: Shenmen of the brain area.

When fire and second fire joins with the upward left energy cycle, this state occurs.

Schizophrenia.

Anti-social, negative thoughts, one does not care about self-respect, laughing without any reason, worrying, etc., are the signs.

Important point.

GV 20, H-7,X-8, ST-10

Ear acupuncture: Shenmen. When fire and second fire elements join with the right side energy cycle, this state occurs.

7.3 Disorders of Soft Tissues, Muscles, Worms and Joints

Cervical Spondylosis.

Important points: GV 20,GB 20.

GV 14, GB 39, X-21 (affected area) U-B 11,(suitable for bone) LU-7.

When the cervical pain is severe, the SI 6 or SI 3 points must be stimulated with force by hand, using the needles, to get immediate relief.

Backache.

Important points: GV 20, GV 2, GV-3, GV-4, UB-23

UB 28,X-21 (affected area) UB 40, ST 44.

When the earth and fire elements join with wood, this state occurs.

Frozen Shoulder.

This oc curs mainly if the supraspinatus tendinitis gets affected. It hurts when the hand is moved. If the left shoulder is affected, it is due to earth and water elements which are connected to wood and fire along with the downward right cycle.

GV-20, LI-15,TW-14,SI-9, GB-34, LI-4, ST-38.To make the hand more flexible, ST-38 should be stimulated heavily.

If the right side of the first fire, second fire, wood elements would join the lower side right side cycle.

Common points to observe while treating any type of joint pain.

Stimulate the pain area.

Use the nearby points.

Use the points suitable for the tissues: UB-11, GB-34

Use pain relieving points: SI-4,ST-14.

You must remember the points which would make the patient calm: GV-20,H-7,X-6.

You should use the point to increase the immunity: GV-20,GV-11.

Should stimulate the point to prevent inflammations.

If the right-side joints are affected, then it is due to the condition of the fire, metal and wood elements joining together with the lower side right cycle.

If the left joints are affected, then with the wood and earth elements, the wood energies join the right side lower cycle.

7.4 Diseases of the Nervous System

Front Side Headache

X-1,X-3,GB-14,ST-8,GV-20, LI-4,SI-10

Ear acupuncture: Shenmen

Since the fire energy of the right lower side energy cycle joins the right upward cycle, these diseases occur.

Insomnia.

GV-20, X-8,X-9, X-6,H-7,P-6. This occurs when the left side energy, second fire joins with the lower side energy of the right side.

Bell's Palsy Important Points

GV-20,X-6,ST-4, ST-5, SI-18,GB-14, X-36.

Right side

All the three earth, fire and wood energies in the wood element join the downward right-side element energy to create this disorder.

Left side

Earth, fire and wood energies of the wood element join the downward right-side element energies to form this state.

Migraine (with vomiting)

GV-20, GB-20, TW-23, ST-8, GB-8, LI -4, ST-44,LI-11, LIV-3.

Right Side

Fire joins with the upward right-side energy element.

Left side

Fire joins with the upward left-side energy element.

7.5 Common Cold, Allergic Rhinitis

Common Cold

Caused by the virus.

Diseases caused in the inner nasal skin along with allergic conditions with undesirable reactions

Suffering increases with sneezing.

Important point

GV-20, GV-14, GB-20,SI-19,LI-20,LI-4,SP-10(Suitable for allergies).

When the metal and downward energy elements, along with the water element join the upward right and left energy elements, this problem occurs.

Sinusitis

Diseases of the sinuses (the hollow cavities of the skull). Common cold and fever may affect.

Important points

GB-14, X-3, LI-20, LI-4, LI-11, SP-10

When metal, water and fire, along with the downward right side energy cycle is joined with the right and left side upward energy elements, this condition will occur.

Bronchial Asthma

In general, asthma is a condition caused by an infection, allergy and emotional stress of a person.

Important points

GV-20, CV-22, CV-17, X-17, UB-13, UB-13, LU-6, LU-9, SP-10, K-3.

Ear acupuncture

Dingchuvan ling point.

When the metal, wood and water elements along with the downward left side energy cycle join with the right and left upward energy elements, this condition occurs.

7.6 Gynaecological Diseases and Obstetrical Disorders

Irregular Menstruation

Excessive bleeding, less bleeding, extended bleeding for many days or bleeding for very few days, etc.

Important points

GV-20, CV-4, CV-6, CV-3, SP-6, GB-21, (Suitable for endocrine glands)ST-36.

When the upward energy cycle combines with the right-side downward energy cycle ,these problems occur.

Delayed Menstruation

Important points

ST-36,SP-4,LI-4,Painful menstruation, Dysmenorrhea.

Important Points

GV-20,CV-4,CV-6,GV-3, GV-4, SP-6, UB-40, LI-4, ST-44, GB-21, LIV-8, Sp-8.

Ear acupuncture

Ovary, Shenmen

When wood and the left side downward energy element join with the right side downward energy this condition occurs.

Leucorrhoea: Important points

CV-2, CV-6,UB-23, UB-25, UB-40, GV-14, GV-20

Ear acupuncture

Ovary, uterus

The mental and right side upward energy cycle joins the right side downward energy cycle to create this problem.

Location Deficiency

(Agalactia or agalactorrhea; hypogalactia or hypogalactorrhea)

Important points

CV-17, P-6, SP-6

When the metal and fire elements join the right side upward energy, then this disorder occurs.

Delivery Without Labour Pain

One should start acupuncture treatment in the second stage.

First, one should use GV-20. Then puncture SI-4 on both hands and stimulate. Then start with hand stimulation. Then use electrical stimulation. SP-6 should be pointed on the right leg.

When the wood element joins the right side downward energy cycle, this state occurs.

Neima

This does not come under any track or meridian. This exists inside the legs (medical aspect). That is between the knee joint and the ankle joint.

One can use an electrical stimulant with a bearable amount.

Benefits

During delivery time no labour pain

Very less bleeding

It does not affect the uterine contraction.

Above 90% of women are benefited.

Acupuncture points on the ear

Diagram

Ear Acupuncture

5000 years before, a method of identifying diseases and treating them was practised by the Chinese, and based on this, they invented many points on the ear to cure many diseases.

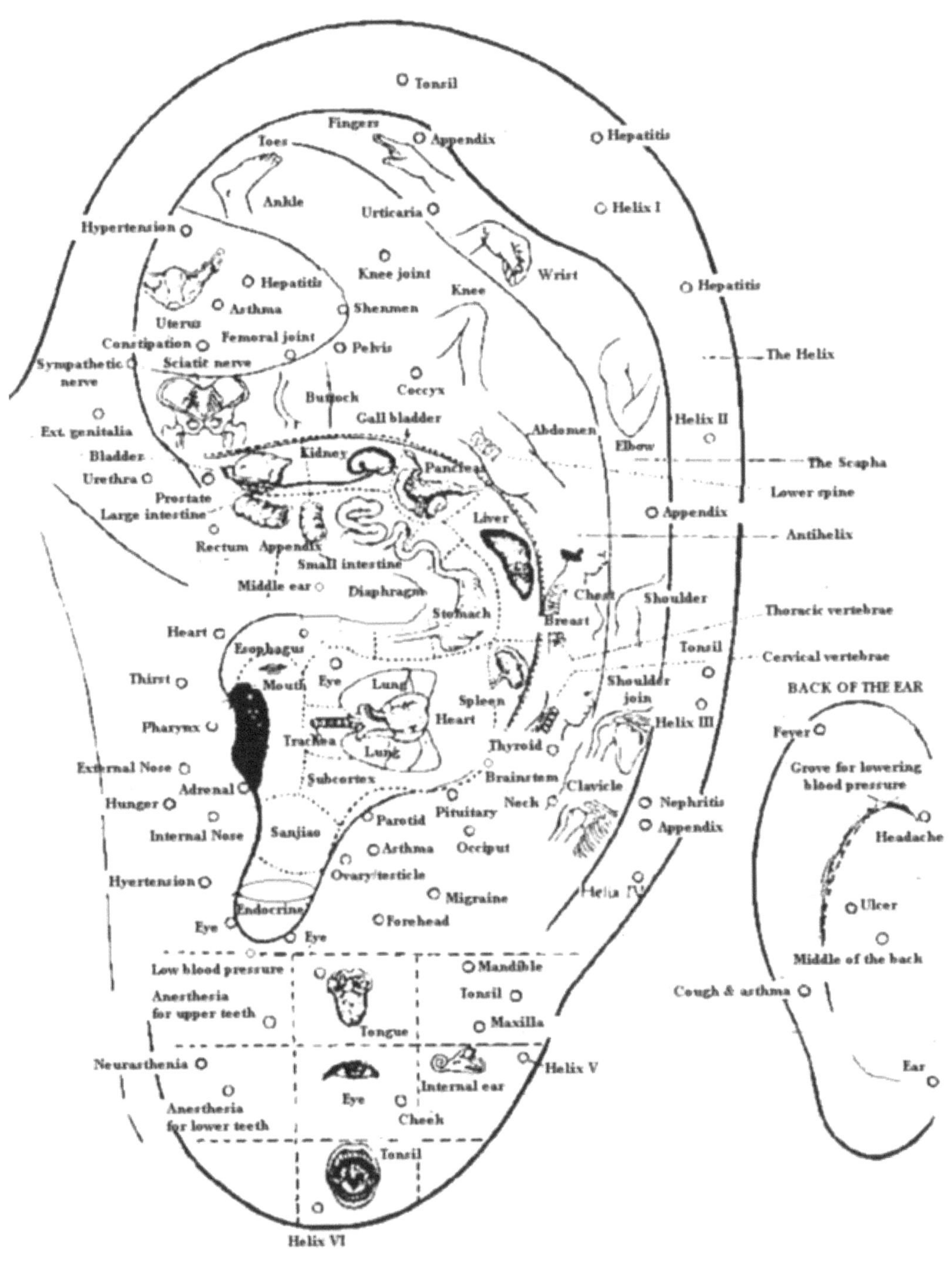

7.1 Diagram of the Ear Acupuncture

This is called Ear Acupuncture. Twelve meridians and their related organs are connected to the ear.

Advantages

Almost all diseases can be cured.

One can use head and body acupuncture along with ear acupuncture.

Immediate relief.

Easy and cost-effective method.

Can control and cure diseases.

There are suitable points on the ear for using acupuncture and Anaesthesia.

Anatomy of the Ear

Principles to Be Followed in the Ear Acupuncture

Filiform or press needles should be used on the skin at the selected point. One should not pierce deeply.

You can use an electrical stimulator.

You should not screw the needle with your hands.

The needles can stay for 20to 30 minutes. After treatment for 7to 10 days, you should discontinue for a week and then you can start treatment again.

Can use press needles using the ad plaster and can have them for 3 to 5 days continuously without removing them.

Important Points in Usage

1. Shenmen
2. Sympathetic
3. Heart
4. Lung
5. Stomach
6. Spleen
7. Hot point
8. Face and jaw bone
9. Inner ear portion
10. Ear Apex

7.7 Scalp Acupuncture

Dr. Jiao Shun Faof China introduced scalp acupuncture to the world between 1966 and 1971. He was the first one to introduce this method, which he demonstrated in a hospital in northern China, along with his juniors. He invented this method by clubbing ancient Chinese acupuncture and the research conducted in neurology. By using this method, one can cure cerebral shock and paralysis due to head injury, etc.

The functioning of this method is not yet explained. Research is still being conducted. According to Chinese research, all the nerves running through the human organs join in a particular area of the head. This is situated on the top of the skull—on the scalp. Hence, by acupuncturing on the head, all sorts of neuro diseases/disorders can be cured.

Through ear acupuncture, one can cure all the diseases related to the visceral organs. Reflexo therapy (foot acupuncture) cures diseases in children.(Paediatric)

Head and ear acupuncture can be used, along with body acupuncture. Acupuncture anaesthesia is used during surgeries.

The patient affected with paralysis due to Hemiplegia feels a change after a few minutes of acupuncture treatment in the contralateral motor area. After a few minutes, the patient moves his limbs and body, which can be seen within minutes of treatment.

Impressed with this treatment, Japan is conducting research in this school of treatment.

It is understood that there are electromagnetic waves that connect the important areas of the brain and the points on the scalp.

Hence, acupuncture points are related to each area of the brain. This philosophy and the functions of the EEG machine, used on brain-damaged patients are similar to a large extent.

Main indications for scalp acupuncture

- Paralysis, nervous weakness, dumbness, blocked urination and problems due to head injury.
- Oedema in the skull.
- Headache due to head injury.
- Diseases related to spinal cold, tremors and chorea.
- All types of delirium and brain-related problems.
- Delirium due to injury.
- Impotence, pain, urinary problems in children.
- High blood pressure, palpitation, oedema of body inflammation or swelling of the body.

- Asthma, intestinal ulcer, spleen and liver diseases.
- Menstrual disorders in women, excessive bleeding, uterine prolapse.
- Scalp acupuncture for anaesthesia.

Important acupuncture points on the head

Motor Area

Part-1

Pain in the head, legs, one's neck, cervical collar or neck brace, numbness and paralysis.

Part-2

Centre part

Part-3

Face, impaired speech or dumbness, facial palsy, excessive saliva/drooling.

Sensory area

The human body has the nature of creating heat or cold temperatures and pain. This point is helpful in treating facial palsy, trigeminal neuralgia, migraines with numbness on one side of the face, a blocked nose, pain in the jaws, toothaches and stomach-related pain. This point helps to cure all the above-mentioned symptoms.

Chorea tremors control area

This area is considered an important point. This point helps to control chorea tremors, delirium, stiffness of the neck, numbness of the face, trigeminal neuralgia, Parkinsonism, as well as a nervous weakness because of brain fever or strong dosage of medicines. If the pain or problem is on the right side, we must point to the left side and vice versa.

Vaso motor area

Because of either hypertension or hypotension or cerebral oedema, a person may get affected with paralysis on one side. This area is connected to this problem.

Foot motor sensory area

If punctured with a needle in this area, it gives better results for pain, paralysis, numbness, uterine prolapse, bedwetting amongst children, disc prolapse and acute contraction of the back muscles.

Auditory Area

Deafness, humming sound in the ear, vertigo and heaviness in the head can be treated with this point.

Second speech area

This area helps to say words.

Third speech area

This cures impaired speech.

Visual area

To repair the vision, to cure eye diseases.

Equilibrium area

Cerebellar disorders can be treated. This balances the changes happening in the body.

Gastric area

Used to treat stomach disorders, gastric problems, fatigue

Thoracic cavity area

Used to treat chest pain, palpitation, suffocation and asthma.

Reproduction genital area

Used to treat impotence, the ejaculation of sperm, menstruation problem, liver diseases, excessive bleeding and uterine prolapse.

Hepatocystic Area

Used to treat one's liver, gall bladder diseases, one's stomach and chest-related diseases, pain can be treated with this point.

7.8 Acupuncture Therapeutics For G.I Tract Diseases

Indigestion-Dyspepsia

Blotted abdomen with pain, chest burning and belching are the symptoms. The abdomen will be surrounded by gas. The symptoms such as the time during which the pain occurs, whether before or after meals, the duration of pain etc., should be taken into account while treating patients with less digestion or digestive disorder.

Main reasons for digestive disorders

Ulcers in the digestive system, alcoholism, indigestion, chronic digestive disorders, excessive acidity or less acidity can be the main reasons. The changes occurring in the upper abdomen, loss of appetite, vomiting, not being able to eat and no secretion or very less secretion of digestive juices may lead to stomach cancer.

Viral hepatitis and cirrhosis of the liver may occur due to chronic intestinal inflammation or swelling, constipation, abdomen bloating and swelling.

Indigestion may also occur due to vascular disorder, heart problems, urea deposits in the blood, T.B. and tumours.

Apart from all these physical problems, psychological imagination which comes under unknown causes may also induce indigestion. These patients will have heartburn and chest pain.

Major points

CV-6,CV-12,20,ST,H-25,36,UB-20,SP-6

Ear acupuncture

Stomach, Spleen, Shenmen

Head acupuncture

Puncture the stomach-related area for 20 to 30minutes for 10to15 days. During the follow-up (5to7 days) it can be treated.

This condition occurs due to the right side downward energy cycle joining the fire and earth elements.

Diarrhoea

Near points-CV-3,6,12,ST-25

Far points-ST-36,SP-4,6

Alarm points-UB-20,25

When the right side downward energy cycle joins the fire and stomach elements along with the water element, this state occurs.

Stomatitis—Glossitis

Ulcers inside the whole of the mouth, due to many reasons, such as inflamed gums, due to viruses, fungus, bacteria and vitamin deficiency. Due to medicinal allergies, some may develop oral ulcers.

GV 20, 28, 14, LI-11, SP 10, x-10.

When the earth and fire in the downward right side energy cycles join the upward right and left energy cycles, this condition occurs.

Toothache

Main points: LI 4, 20, SI-18, ST-5,6,7.

CV-24, ST-44 (stimulated strongly) with these points can remove the tooth.

When the fire and the right-side downward energy cycle join the upward right and left-side energy cycles, this condition occurs.

Dysphagia (difficult to swallow)

Reasons for dysphagia: Oral ulcer, problems with the food pipe, tonsillitis, abscess or cyst in the throat, hysteria, nervous disorders.

Points: GV-20,CV-17,22,23, P-6

When the second fire, water and wood elements, along with the right and left upward energy cycle joins the downward right side energy, this condition occurs.

Gastric—duodenal ulcer

The ulceration may occur at the mouth of the stomach and the beginning of the small intestine. Sometimes, the ulcer may occur at a certain place in the stomach. Symptoms may be a stomach ache, swelling at times and pain in the right side, if the ulcer is in the mouth of the small intestine.

If the stomach ache occurs half an hour to one hour before meals, then it is considered a stomach ulcer. If the pain occurs two to three hours after eating, then it is considered an ulcer at the junction point where the mouth of the stomach and the mouth of the small intestine join, namely the duodenum.

Points: GV 20, ST 21, 25, 36, ST-6, UB -20, 21, CV 12,P-6.

When the fire and earth elements join with wood and the right side downward energy cycle, this condition occurs.

Flatulence.

The gas stays in the abdomen without getting eliminated.

Reasons: constipation, diarrhoea, any type of block, such as an abscess or cancer.

Points: GV 20,GB 25,26,LIV 3h,13,CV 12,ST 36,SP 6...

When the wood elements join with earth and fire elements, this problem occurs.

Helminthiasis—Amoebiasis, Anorexia

This is spread from one to the other person through food, water, etc. Itching in the anus, diarrhoea, stomach ache, vomiting, anorexia(loss of appetite) anaemia are the symptoms.

Points: GV 20, SP 15, 25, CV 12, ST 36, P-6. Acupuncture was used to cure this condition before the medicines were invented.

When the metal element combines with the right and left side downward energy, this condition occurs.

Diarrhoea—Dysentery.

Points: - GV20,ST 35,36,37,SP 4,6,CV-3,6.

Abdomen ache. For the unbearable abdomen ache, ST 34 must be punctured and tuned fast.

This stops the pain immediately.

Nausea/vomiting: P 6 must be punctured.

High fever: GV 14 should be punctured to reduce the high temperature immediately.

Flatulence: LIV 13, E, GB 25,26 must be punctured.

The second fire and fire elements join with the downward right-side energy cycle along with water. When the fire increases (double the amount), it creates dysentery. When the upward right side energy cycle joins, nausea occurs. When the wood elements become excess flatulence occurs.

Constipation.

Reasons: Food that is not suitable for the body, loss of sleep, eating at odd times, lack of exercise.

Points: ST 25,36,GV 20, SJ 6, CV1.

Prolapse of rectum

Main points: GV 1, GB 34, UB 34, 67

When the fire and earth elements join with the right and left downward energy cycles, this condition occurs.

Genito urinary disorders.

According to the Chinese method, these diseases occur when the energies in the meridians of the stomach, spleen, testis and urinary bladder are affected.

Yin Yang

CV GV

Spleen, testis; Stomach, testis.

Before starting the treatment, an investigation of the system should be done to determine whether there is any sort of growth, the presence of stones, etc.

When fire and water element energies join fire or earth or both, it creates these problems.

Nephritis Pyelitis, pyelonephritis (295)

Reasons: From the urinary bladder, the bacteria travel, affect the testis and produce the symptoms, such as throat hoarseness, headache, backbone pain, oedema of the face and leg and at times bleeding in the urine, vomiting or some changes in the skin. Apart from these, the urea in the urine will be in excess. Blood pressure will become high. At times, because of the medicines to which patients become allergic, it affects the testis as well.

Points:(allergy) GV 20, 4, 3,SP-10.

Important points on which puncture is done: UB-23,25 GB 26, CV-3,4, SP-3, K 3.

When the water and second fire, along with the wood element join with the downward right and left energy cycles, this situation occurs. When the fire becomes excess, bleeding occurs. When the water element is in excess, urea becomes excess.

Infections: GV 14, LI-11.

Oedema of the face, the legs and the body: CV 5,9, UB 20, SP9.

Renal colic(pain in the urinary tract or organs)

This pain occurs suddenly. This is due to the block created by the formation of stones in the testis, the urinary tract or the urinary bladder. Symptoms are sudden, acute, unbearable pain, vomiting and sweat. Symptoms may exist for up to one or two hours.

Points: LI-4, K-5(for pain).This is used when there is pain.

After the treatment, any pain is reduced.

Distance points: ST 36, SP 6, UB 40, K 3.

Nearby points: GV 20,3, UB 23,25,26,32,52.

If vomiting is present, P 6 should be applied for a few days.

When the water, fire and earth elements join the downward right and left energy elements, the stones are formed. When the metal element joins with the abovementioned energies, this state occurs.

Enuresis—nocturnal enuresis: bed wetting

When the sphincter urethane, which is responsible for the control and elimination of urine becomes weak or does not work properly, this condition is called enuresis or bed wetting.

Causes: Diabetes mellitus, fear, psychological problems, urinary bladder stone.

Nearby Points: GV 20, UB 23,38,32

Far points: ST 36, UB 40, SP 18, K3.

Psychological factors.

Points: H7,UB 62, (can apply Moxibustion.)

When treating children, first apply the points on the front of the body. Later, after a few days, one can treat the back of the body.

Spina Bifida: The tail region of the spine will be swollen from birth.

When the second fire, along with the water element works as the right side downward energy cycle, this problem occurs.

When the wood element joins with the left side downward energy cycle and wood energy, the bulge in the tail of the spine forms.

Special Sense—Organs.

Diseases of the eyes.

Myopia—There will be a squint in the eye. Long-sightedness problems will occur. Because of this, there will be a pain in the eye.

Points:

1. GV 20/UB 1/ST—1/GB -1/LI-4 extra—4.
2. extra—4, 7, GB 20,37.
3. Additional points L. I—4, GB 37, LIV 3, UB-58.

Ear: Liver, testis, eye Shenmen.

Head: (Scalp), eye area.

When the cold fire or the second fire joins the right side upward energy cycle in the head region, this condition occurs.

Cataract: Clouding of the eye leads to a decrease in vision. It can affect one or both eyes.

Reasons: Due to age, diabetic mellitus and excess calcium.

If the cataract is fully grown, it is called a mature cataract and if it is not grown fully, it is known as an immature cataract.

When the earth energy element joins with the upward right-side energy cycle, the above condition occurs.

Points: ST:1, GB14, UB2, extra 1,4

Additional points: LI 4, GV20, LIV 3

Ear: Eye side 2, liver Shenmen, head, eye

Glaucoma

This condition causes damage to the eye's optic nerve and is often linked to the build-up of pressure inside your eyes. If untreated, it leads to blindness.

Points: 1: GV20, GB1,20,UB2, ST1

2: ST2, extra 1,3, GB14

When the wood and the earth element energies link with the upward right-side energy cycle of the head, this condition occurs.

Additional points: LI 14, LIV 1,2,3, GV37, UB 18, 58, ST 36

If the headache combines: GV20, LI 4, ST 44

If vomiting occurs with the above disorder: GB6, CV12, ST 36

Ear points: Eye 1, 2 liver, Shenmen, endocrine, oedema points.

Head points: Vaso motor a reason both sides, eye area

Acute Conjunctivitis

This occurs due to external infections, such as germs in the air, bacteria, viruses and dust in the air.

When the earth and air elements' energies link with the upward right-side energy cycle of the head, this condition occurs.

Reddened and swollen eye: Chemosis

The reason for Ophthalmia Neonatorum, which is swelling of the eye in newborn babies is due to venereal diseases. The redness in the eye may occur due to glaucoma, whooping cough, ulcer in the cornea of the eye, etc.

Important points: 1. GV20, GB20, ST1, extra 2

2. UB1, UB 2, GB1, 14,17, TW23, LI14, LI1,11,CV14, LIV3,SP6

Ear acupuncture: Liver, spleen, Shenmen

When the wood and fire element energies link with the upward right-side energy cycle of the head and the downward right-side energy cycle of the head, this condition occurs.

Night blindness: Vision impaired after sunset.

Reason

Vitamin A deficiency. This affects the eyes and the skin.

Important point: GB 1, 14,20, ST-1, TW-25, UB-1.

Supporting points: SI 4, LIV 3 and GB 37.

Ear acupuncture: Eye I, II, liver, Shenmen.

Head acupuncture: Eye area.

Nutritious food and vitamin A must be given to the patients.

When the left-side upward energy cycle, along with wood joins with the right-side upward energy, this condition occurs.

Optic Neuritis.

Damage of the optic nerve. In this condition, eyesight will be reduced gradually and, in the end, the patient will become blind.

Either one or both eyes may get damaged. Oedema may be present. This may be caused due to sclerosis, diabetes, alcoholism and accidents due to chemicals.

CV-1,2, ST-1, Extra-1,3.

GB-1, 14, GT 20, Extra-2, 4, LI-4, LI-11, GV 14, GB 20,LIV-3

Ear: Eye I and II, Liver, sub cortex.

Head: Eye area.

Vitamin B1 andB12 can be supplemented.

When the fire and earth elements join with the right-side upward energy cycle, this condition occurs.

Colour blindness

This condition is hereditary. This affects men more than women. The green, blue and red colours cannot be seen.

Points: GV 20, GB -1, G 20, UB 2, TW 23, LI -14, LIV 3, Extra 7

Ear: I, II Shenmen, liver.

When the right-side downward energy, along with water joins the right-side upward energy this condition occurs.

Photophobia

Reasons:

Irritation in the eye, eye pain because of dirt falling in the eye, a wound in the eye from getting hit or so, soreness in the eye and glaucoma.

Points: GV 20, GV20, Extra 2, UB 1, Extra 1,4, ST 2 LI 4, LI 11, GB 37, LI 11, GB 37, LIV 3.

Ear: Eye I, II liver Shenmen.

When the second fire, along with the right-side downward energy joins the right-side upward energy cycle, this condition occurs.

Optic Atrophy.

Reason:

Venereal diseases, neurotoxins, tobacco, glaucoma, tuberculosis, leprosy and nutrition deficiency.

Points: 1. GV 20, UB 1, ST 1, Extra 1, Extra 7.

2. Extra 34, GB 1,14, UB 2, LI 4, SI 6, ST 6, LIV 3, UB 1, 23, GV37.

When the earth, fire and wood join the right-side upward energy cycle to form this condition.

Ear: eye I, II liver, Shenmen.

Head: vision area.

The treatment must be given for a longer duration.

Ear-related Diseases.

The Triple Warmer and the Gall Bladder meridian travel around the ear. Hence, if the needle is used in these meridians, then the diseases get cured. Apart from this, the small intestine meridian is also related to this area.

Diseases which are cured: deafness, dumbness, noises in the ear, dizziness.

Deafness

Reasons: Block in the ear path, excessive wax deposit, abscesses, damaged eardrums and nervous problems related to the ears. Due to strong dosages of some medicines, deafness may occur.

Points:

Nearby points: TW 17, 21, SI 19, GB 2

Far Points: LI 4, SI 3, GB 41, TW 3

Ear point: inner ear, Shenmen—testis.

Dumb

Reasons:

Congenital, skull injury, mumps, excessive doses of strong medicines, sudden shock and fear.

In Europe and the United States, through acupuncture treatment, many dumb people have been made to talk.

Important points.

The GV 15 is a very dangerous point to handle. It should be used only by an experienced acupuncture doctor.

When the fire and second fire element energies join the right-side energy cycle in the head.

Noises in the ear.

Reasons:

Problems in the inner ear, nerves around the ears getting impaired, chronic infection and puss formation, bleeding in the ear, ear injury, circulation disorders or vascular disorders.

Important points: Nearby points: x 7, TW 17, 21 GB 2, SI-19.

Far Points: GB 41, TW 3,5

Nearby points: TW 21, SI 19, GB 2

Far points: TW 3, 5,17, GB 41, SI 4, GV 14, SP 6

When the right-side downward energy cycle, along with fire and wood elements joins the right-side upward energy cycle, this condition occurs.

7.9 The Points Which Are Used Often in Acupuncture Treatment

LU	**Lung meridian (LU 2,5,6,7,10)**
LI	**Large intestine meridian(LI,3,4,11,15,18,20)**
ST	**Stomach meridian (ST I,3,6,7,31,36,39,40,43,44)**
H	**Heart meridian(H—2,3,5)**
SP	**spleen meridian (SP-3,4,6,9,10,13,15)**
SI	**Small intestinal meridian(SI-3,6,9,15,18)**
UB	**urinary bladder meridian(UB-2,18,25,30,31,32,33,57,60,64)**
K	**Kidney meridian (K-1,3,4,6,7)**
P	**Pericardium meridian (P-4,6)**
TW	**Triple warmer meridian(TW-3,5,6,8,17)**
GB	**Gall bladder meridian (GB-2,8,14,20,26,27,28,30,34,36,38,39,41,43)**
LIV	**Liver meridian (LIV-3,6,13)**

Extraordinary points

Head and neck point.

*EX-1,2,3,4,5,6,7,8,9,10,11,12,13.

Below the neck point.

EX-14,15,16,17,18,19,20,21

Points on the hand.

Ex-22,23,24,25,26,27,28,29,30

Points on the leg.

Ex-31,32,33,34,35,36

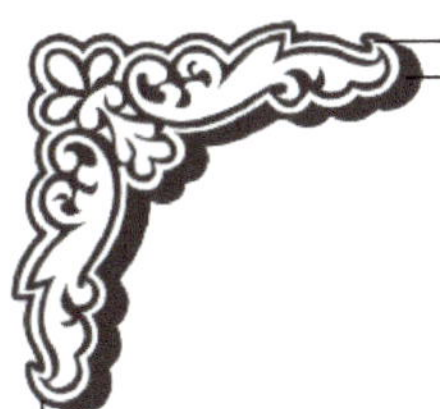
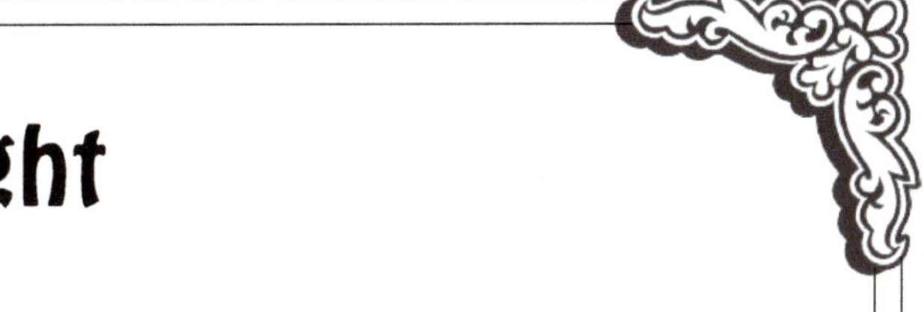

Part Eight

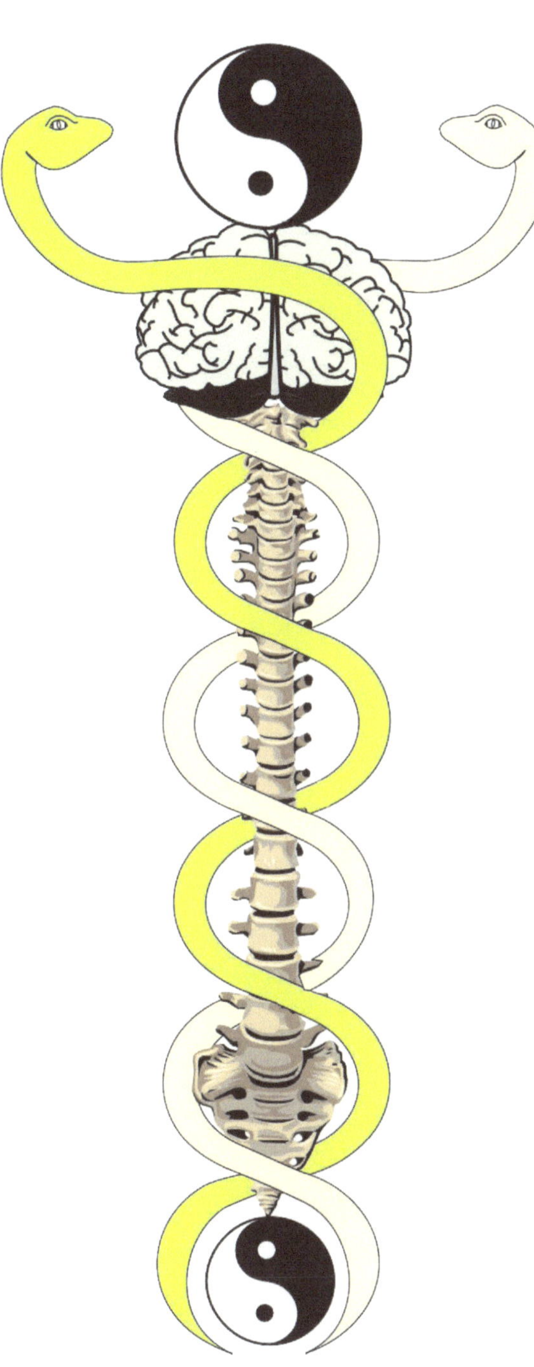
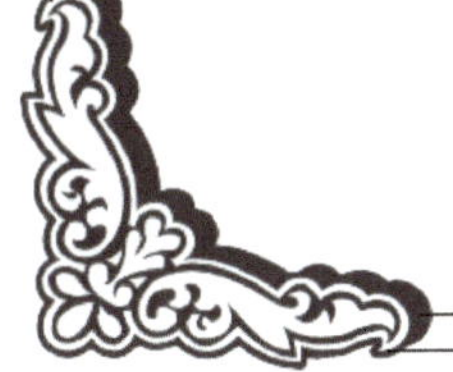

The Six Tastes and the Related Organs.

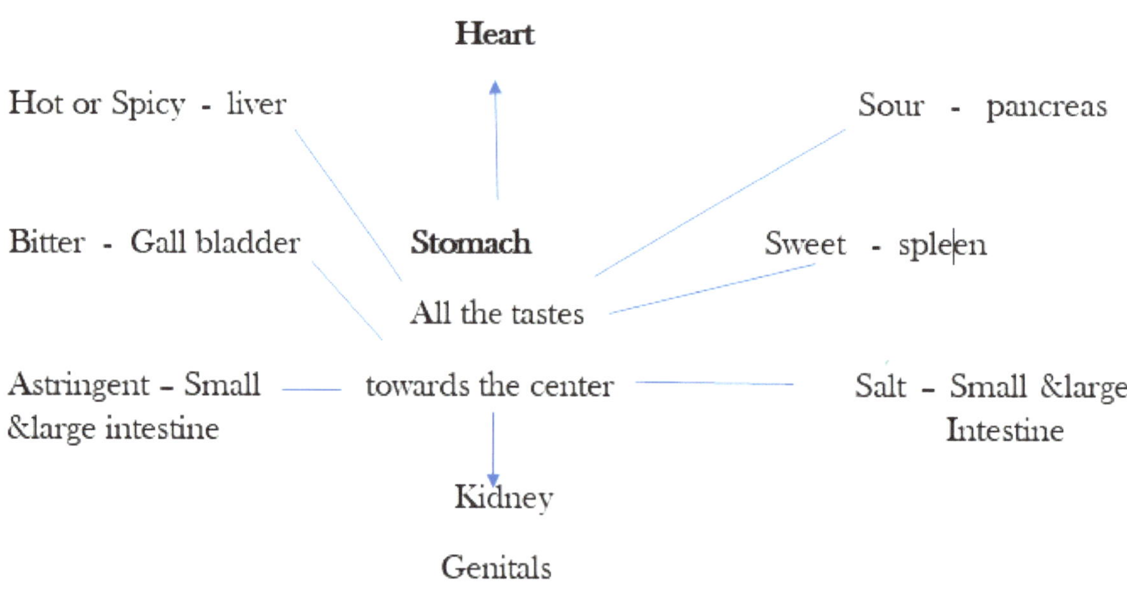

Genitals

Download action of

All the six tastes.

6 Tastes	
⊓	T
✓	Λ
✓	m

12 Tastes			
⊓	T	⊥	⊔
✓	Λ	V	^
✓	m	ш	^

18 Tastes		
⊓ T	⊓ T ⊔ ⊥	⊥ ⊔
✓ Λ	✓ Λ ^ V	V ^
✓m	✓m ^ш	ш ^

⊓ Hot	⊓T Hot,Sour	T Sour
⊓ ✓ Hot, bilter	⊓ ✓ Hot, sour TΛ bilter,sweet	TΛ Sour sweet
✓ Bitter	✓ Bitter, Sweet Λ	Λ Sweet
✓ ✓ Bilter, Astringent	✓✓ Λm Bilter sweet Astringent Salt	Λm Sweet Salt
✓ Astringent	✓m Astringent salt	m Salt
✓ ⊓ Astringent, Hot	✓✓ mT Astringent, salt Hot sour	mT Salt sour

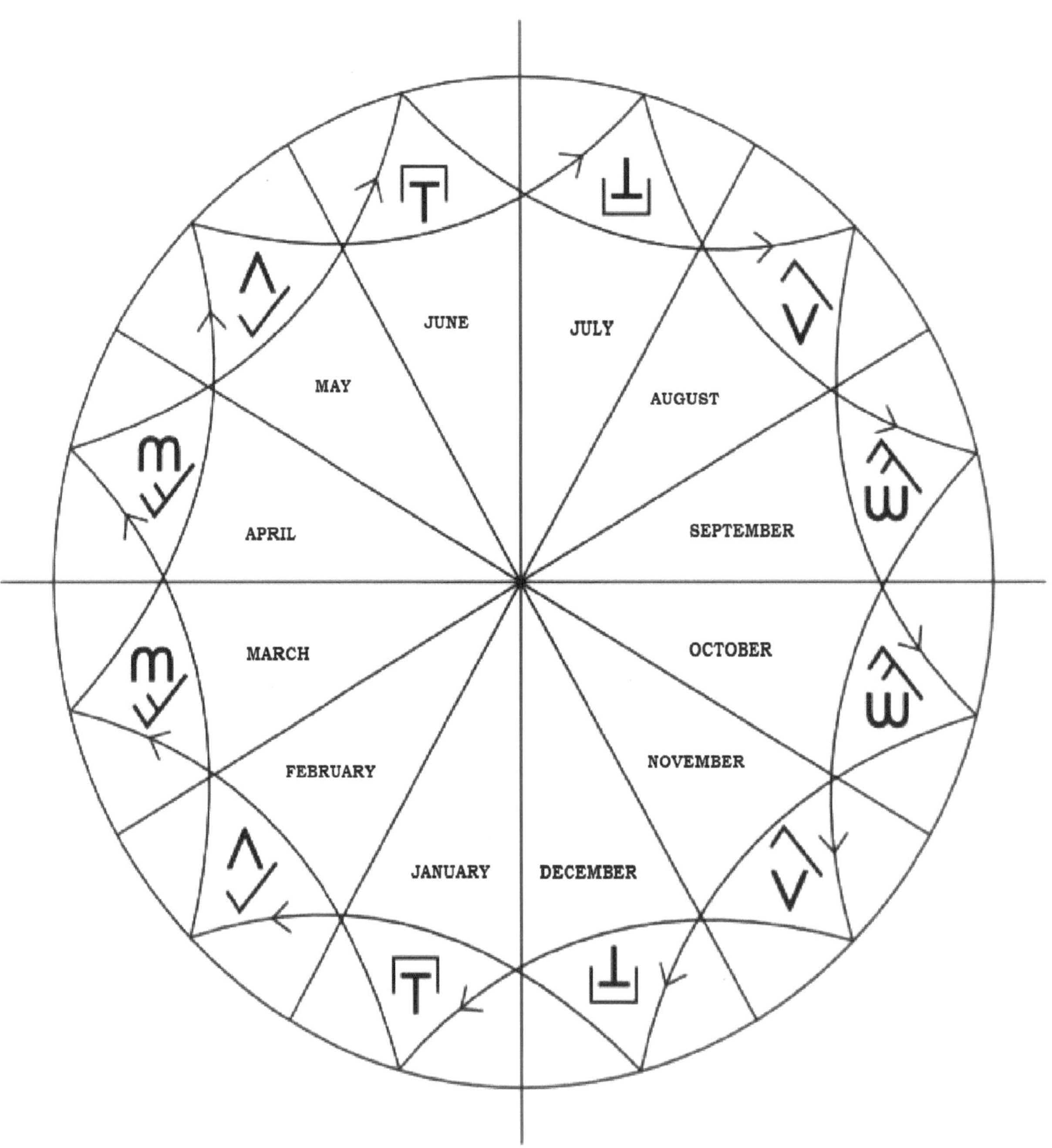

Figure 8.1 The Relativity Between the Six Elements and the 12 Months of a Year

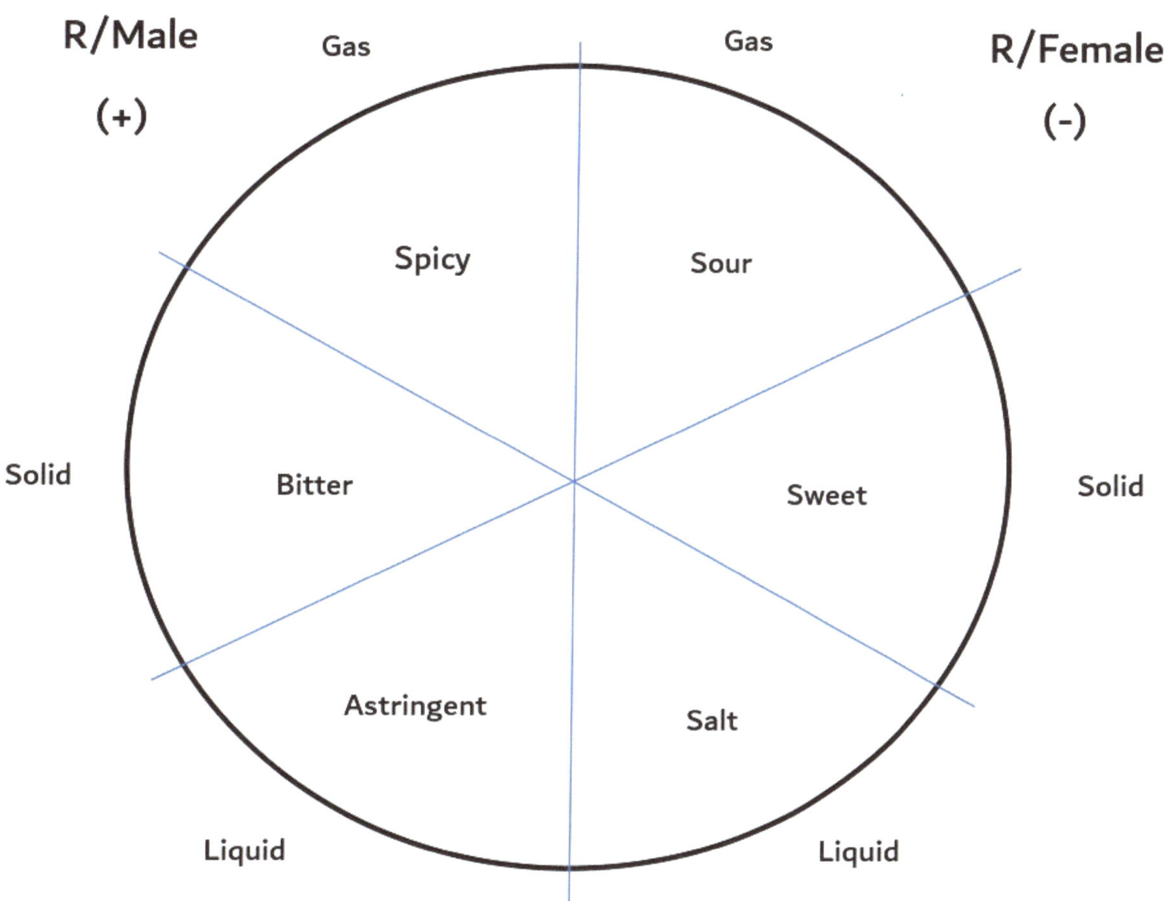

Figure 8.2 Six Tastes—Right/Left

The 24 Hours Cycles of the Six Tastes

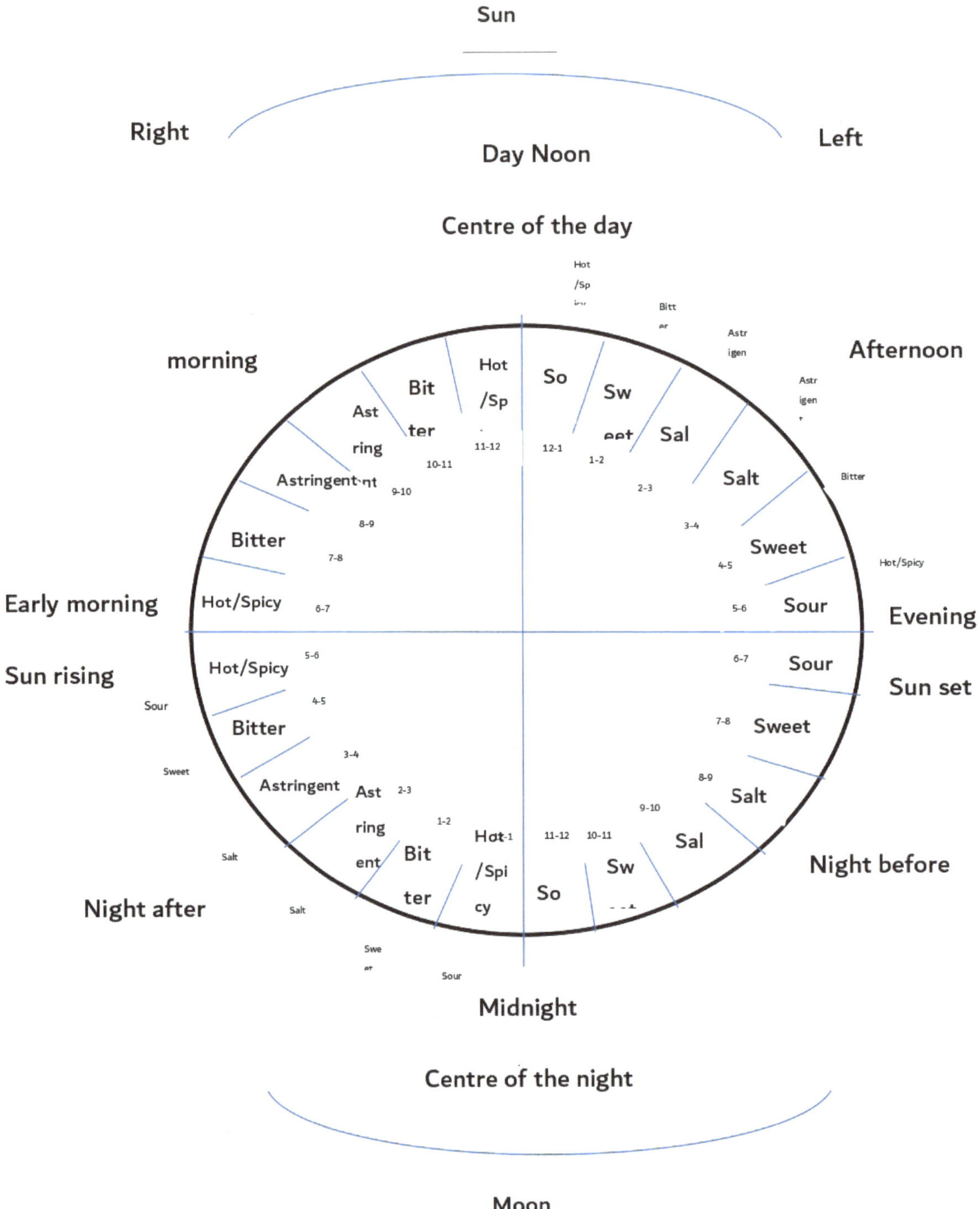

Figure 8.3 Six Types of Tastes-24-in State of Four Segments

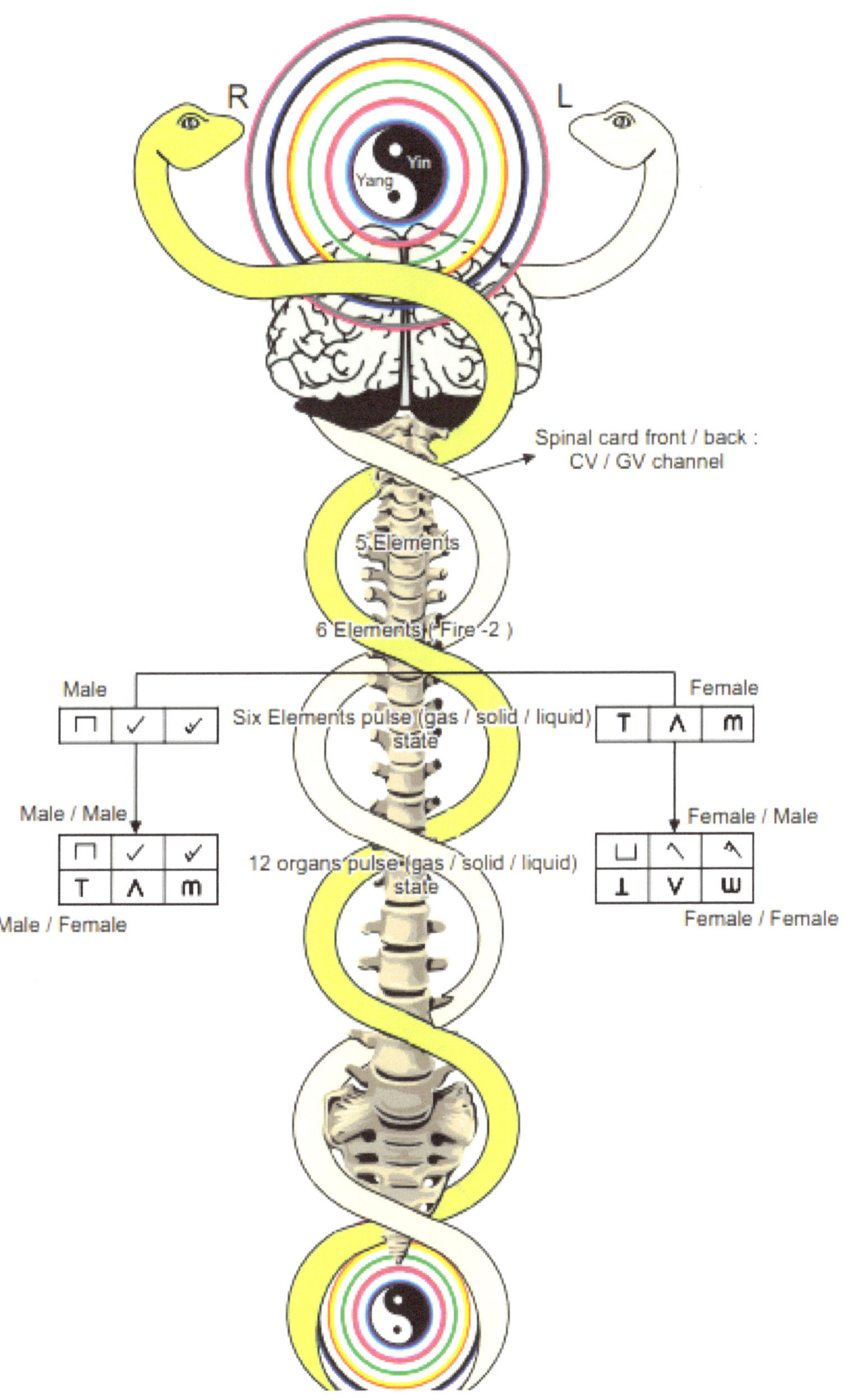
R
L
Yin
Yang
Spinal card front / back :
CV / GV channel
5 Elements
6 Elements (Fire -2)
Male
Female
Six Elements pulse (gas / solid / liquid) state
Male / Male
Female / Male
12 organs pulse (gas / solid / liquid) state
Male / Female
Female / Female

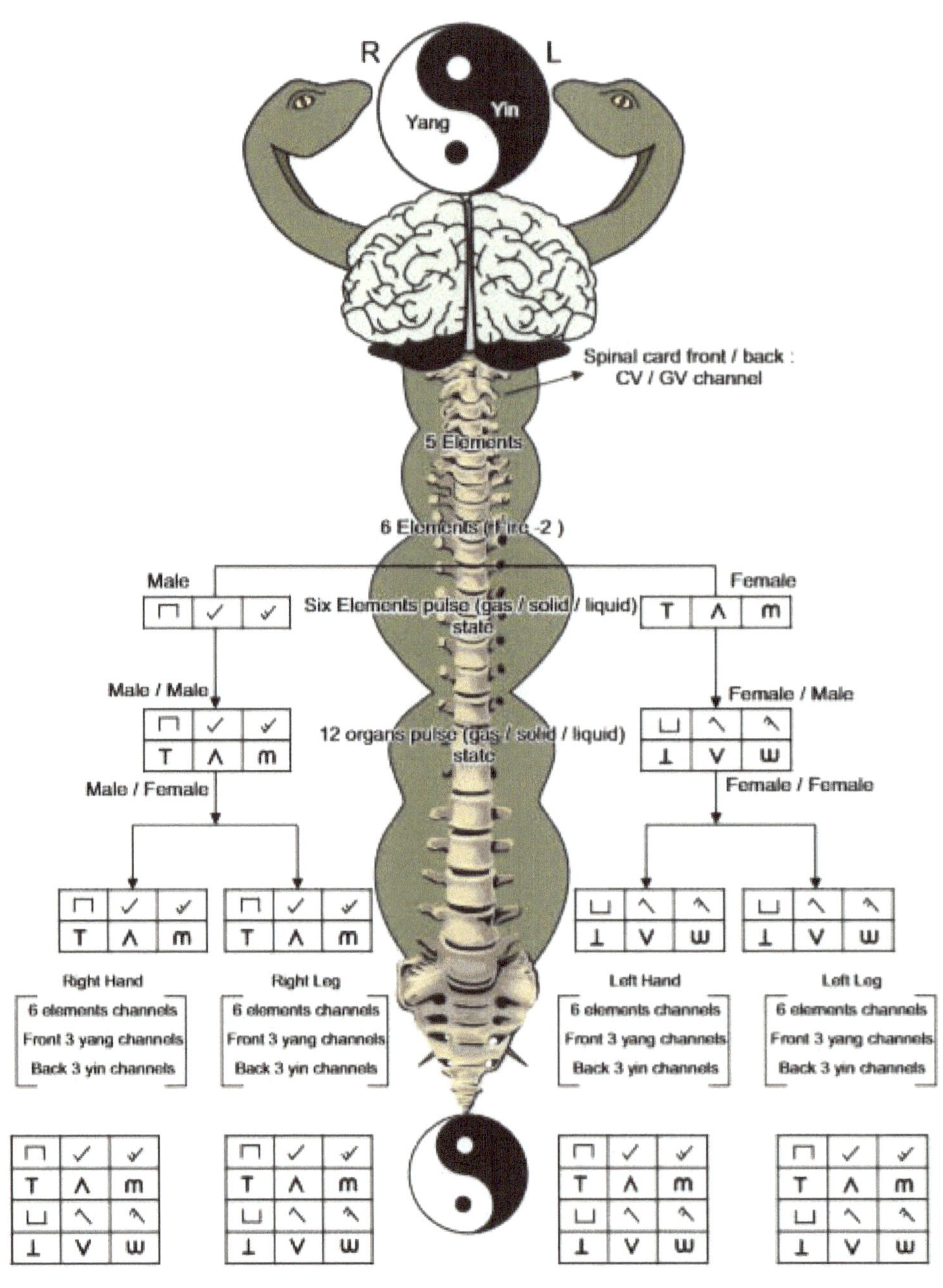
R
L
Yang
Yin
Spinal card front / back :
CV / GV channel
5 Elements
6 Elements (Fire -2)
Male
Female
Six Elements pulse (gas / solid / liquid) state
Male / Male
Female / Male
12 organs pulse (gas / solid / liquid) state
Male / Female
Female / Female
Right Hand
6 elements channels
Front 3 yang channels
Back 3 yin channels
Right Leg
6 elements channels
Front 3 yang channels
Back 3 yin channels
Left Hand
6 elements channels
Front 3 yang channels
Back 3 yin channels
Left Leg
6 elements channels
Front 3 yang channels
Back 3 yin channels

The new invention of five elements
five cycles in Acupuncture / Acupressure

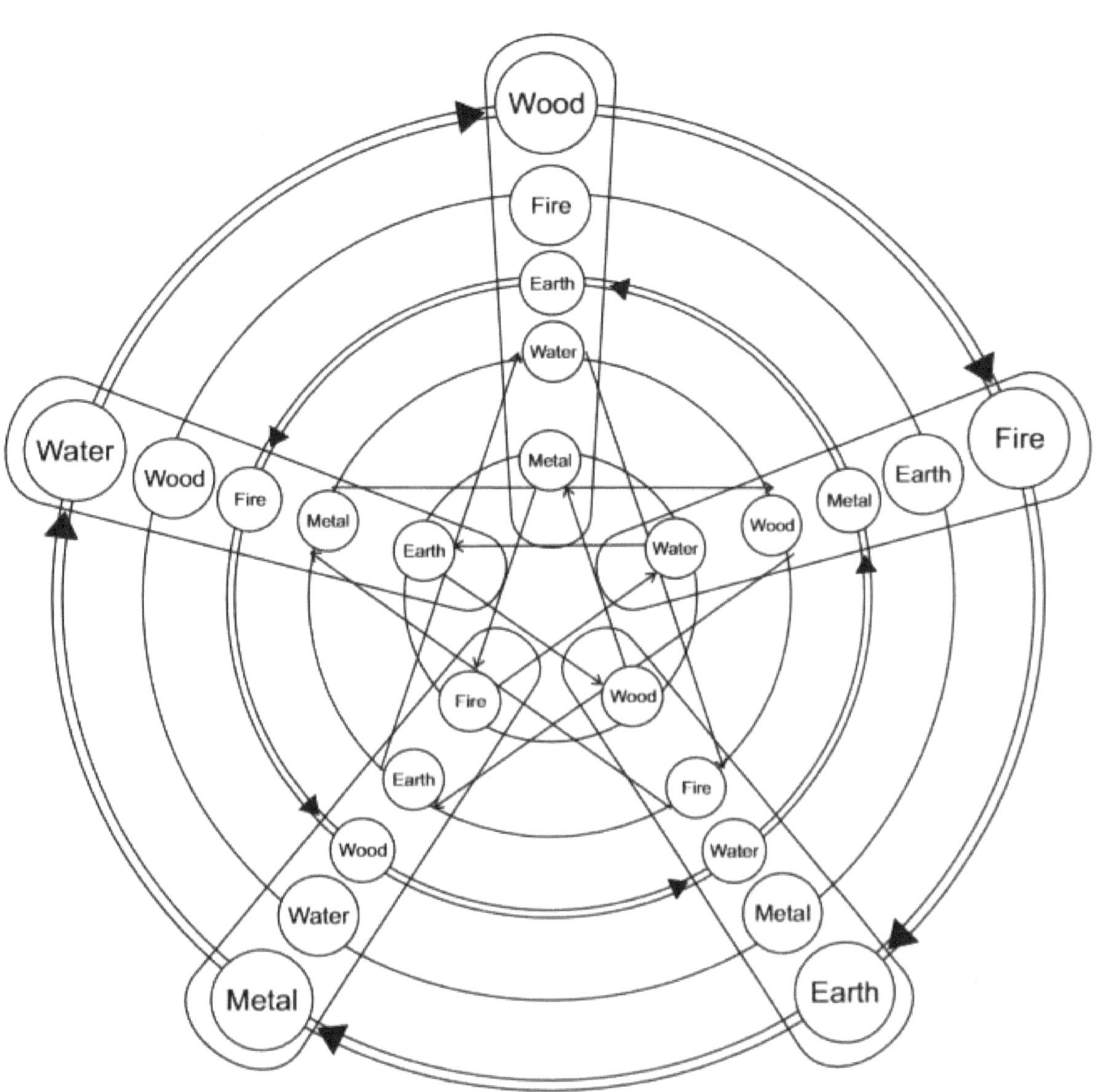

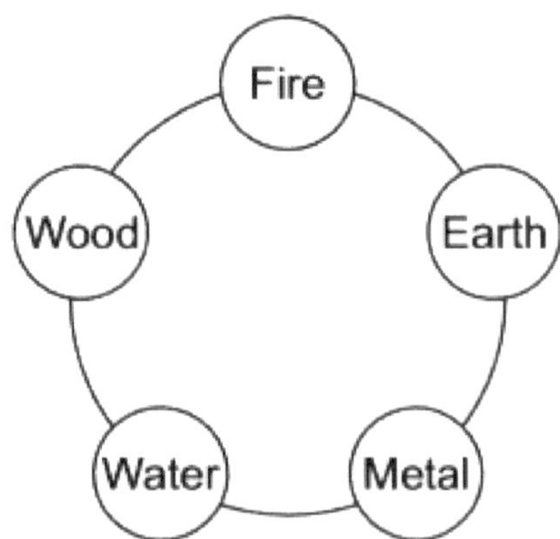
Self Cycle
Fire
Earth
Metal
Water
Wood

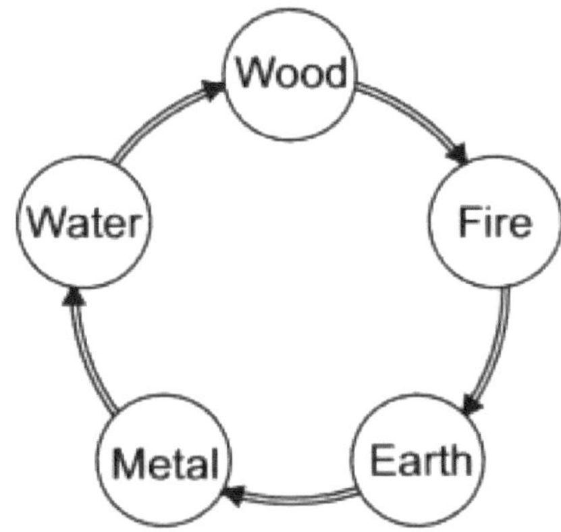
Enlargement Cycle
Wood
Fire
Earth
Metal
Water

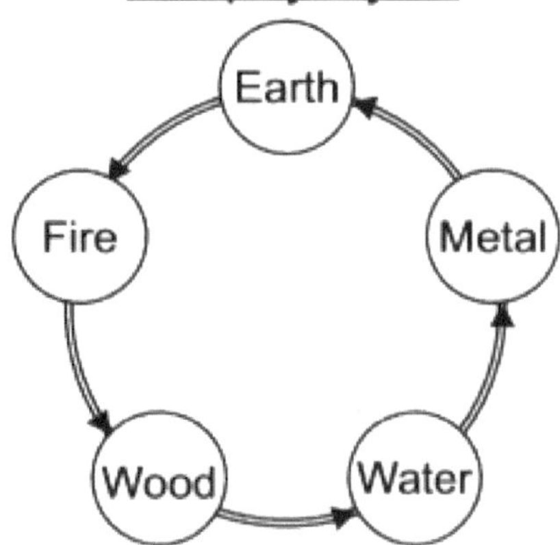
Atrophy Cycle
Earth
Metal
Water
Wood
Fire

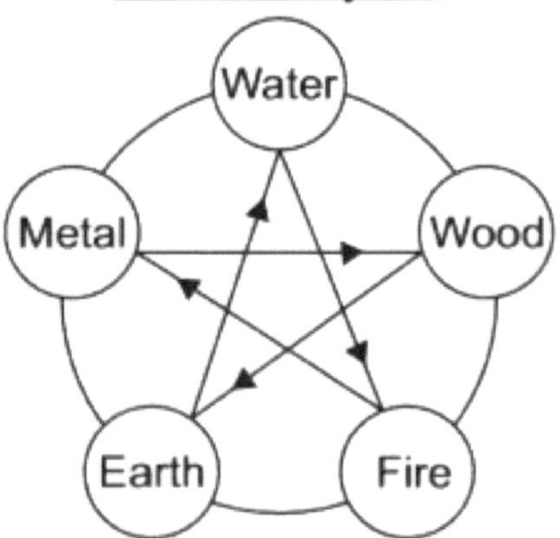
Control Cycle
Water
Wood
Fire
Earth
Metal

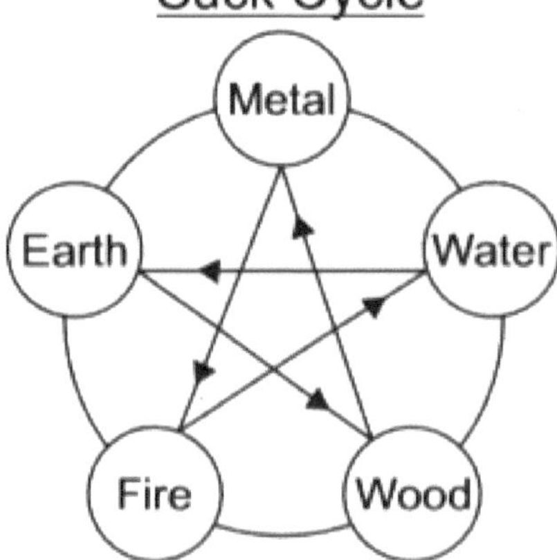
Suck Cycle
Metal
Water
Wood
Fire
Earth

CYCLES BASED ON TASTES

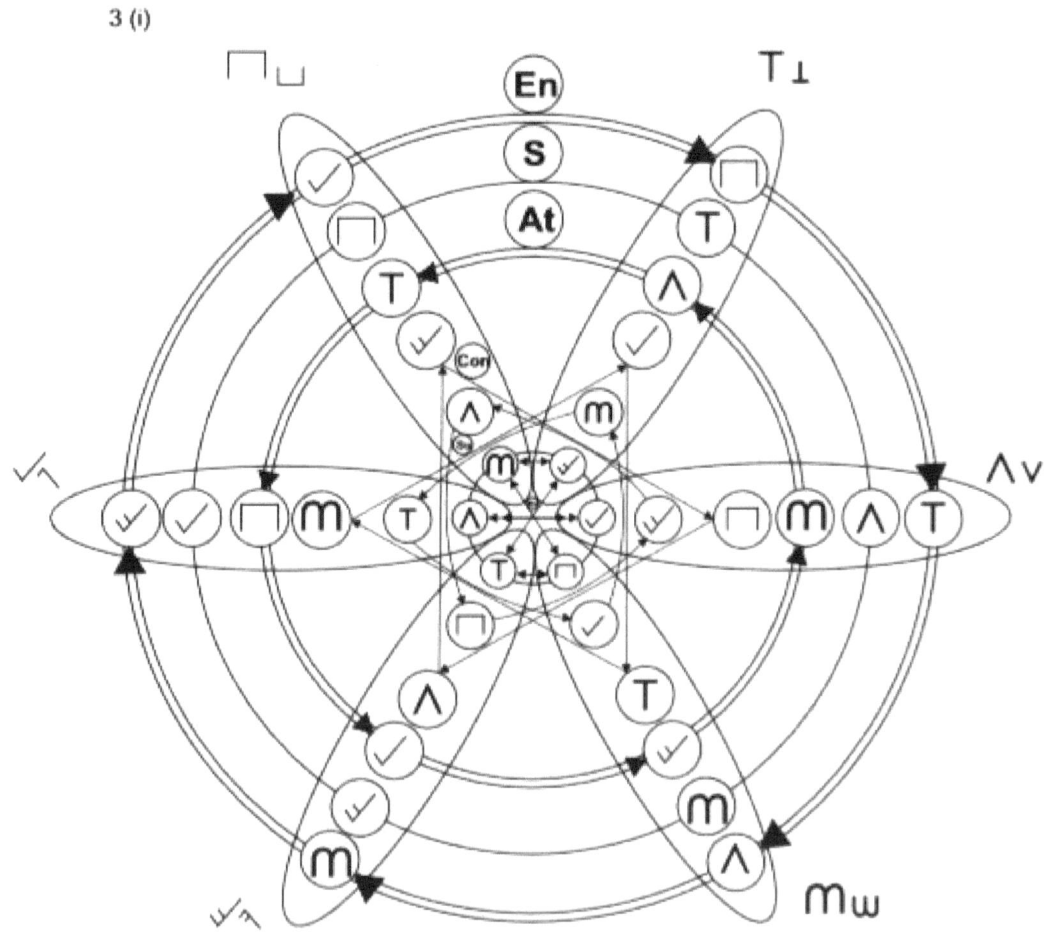

Single :

En – Enlargement cycle (Single)
Se – Self cycle
At – Atrophy cycle
Con – Control cycle
Su – Suck cycle
Ba – Balance cycle

Double

Self + Enlargement
Enlargement + Atrophy
Atrophy + Control
Control + Suck
Suck + Balance
Balance + Self

Trible

Self + Enlargement + Atrophy
Enlargement + Atrophy + Control
Atrophy + Control + Suck
Control + Suck + Balance
Suck + Balance + Self
Balance + Self + Enlargement

Four

Self + En + At + Con
En + At + Con + Su
At + Con + Su + Ba
Con + Su + Ba + Self
Su + Ba + Self + En
Ba + Self + En + At

Five

Se + En + At + Con + Su
En + At + Con + Su + Ba
At + Con + Su + Ba + Se
Con + Su + Ba + Se + En
Su + Ba + Se + En + At
Ba + Se + En + At + Con

Six

Se + En + At + Con + Su + Ba = Table ⊓
Se + En + At + Con + Su + Ba = Table ✓
Se + En + At + Con + Su + Ba = Table ✓
Se + En + At + Con + Su + Ba = Table T
Se + En + At + Con + Su + Ba = Table Λ
Se + En + At + Con + Su + Ba = Table m

These cycle will combine in patents as above stated.
Accordingly the treatment will be given.

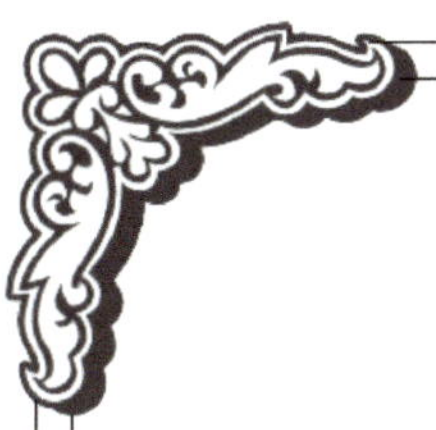
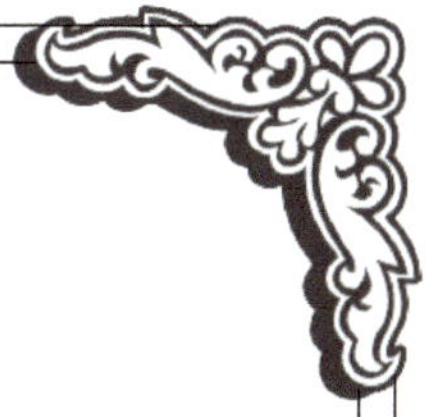

Part Nine

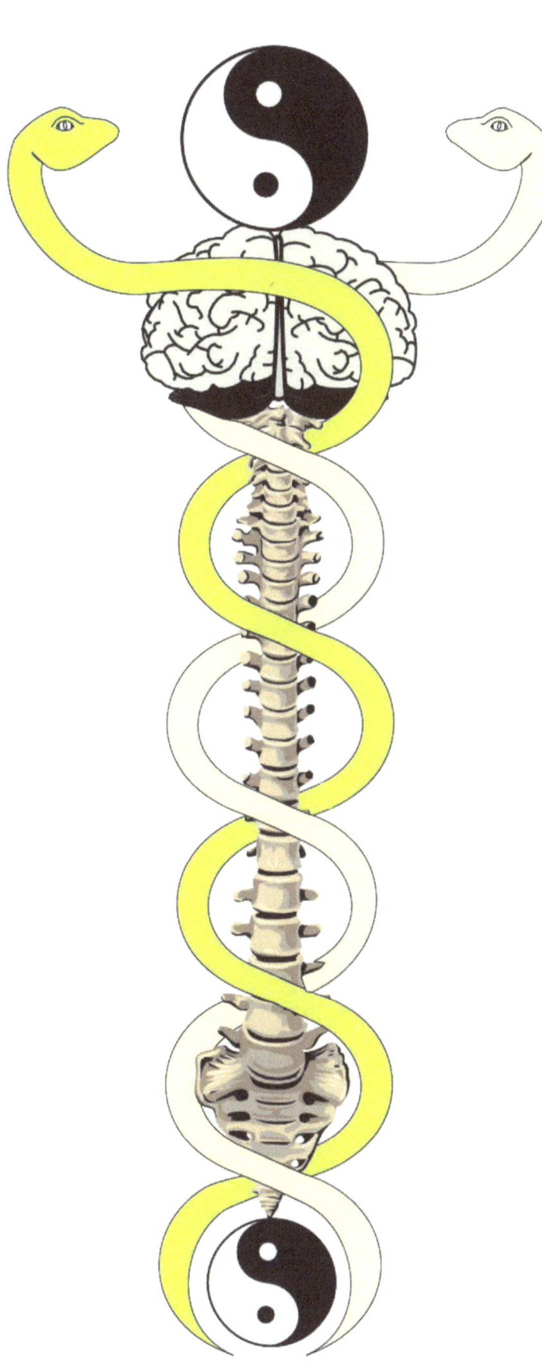

SIX ELEMENTS ENERGIES EXPANSION

YANG ±

3 (ii)
6 Elements

RIGHT SIDE
MALE (+)
FEMALE (+)

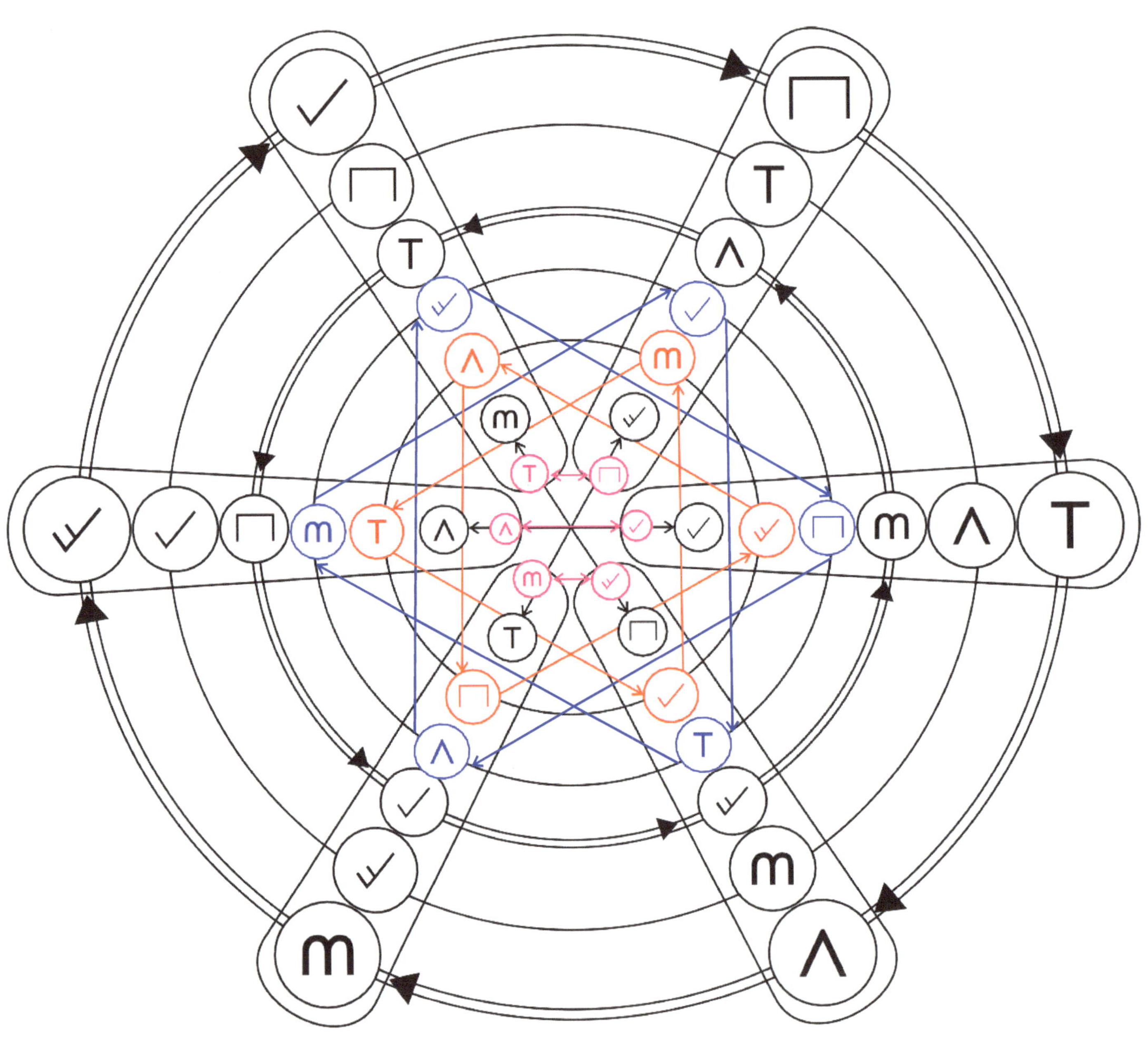

YANG ±

Self Cycle
Metal
Wood
I Fire
Earth
II Fire
Water

Enlargement Cycle -1
Metal
Wood
I Fire
Earth
II Fire
Water

Atrophy Cycle -1
Metal
Wood
I Fire
Earth
II Fire
Water

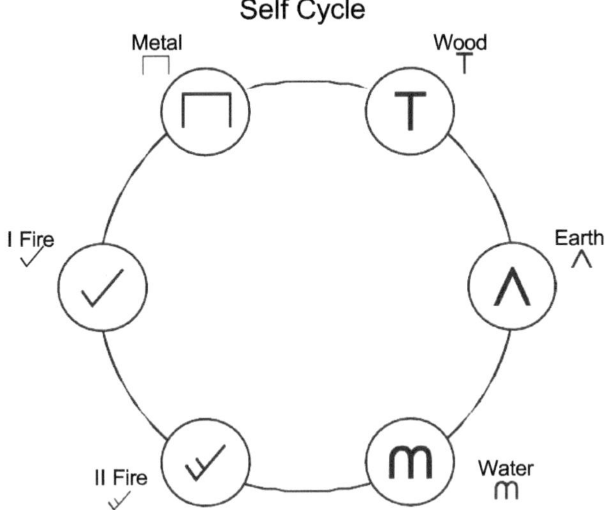

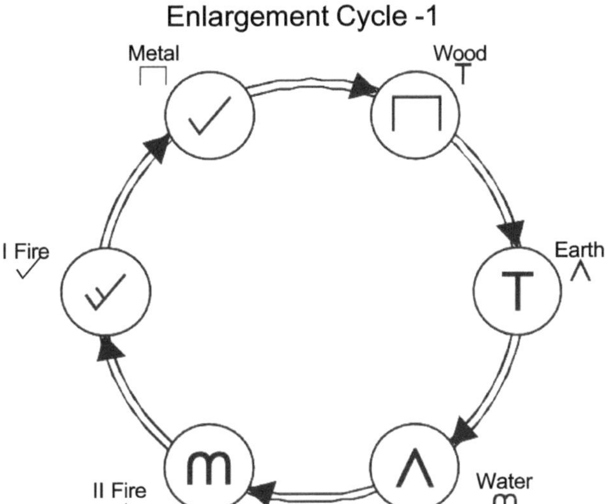

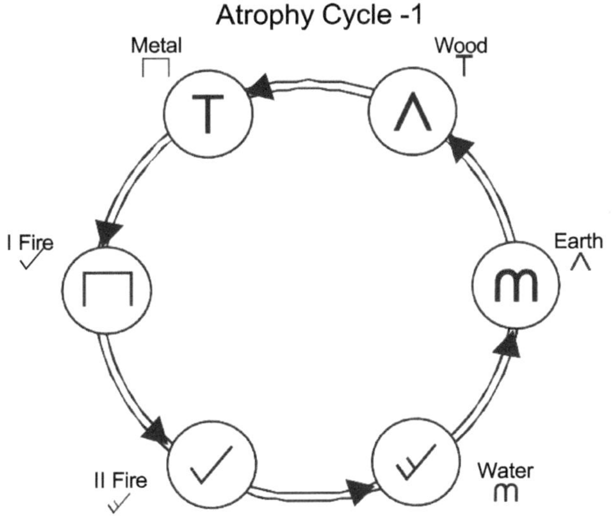

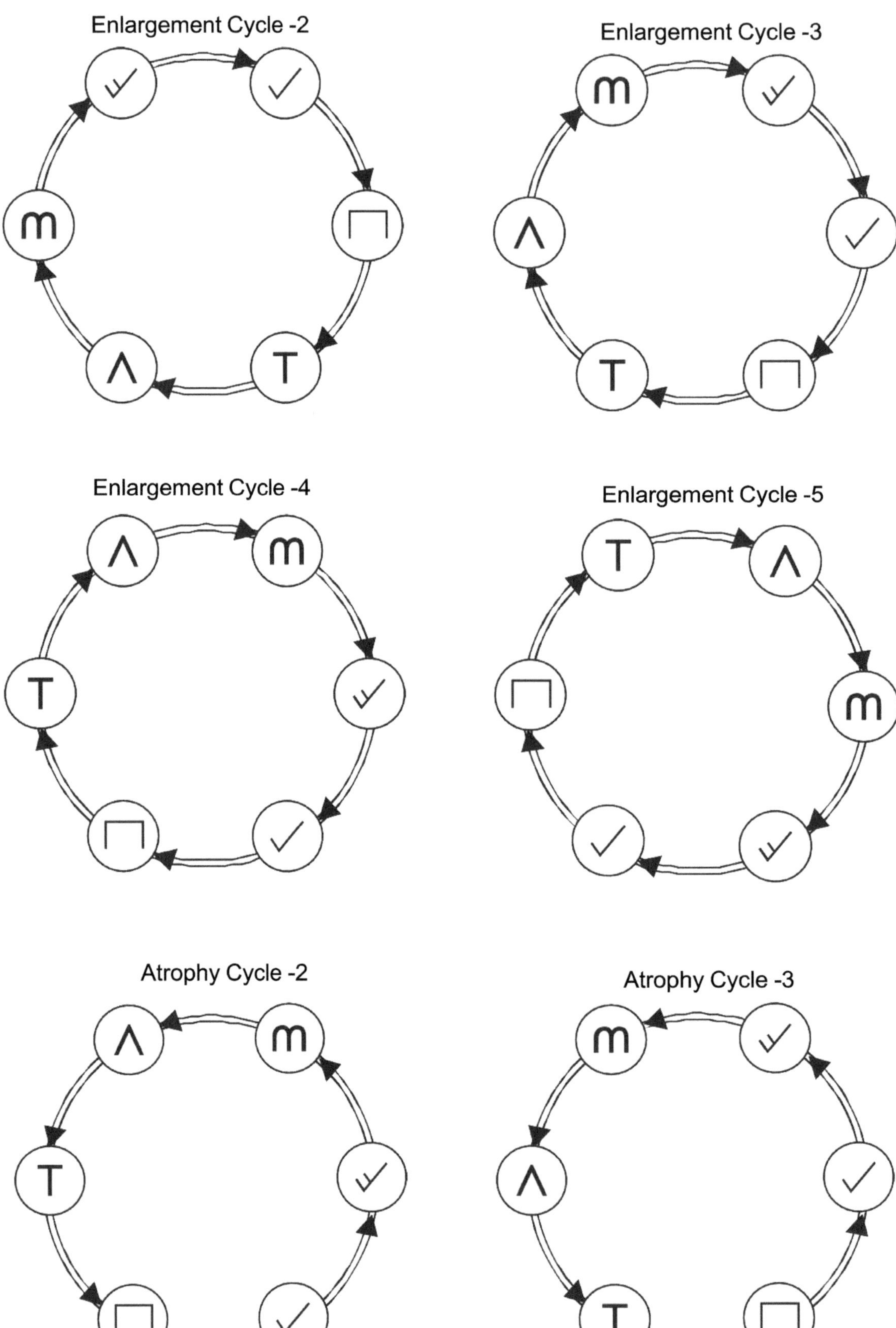
Enlargement Cycle -2
Enlargement Cycle -3
Enlargement Cycle -4
Enlargement Cycle -5
Atrophy Cycle -2
Atrophy Cycle -3

YANG ±

Atrophy Cycle -4

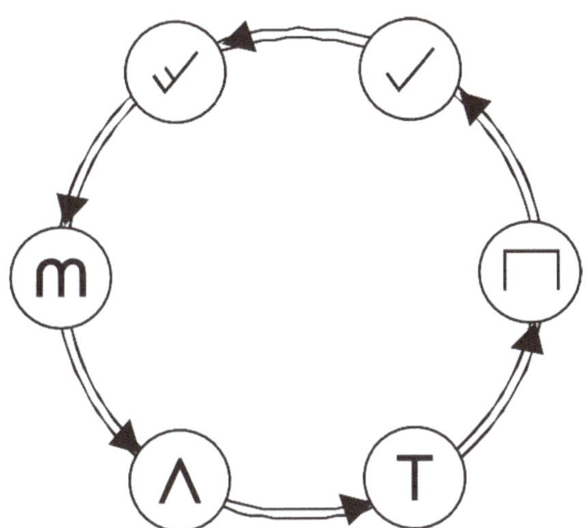

Atrophy Cycle -5

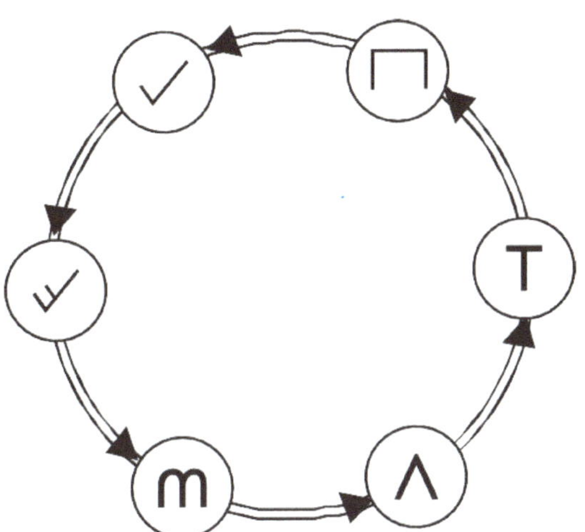

Control Cycle

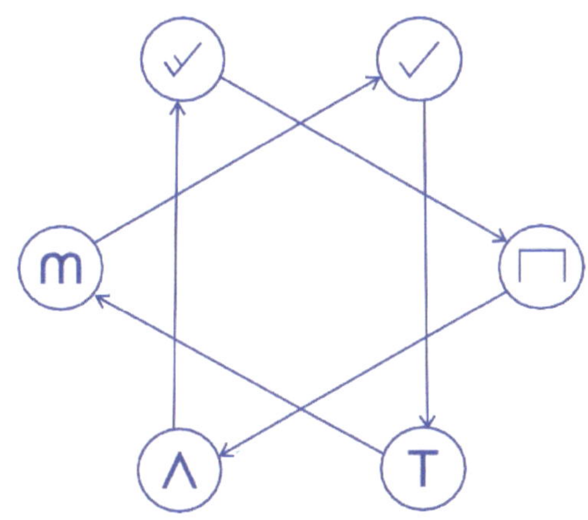

Suck Cycle

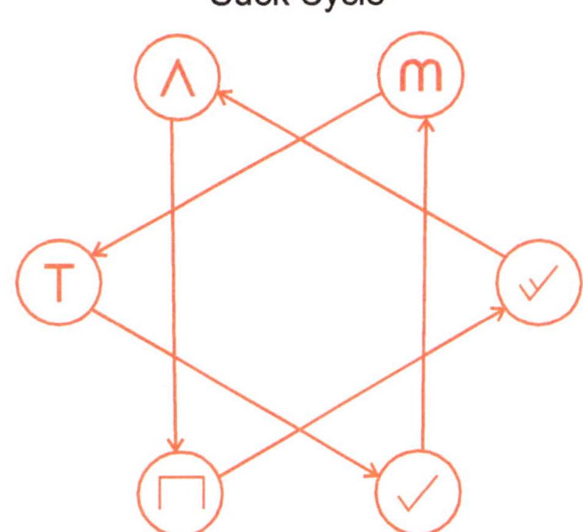

Balance Cycle

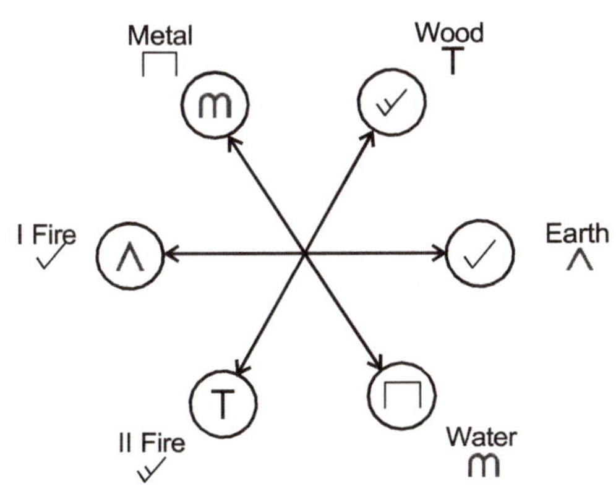

Husband & Wife Cycle

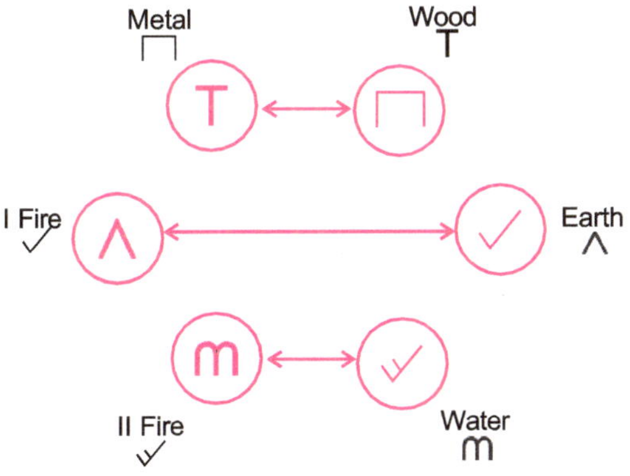

LEFT SIDE MALE AND LEFT SIDE FEMALE ENERGY CYCLEING

YIN ±

LEFT SIDE
MALE (-)
FEMALE (-)

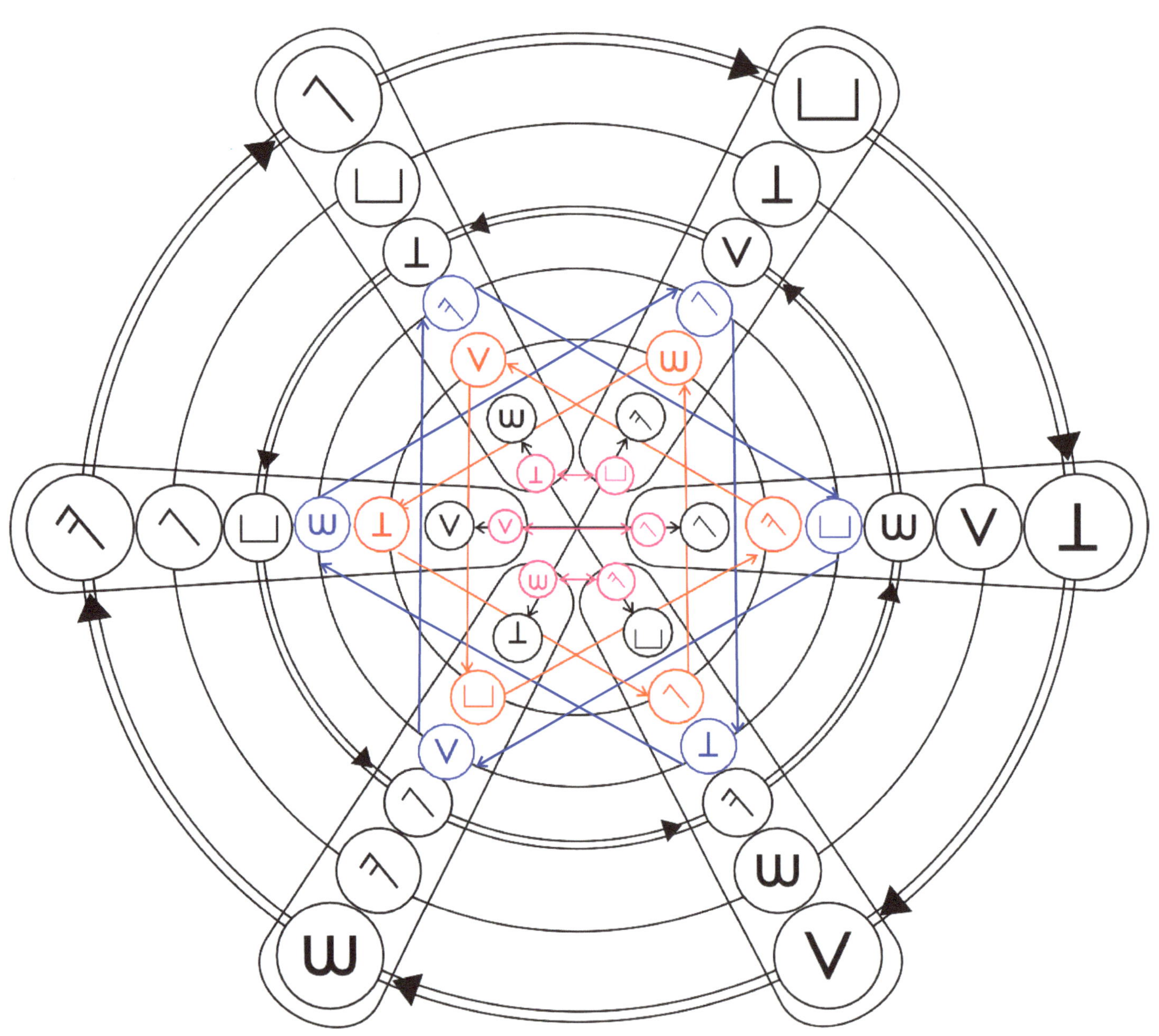

YIN ±

Self Cycle

Metal -

Wood -

Earth -

Water -

II Fire -

I Fire -

Enlargement Cycle -1

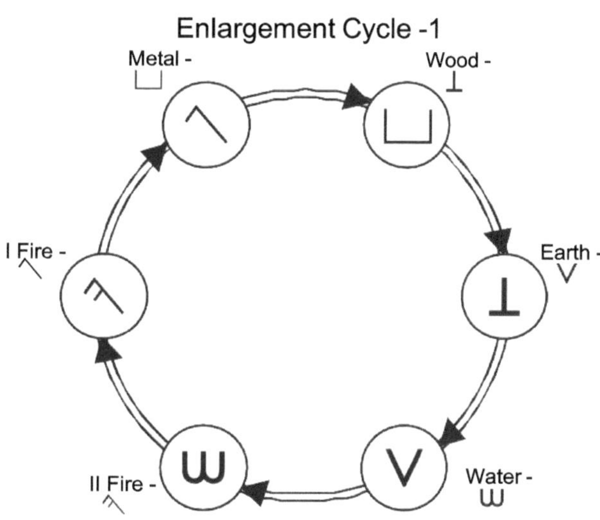

Atrophy Cycle -1

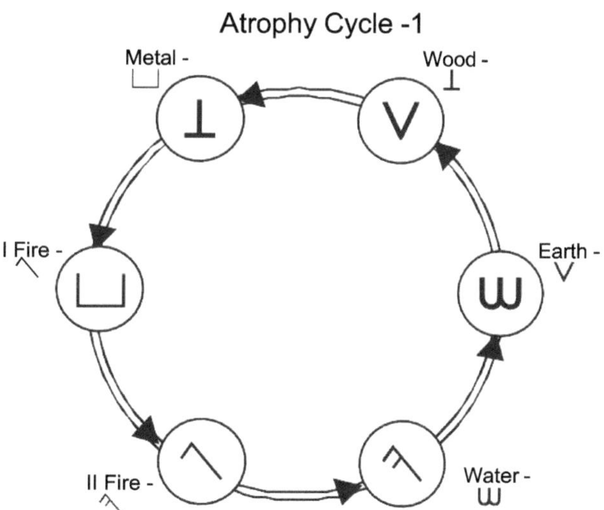

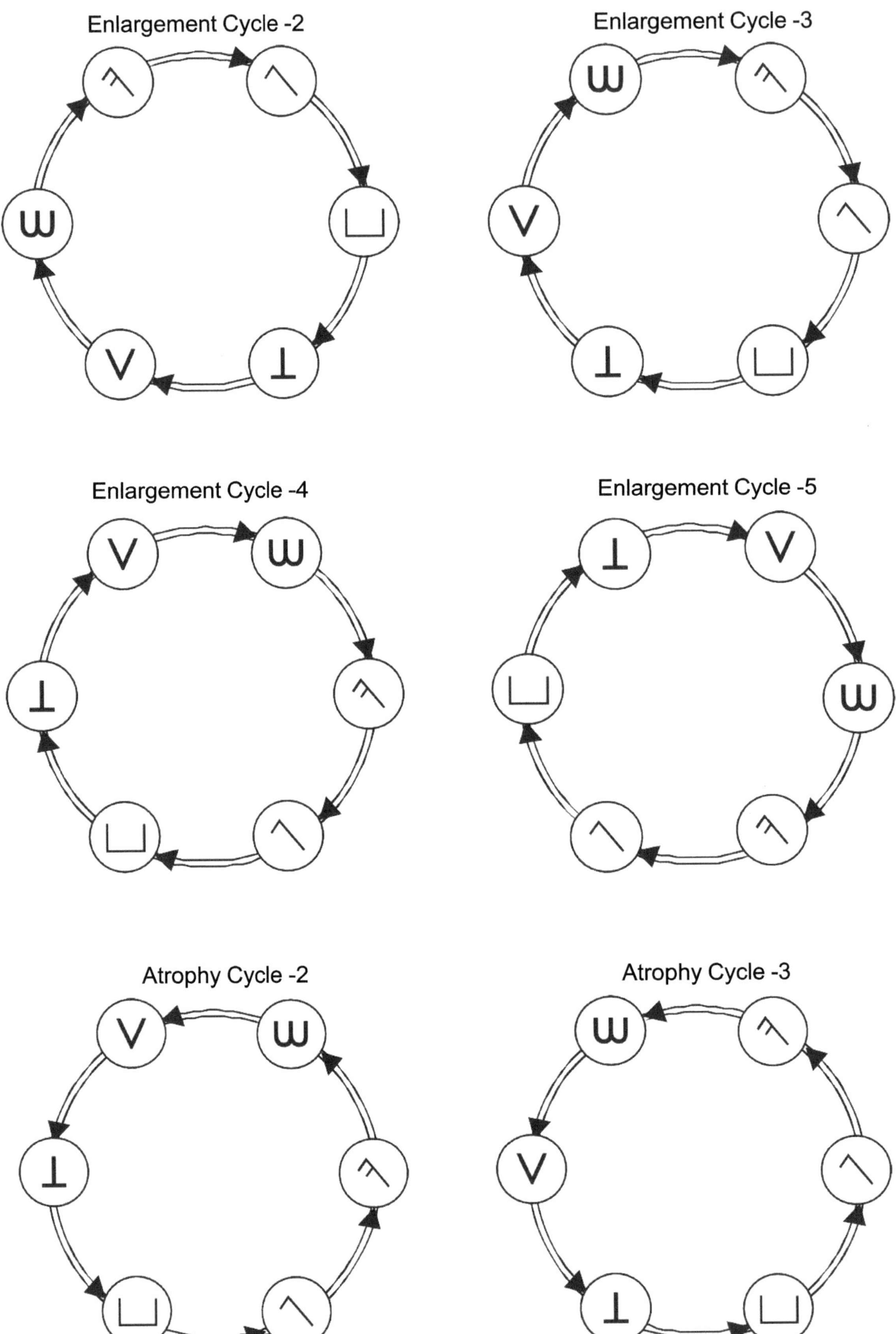
Enlargement Cycle -2
Enlargement Cycle -3
Enlargement Cycle -4
Enlargement Cycle -5
Atrophy Cycle -2
Atrophy Cycle -3

YIN ±

Atrophy Cycle -4

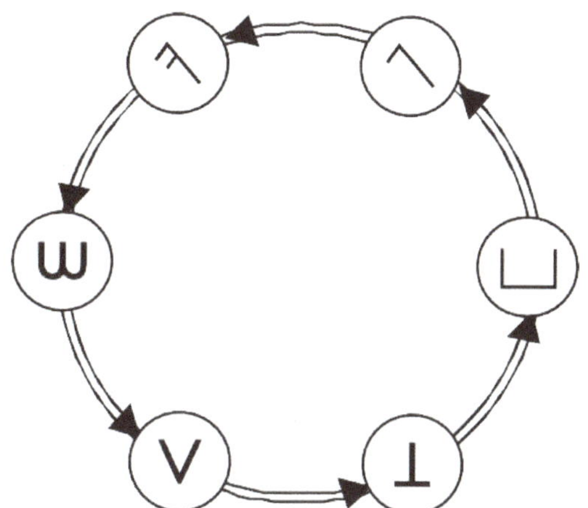

Atrophy Cycle -5

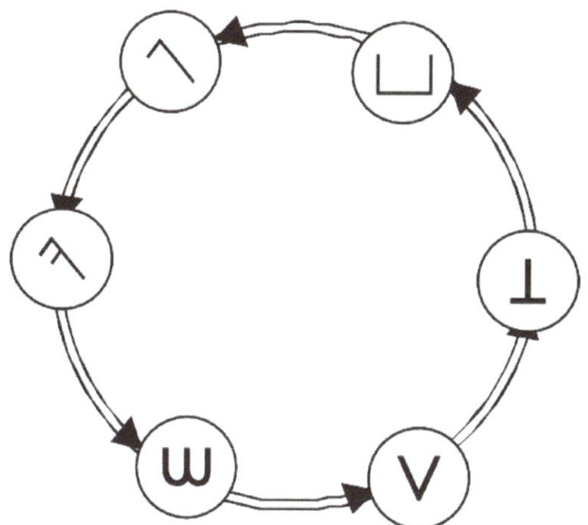

Control Cycle

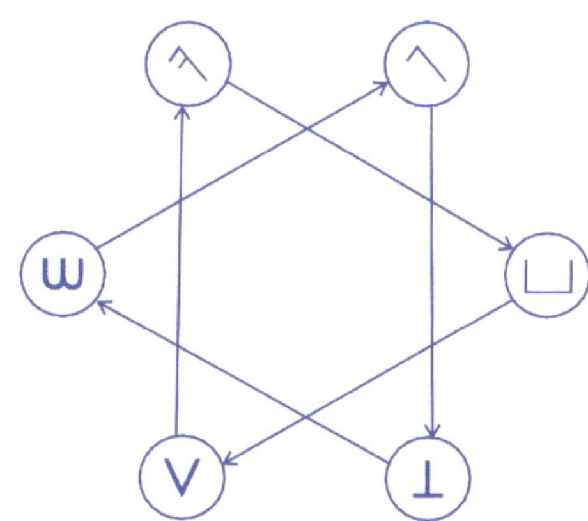

Suck Cycle

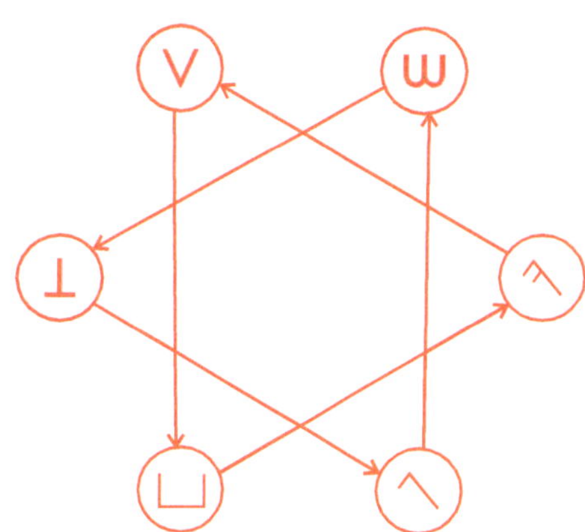

Balance Cycle

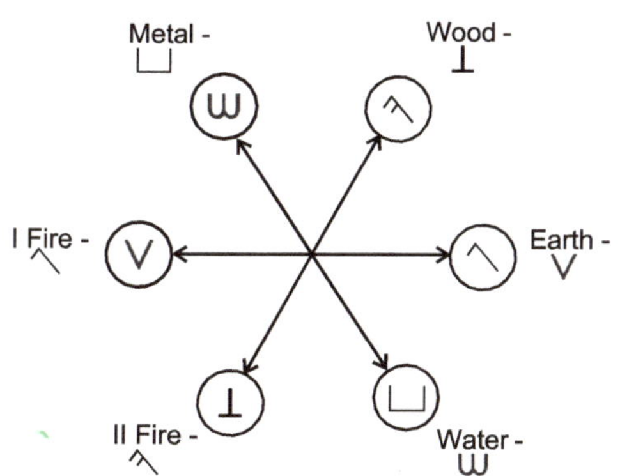

Husband & Wife Cycle

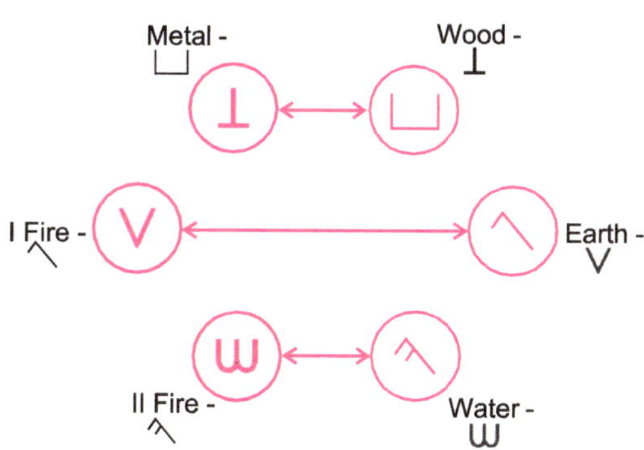

RIGHT SIDE MALE AND LEFT SIDE FEMALE ENERGY CYCLEING

YANG (+) YIN (-)

MALE (+) FEMALE (-)

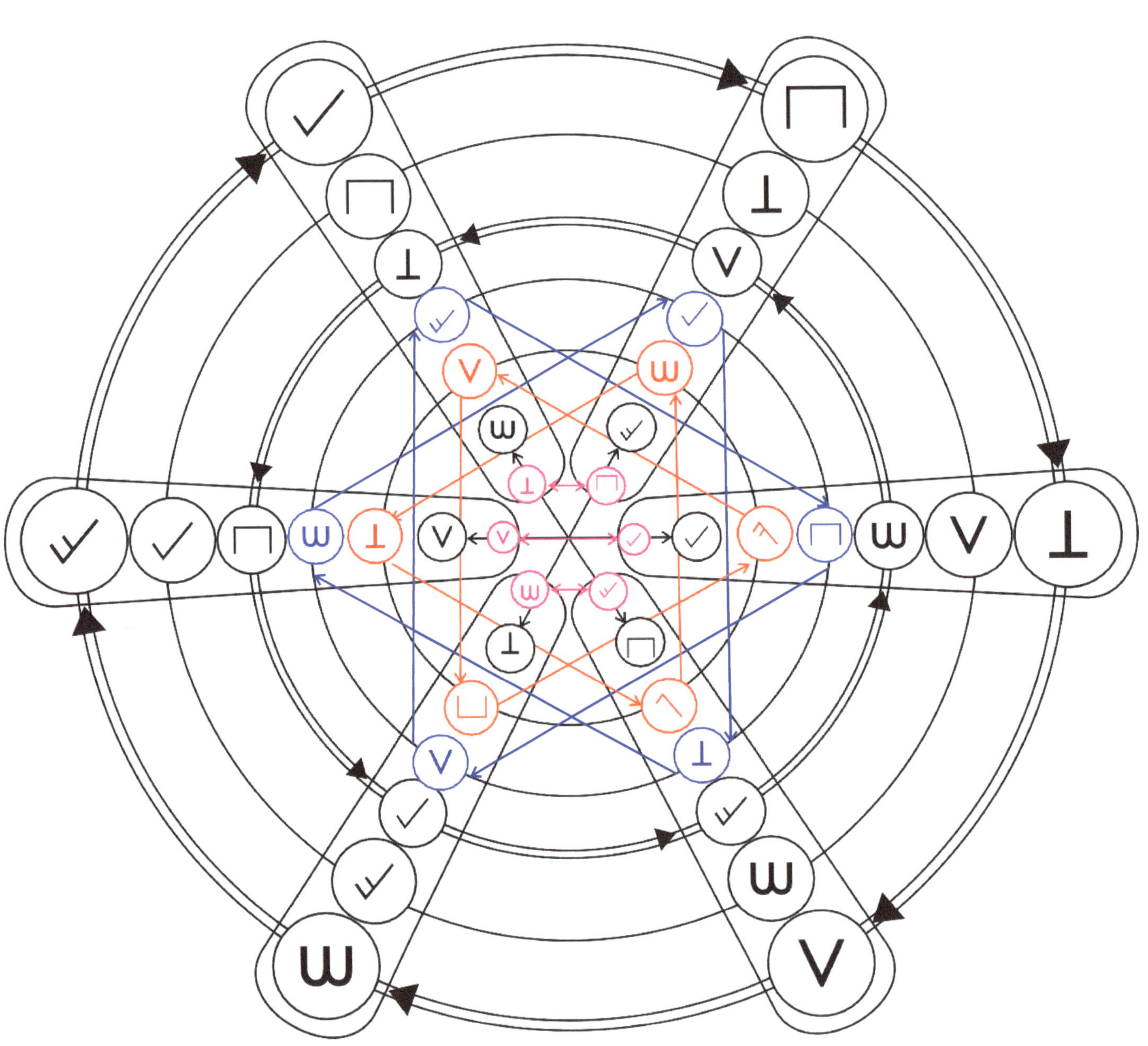

YANG (+) YIN (-)

Self Cycle
Metal +
Wood -
I Fire +
Earth -
II Fire +
Water -

Enlargement Cycle -1
Metal +
Wood -
I Fire +
Earth -
II Fire +
Water -

Atrophy Cycle -1
Metal +
Wood -
I Fire +
Earth -
II Fire +
Water -

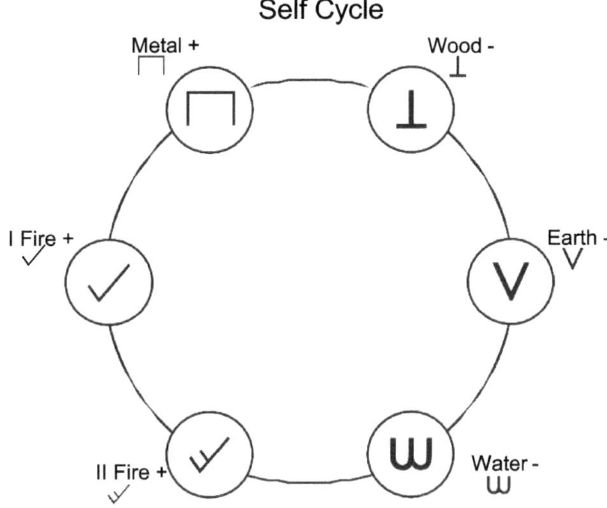

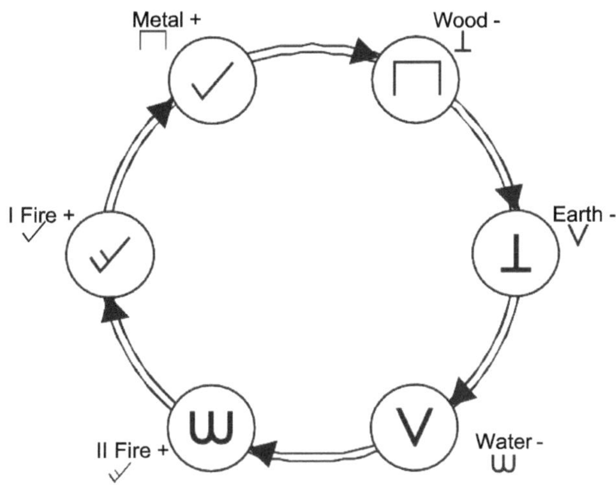

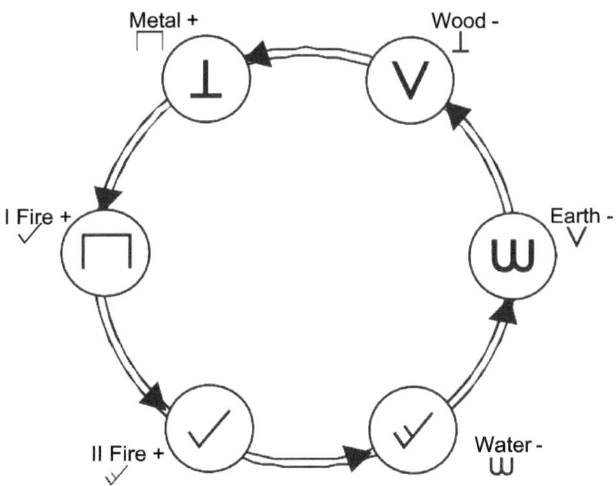

YANG (+) YIN (-)

Enlargement Cycle -2

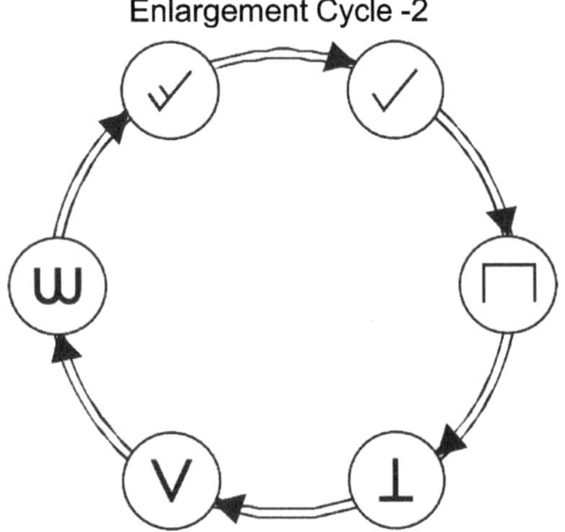

Enlargement Cycle -3

Enlargement Cycle -4

Enlargement Cycle -5

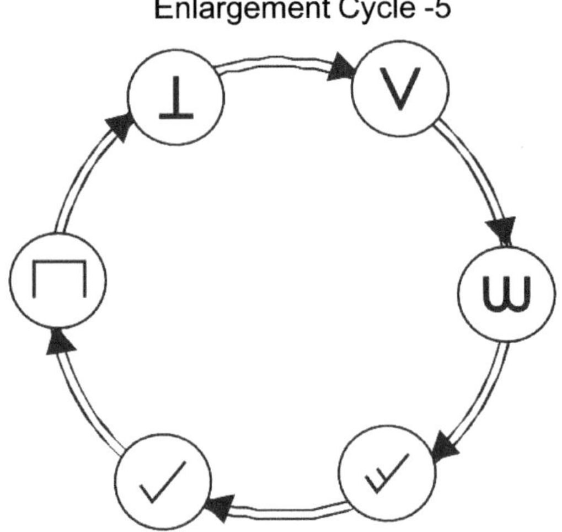

Atrophy Cycle -2

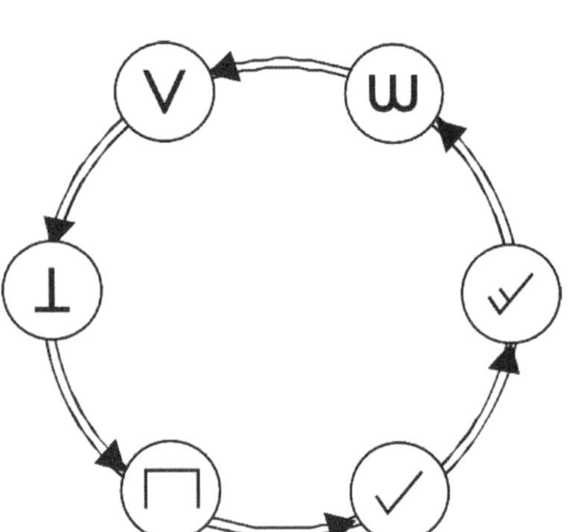

Atrophy Cycle -3

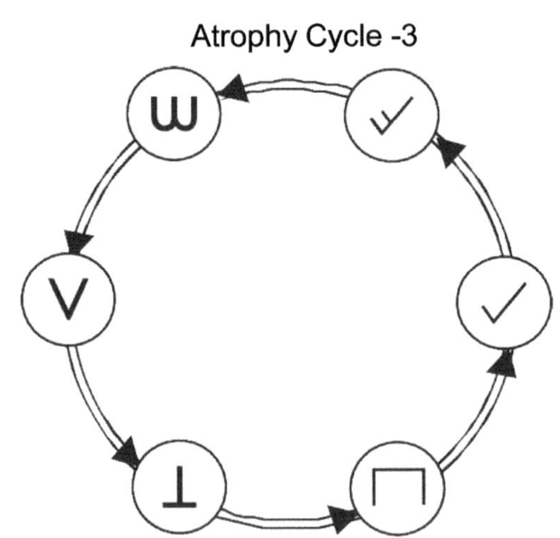

YANG (+) YIN (-)

Atrophy Cycle -4

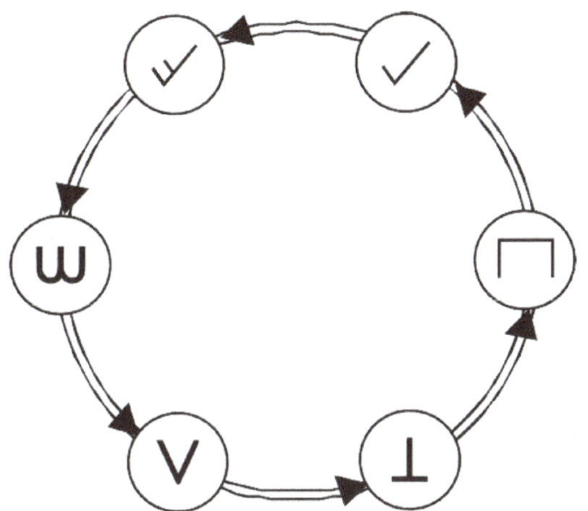

Atrophy Cycle -5

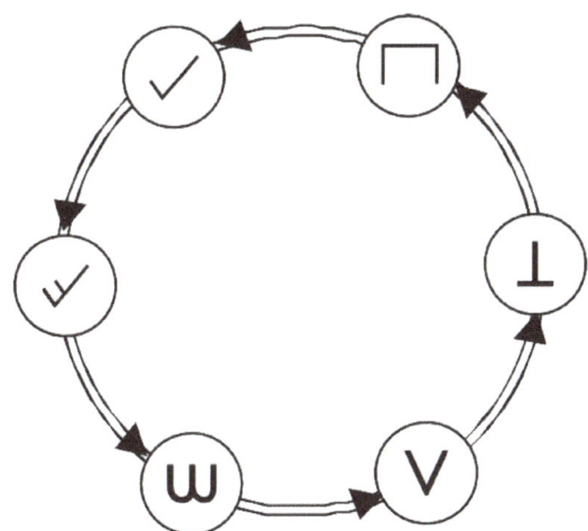

Control Cycle

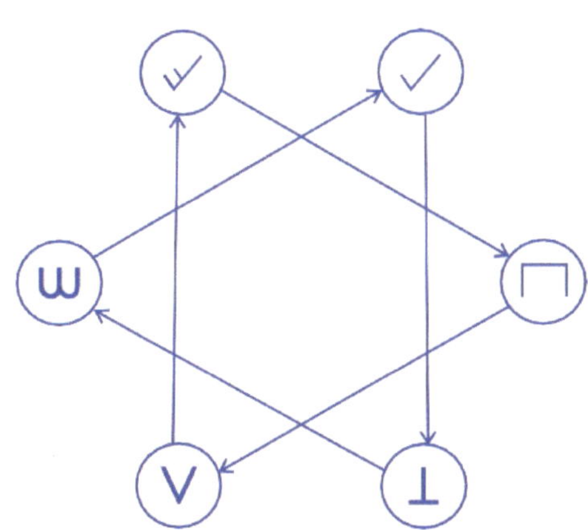

Suck Cycle

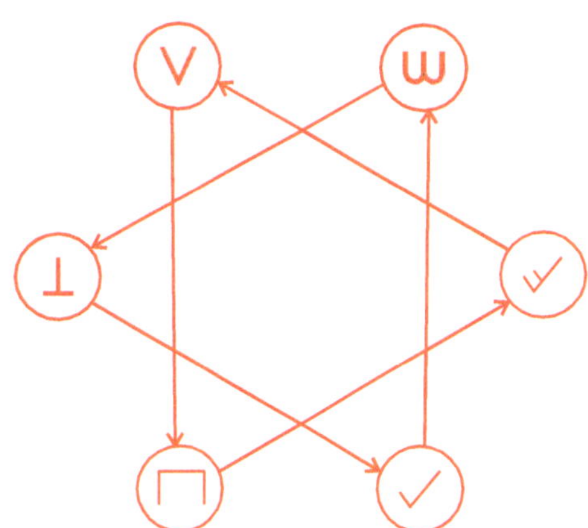

Balance Cycle

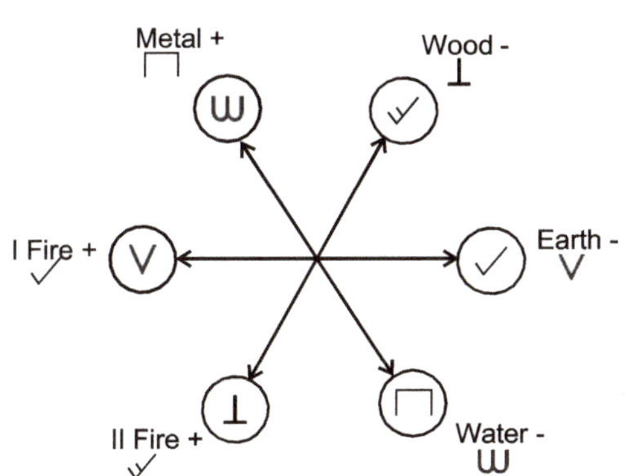

Husband & Wife Cycle

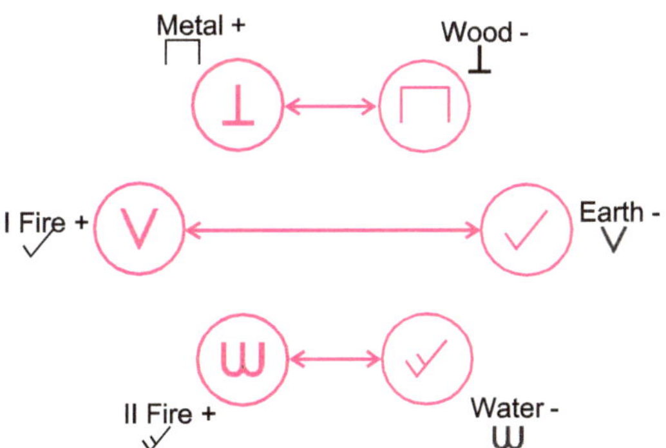

RIGHT FEMALE AND LEFT MALE - ELEMENTS ENERGY CYCLING

YIN (+)	YANG (-)
FEMALE (+)	MALE (-)

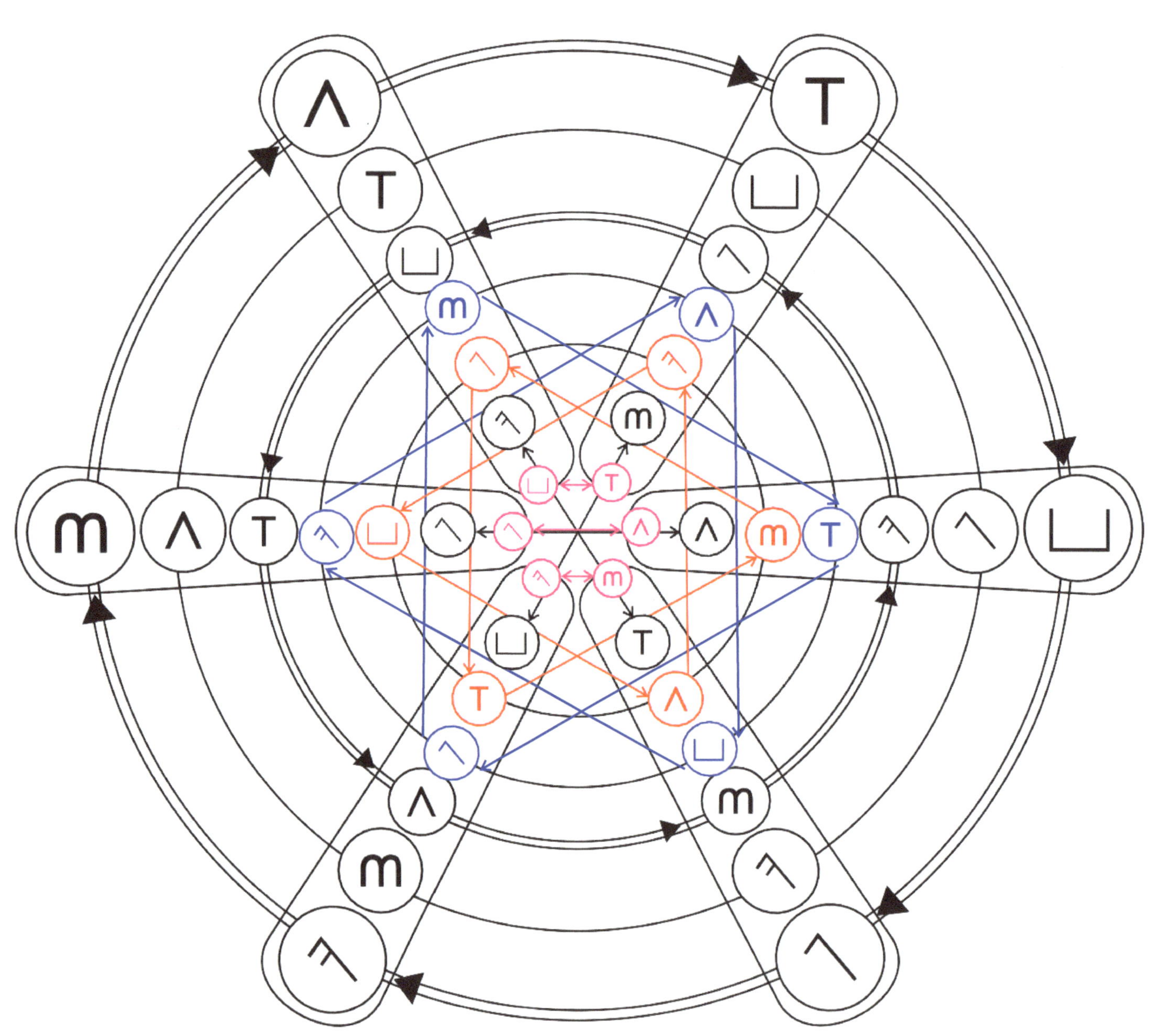

FEMALE (+) MALE (-)

Self Cycle
Wood +
Metal -
I Fire -
Earth +
Water +
II Fire -

Enlargement Cycle -1
Wood +
Metal -
I Fire -
Earth +
Water +
II Fire -

Atrophy Cycle -1
Wood +
Metal -
I Fire -
Earth +
Water +
II Fire -

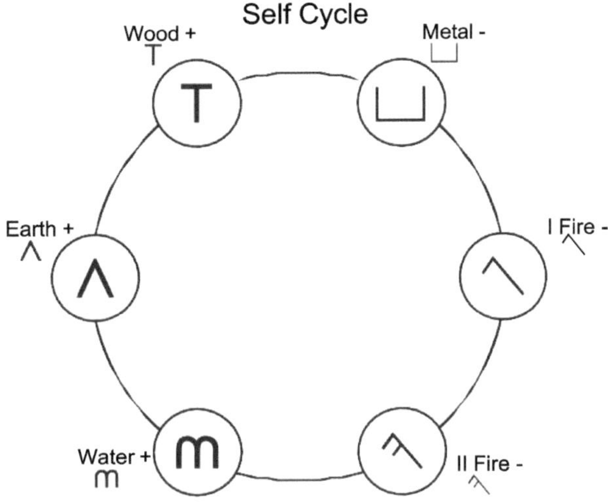

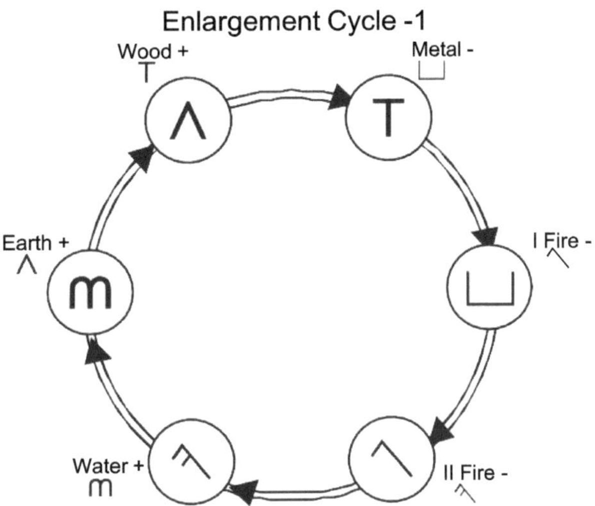

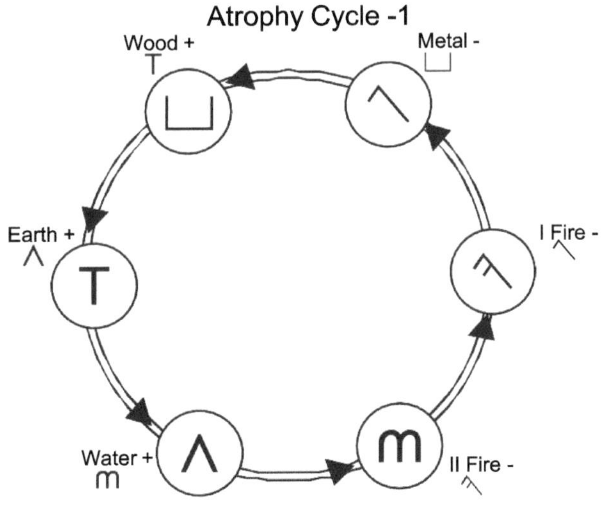

FEMALE (+) MALE (-)

Enlargement Cycle -2

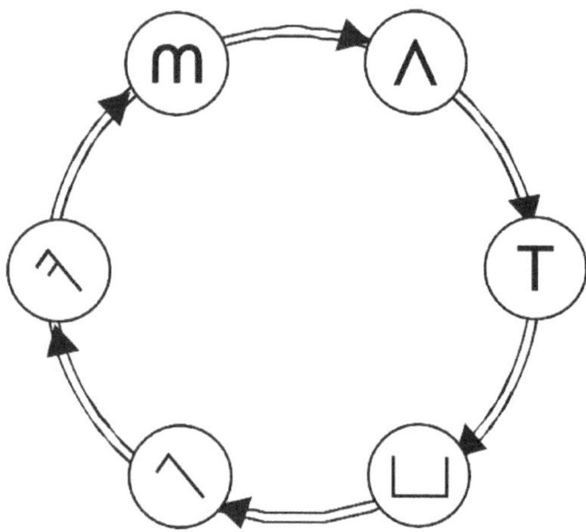

Enlargement Cycle -3

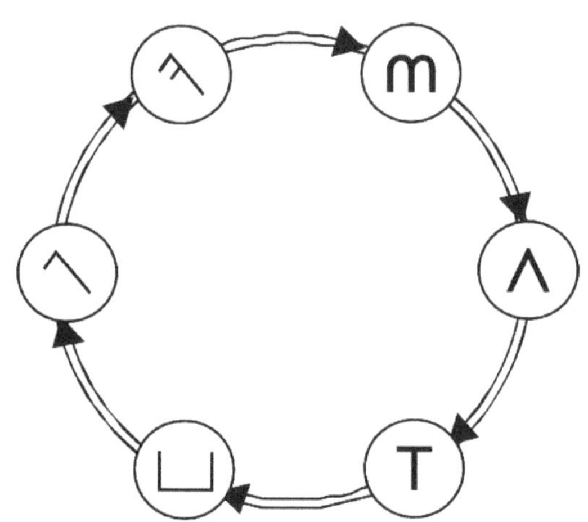

Enlargement Cycle -4

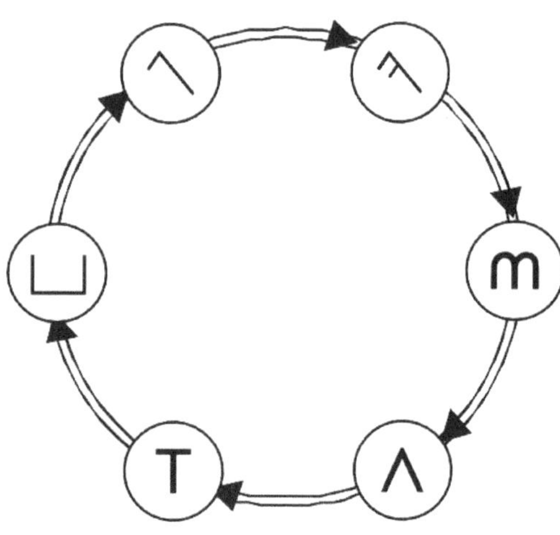

Enlargement Cycle -5

Atrophy Cycle -2

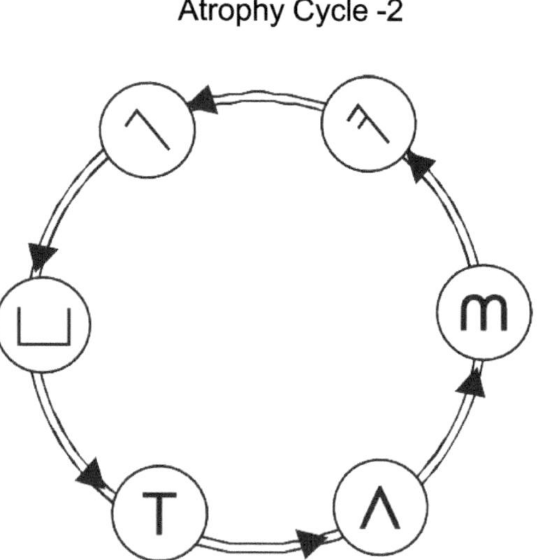

Atrophy Cycle -3

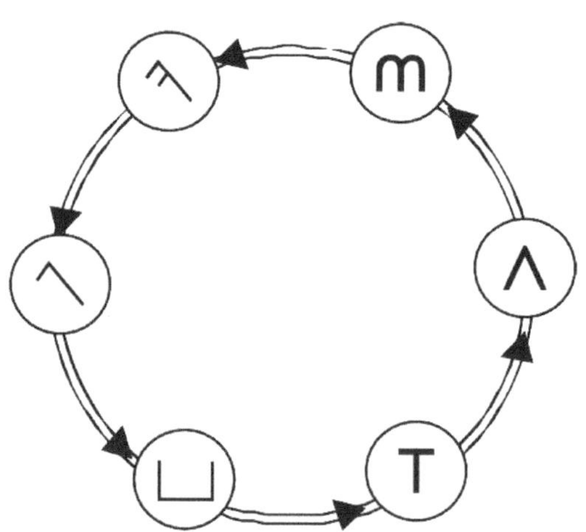

FEMALE (+) MALE (-)

Atrophy Cycle -4

Atrophy Cycle -5

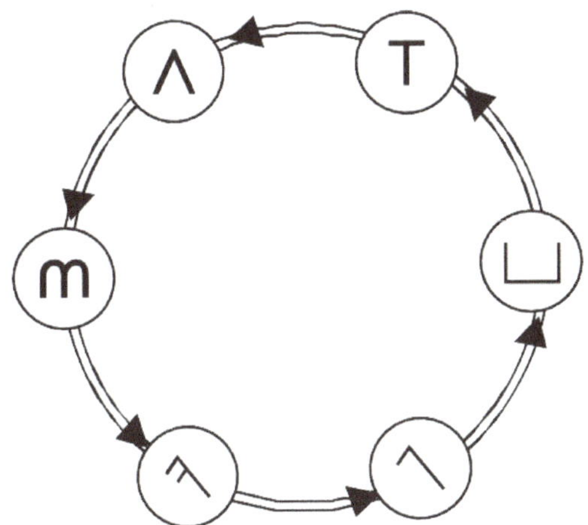

Control Cycle

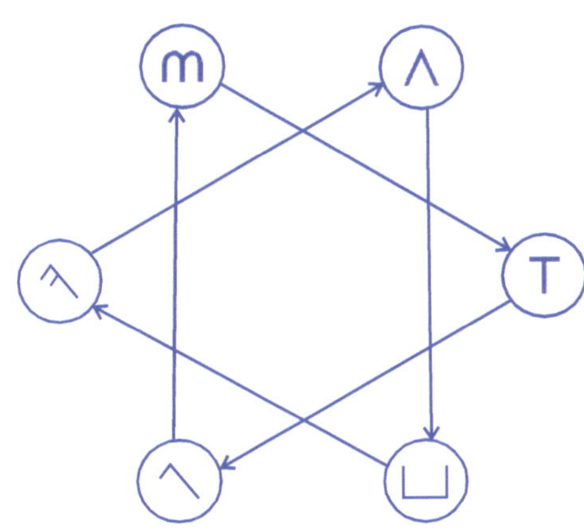

Suck Cycle

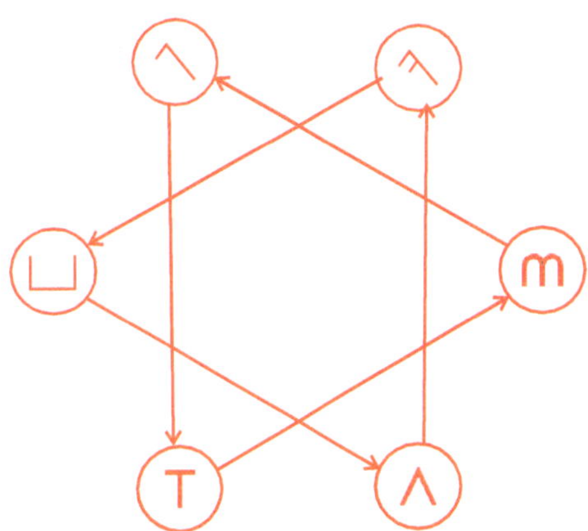

Balance Cycle

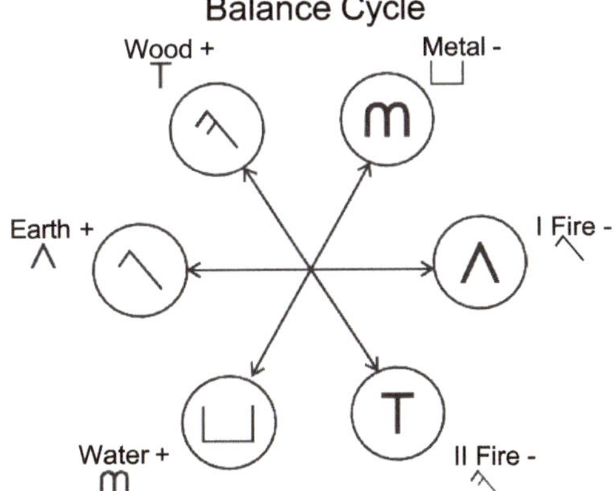

Husband & Wife Cycle

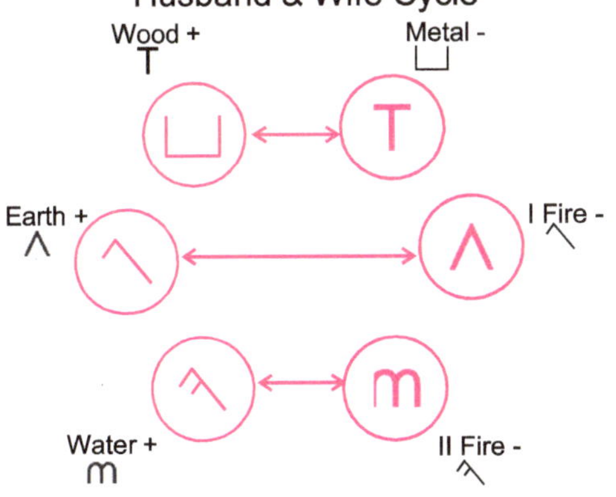

MALE (+) AND MALE (-)

YANG (+)	YANG (-)
MALE(+)	MALE (-)

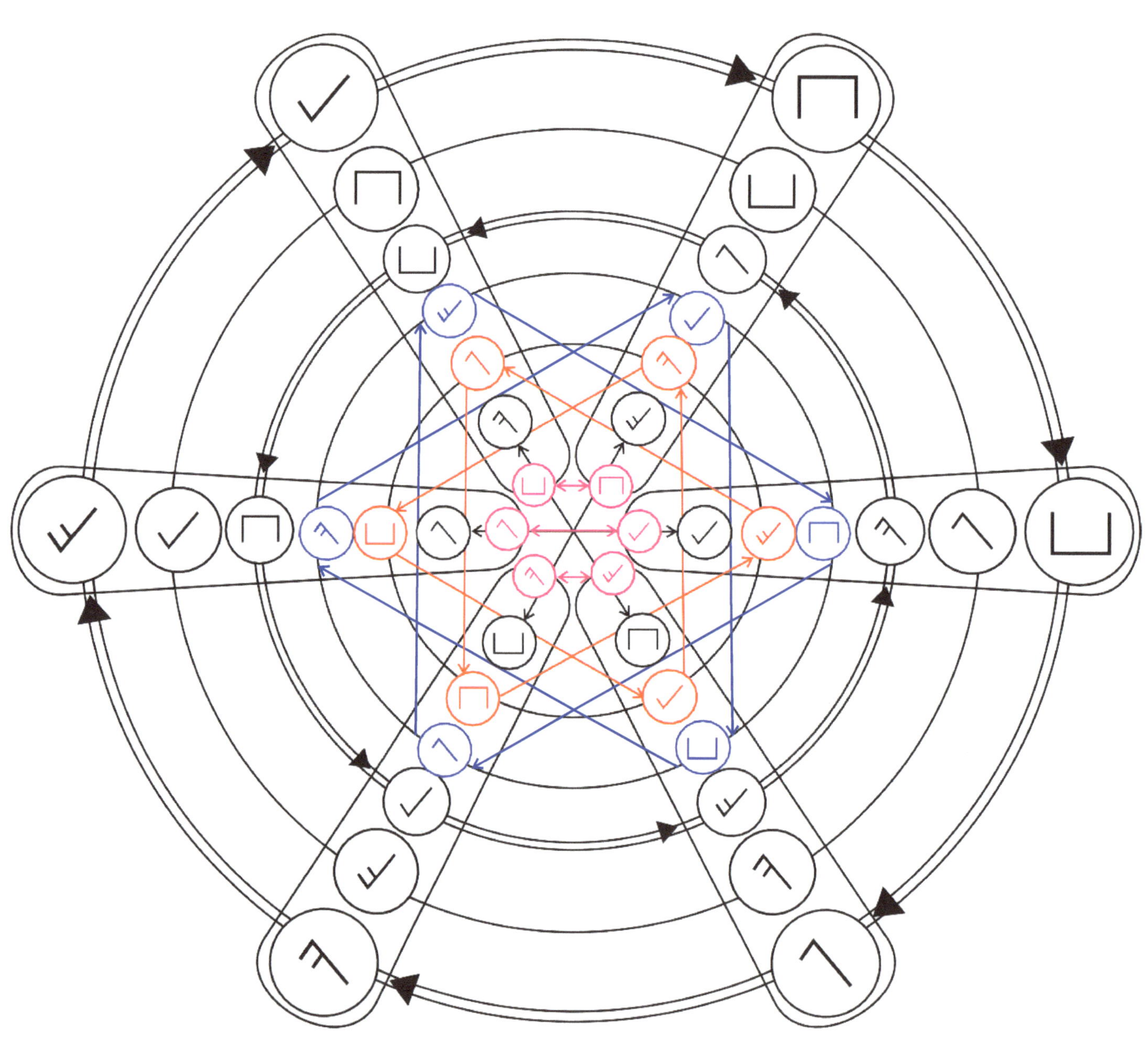

YANG(+) YANG (-)

Self Cycle
Metal +
Metal -
I Fire +
I Fire -
II Fire +
II Fire -

Enlargement Cycle -1
Metal +
Metal -
I Fire +
I Fire -
II Fire +
II Fire -

Atrophy Cycle -1
Metal +
Metal -
I Fire +
I Fire -
II Fire +
II Fire -

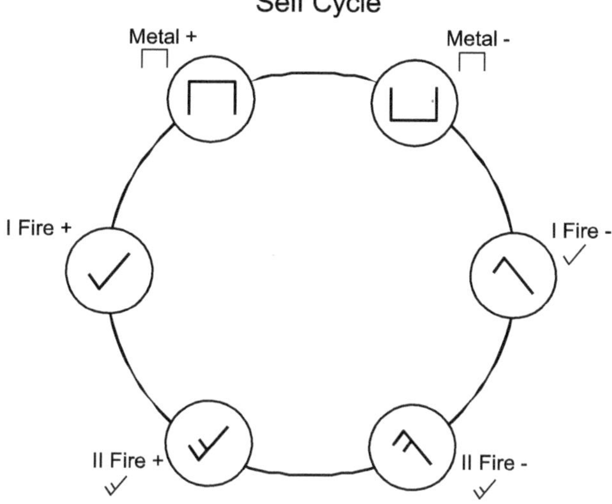

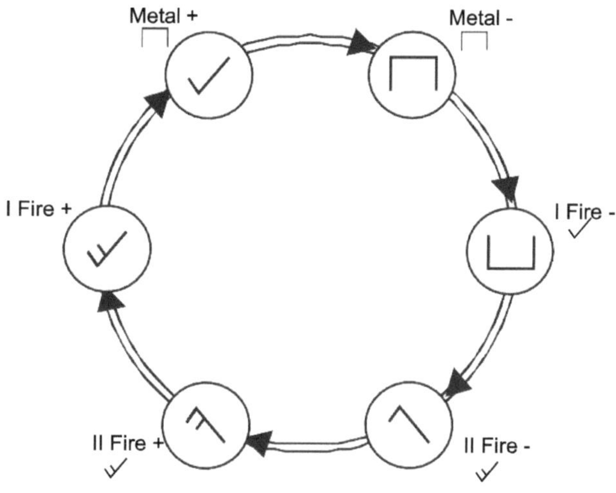

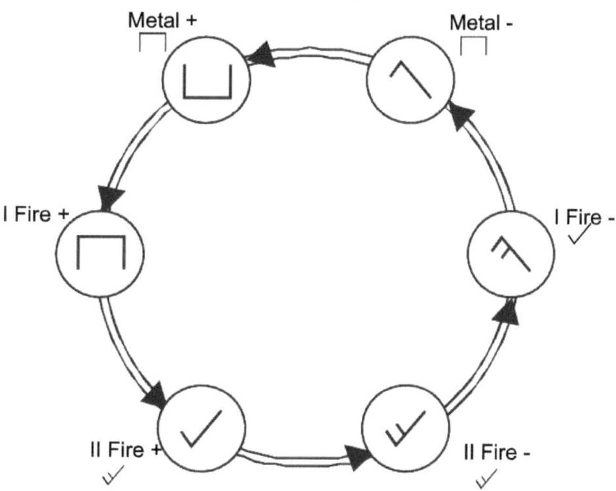

YANG(+) YANG (-)

Enlargement Cycle -2

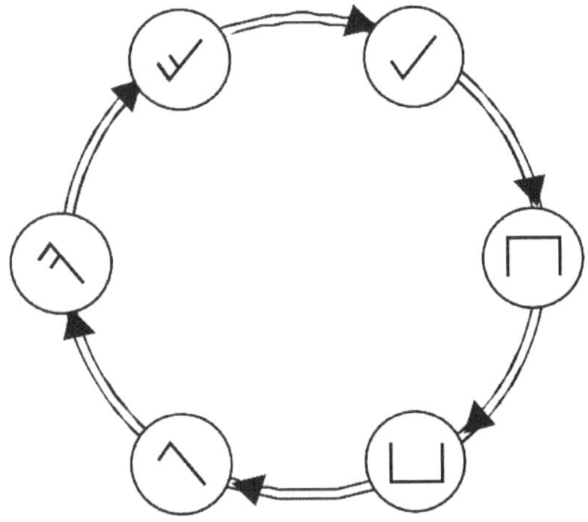

Enlargement Cycle -3

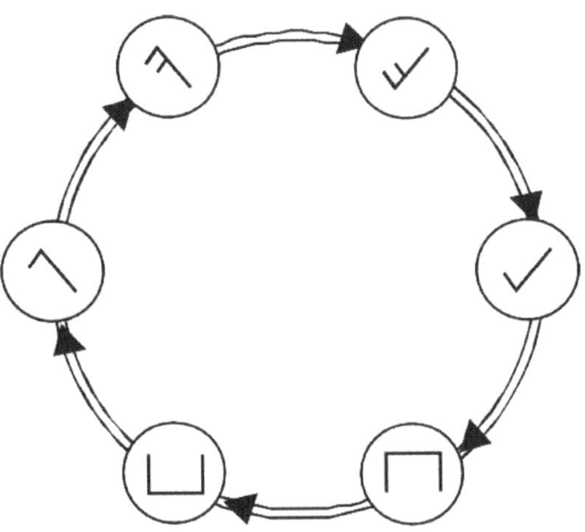

Enlargement Cycle -4

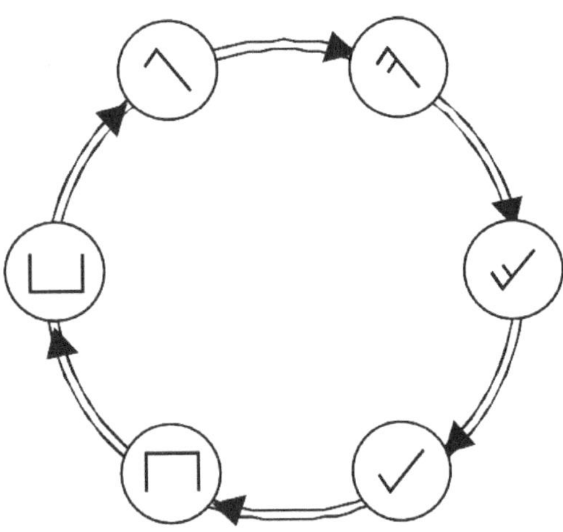

Enlargement Cycle -5

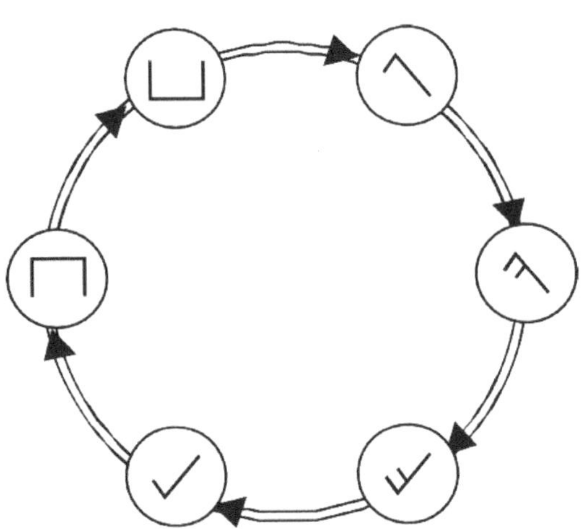

Atrophy Cycle -2

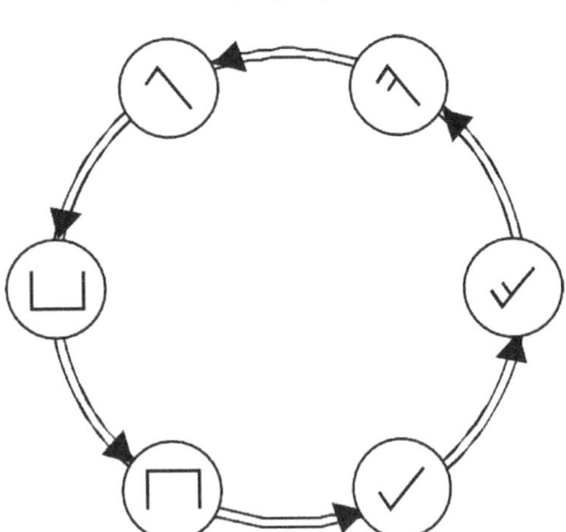

Atrophy Cycle -3

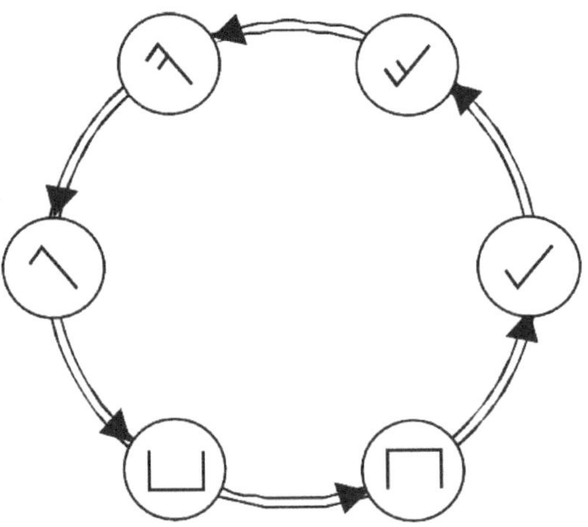

YANG(+) YANG (-)

Atrophy Cycle -4

Atrophy Cycle -5

Control Cycle

Suck Cycle

Balance Cycle
Metal +
Metal -
I Fire +
I Fire -
II Fire +
II Fire -

Husband & Wife Cycle
Metal +
Metal -
I Fire +
I Fire -
II Fire +
II Fire -

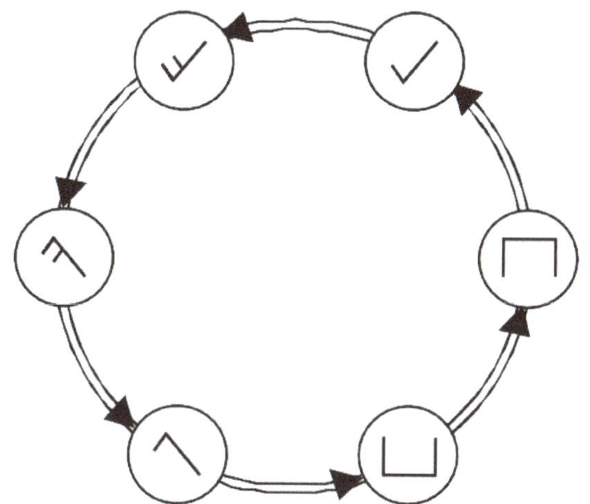

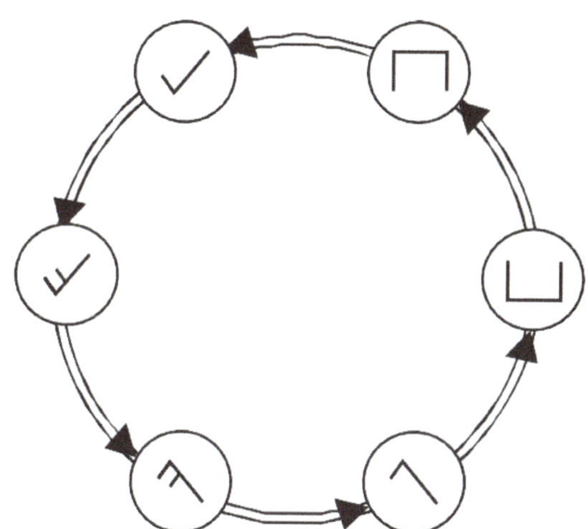

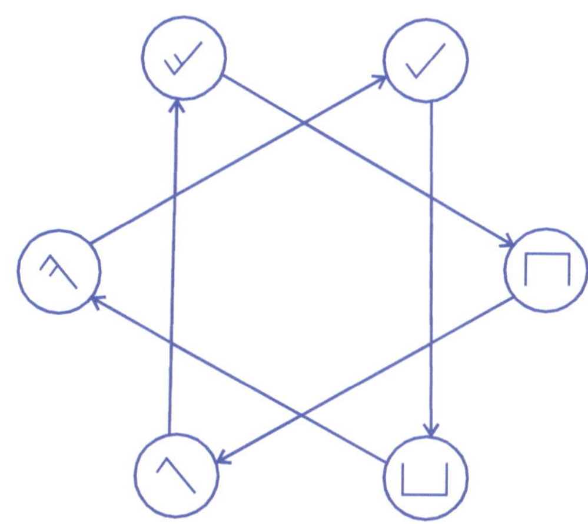

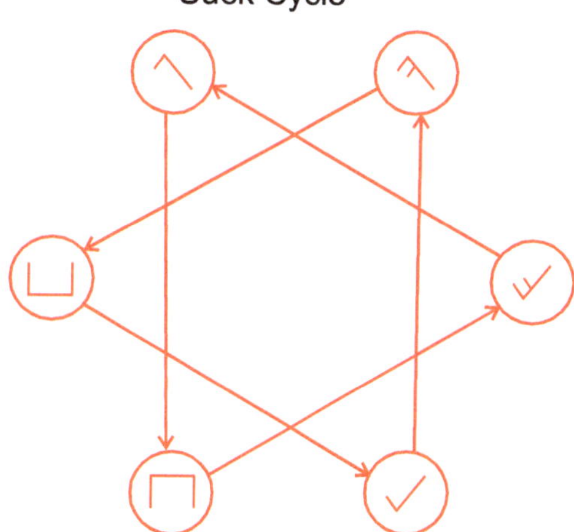

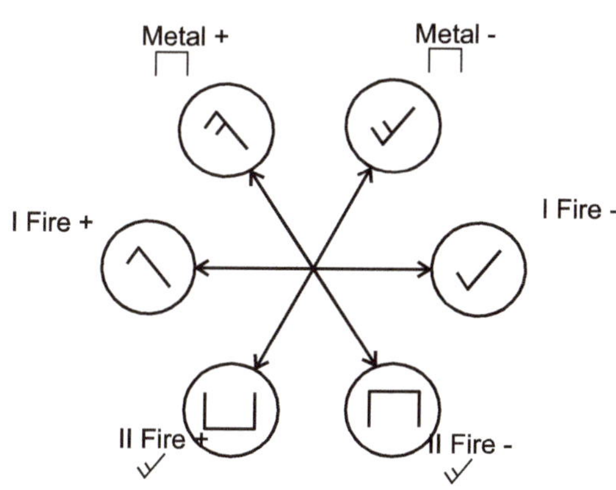

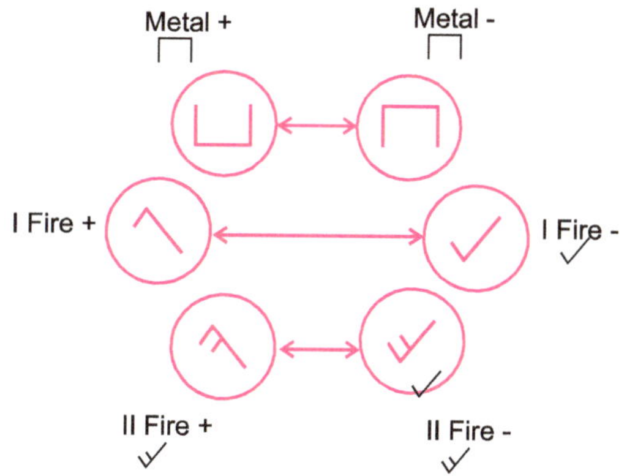

FEMALE (+) AND FEMALE (-)

YIN (+) FEMALE (+)

YIN (-) FEMALE(-)

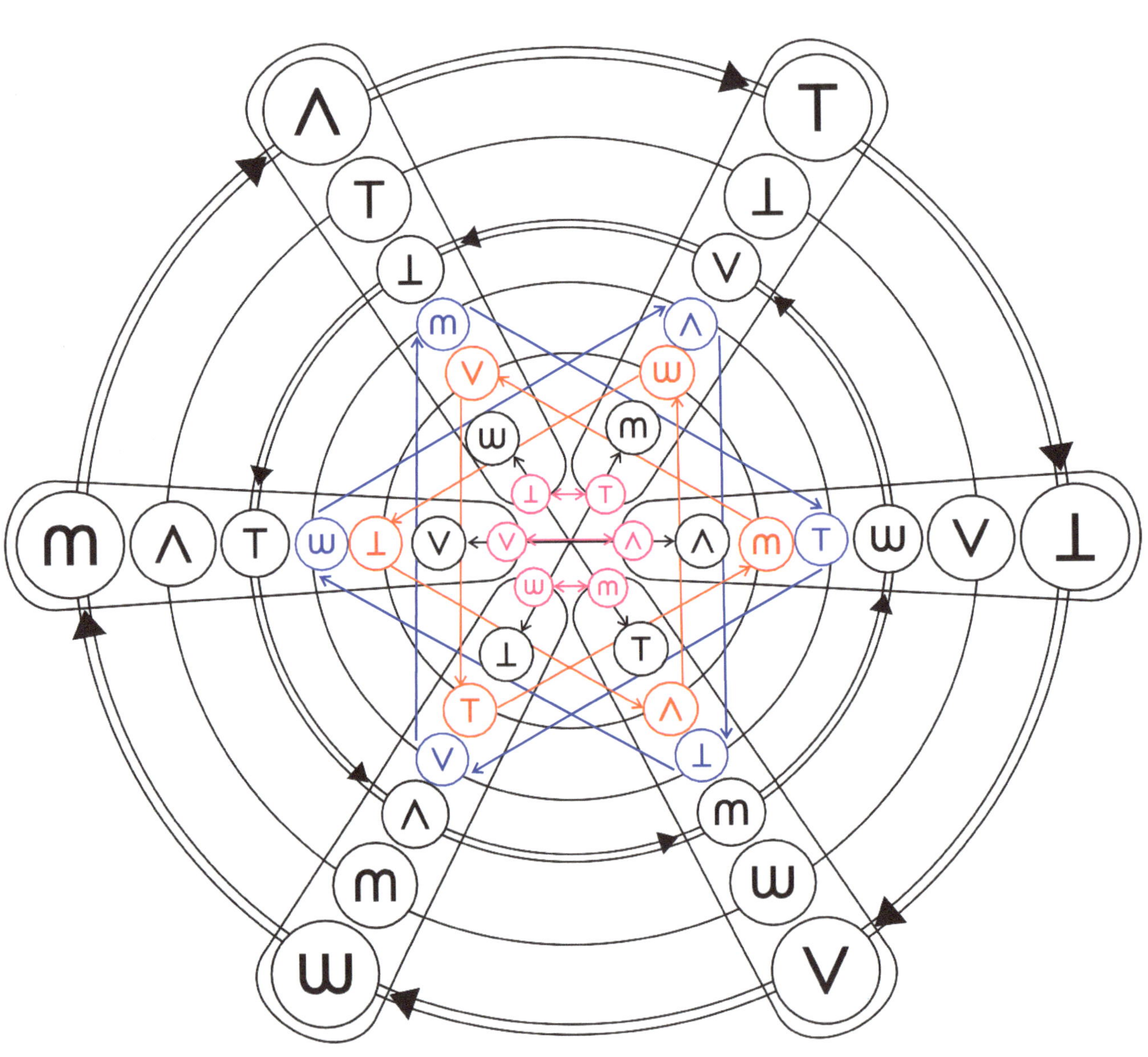

YIN (+) YIN (-)

Self Cycle
Wood +
T
Wood -
⊥
T
⊥
Earth +
Λ
Λ
Earth -
V
V
Water +
m
m
ω
Water -
ω

Enlargement Cycle -1
Wood +
T
Wood -
⊥
Λ
T
Earth +
Λ
m
Earth -
V
⊥
Water +
m
ω
V
Water -
ω

Atrophy Cycle -1
Wood +
T
Wood -
⊥
⊥
V
Earth +
Λ
T
Earth -
V
ω
Water +
m
Λ
m
Water -
ω

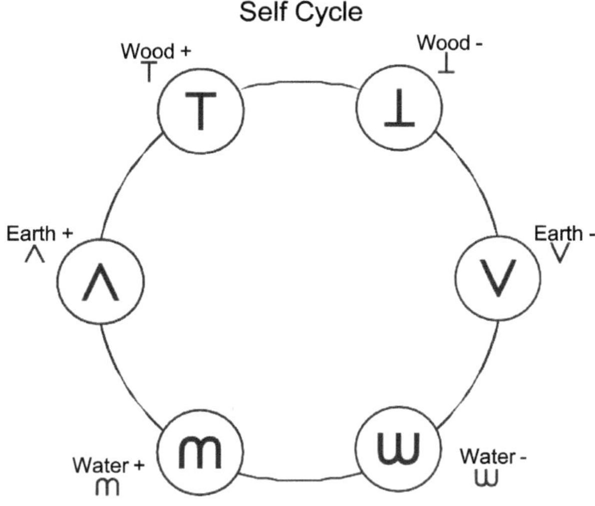

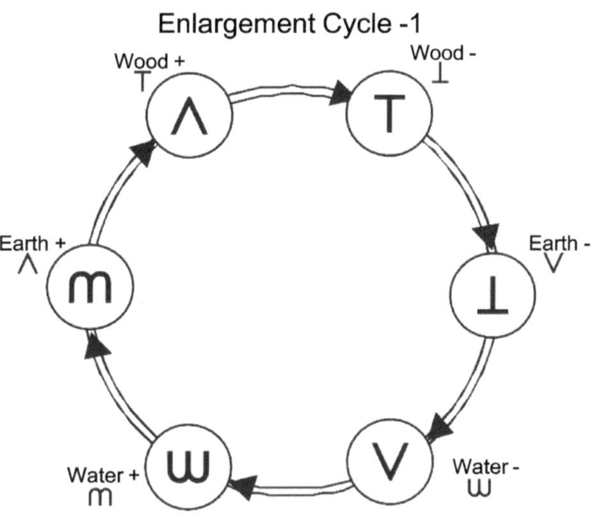

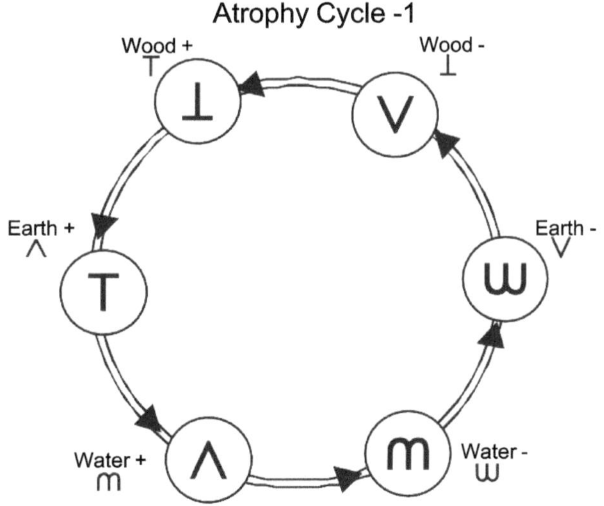

YIN (+) YIN (-)

Enlargement Cycle -2

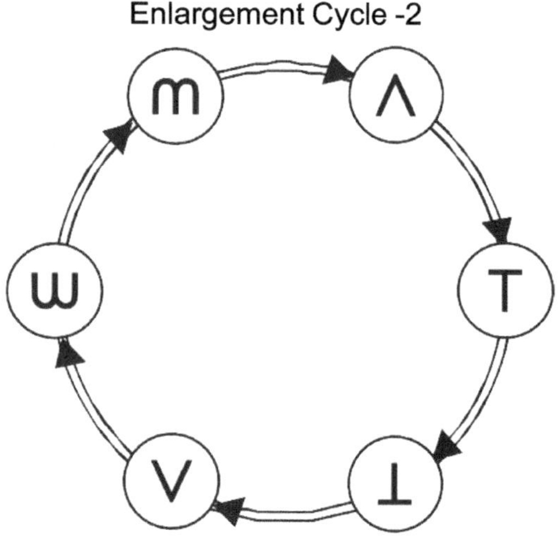

Enlargement Cycle -3

Enlargement Cycle -4

Enlargement Cycle -5

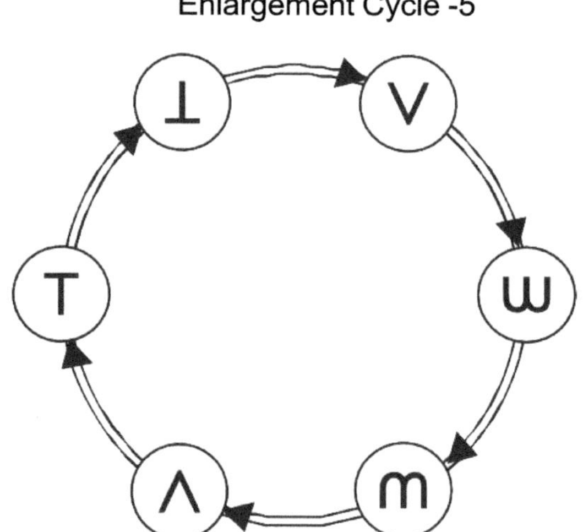

Atrophy Cycle -2

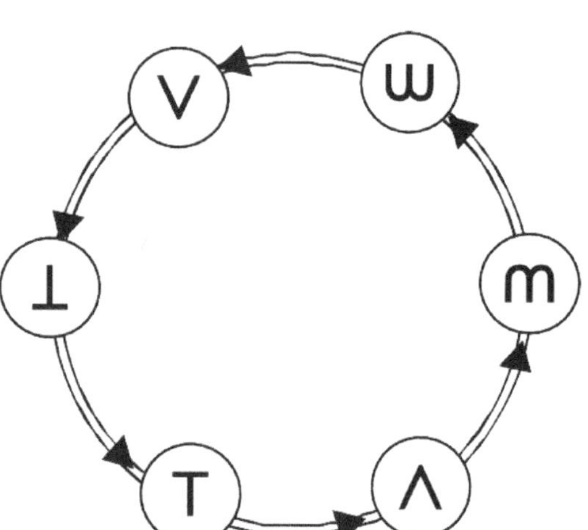

Atrophy Cycle -3

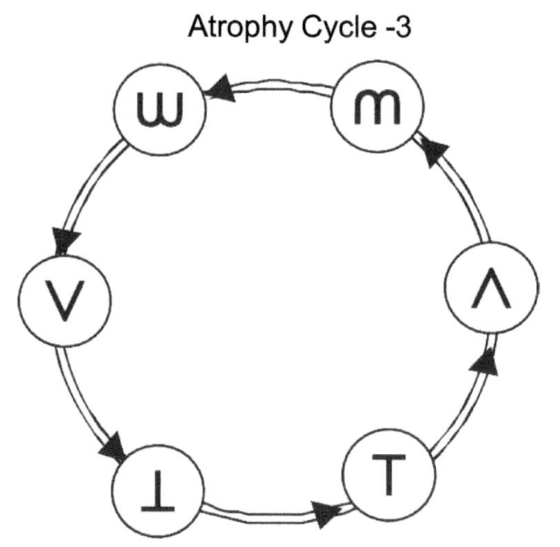

YIN (+) YIN (-)

Atrophy Cycle -4

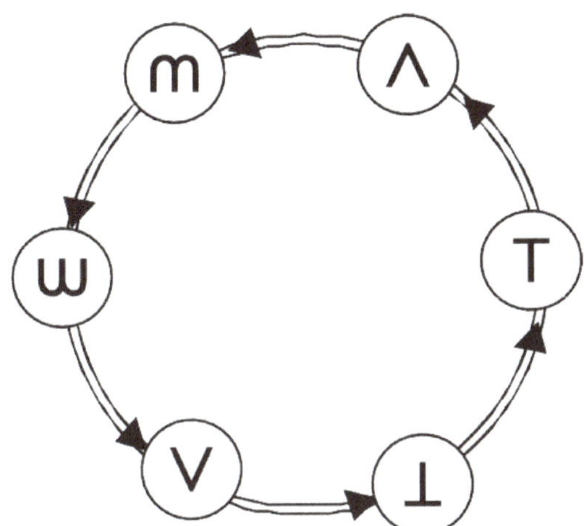

Atrophy Cycle -5

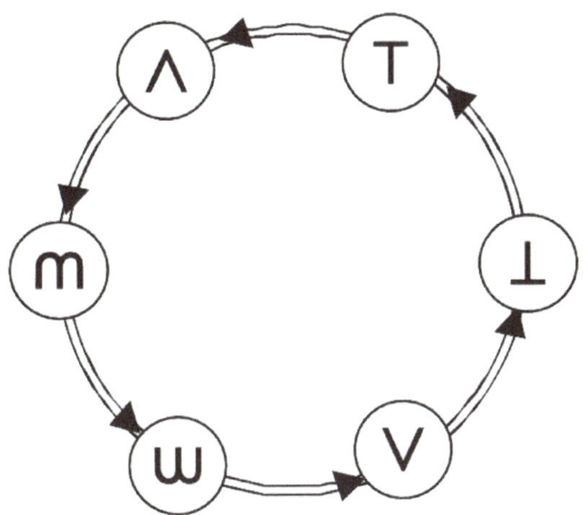

Control Cycle

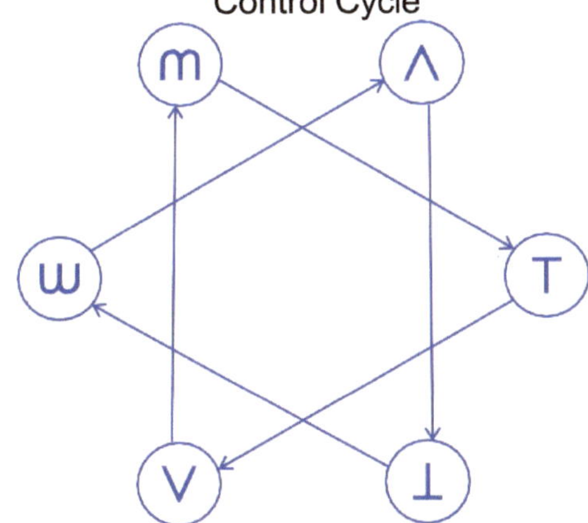

Suck Cycle

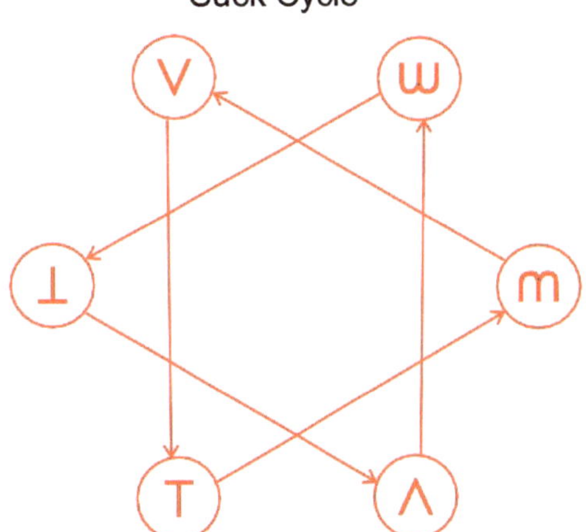

Balance Cycle

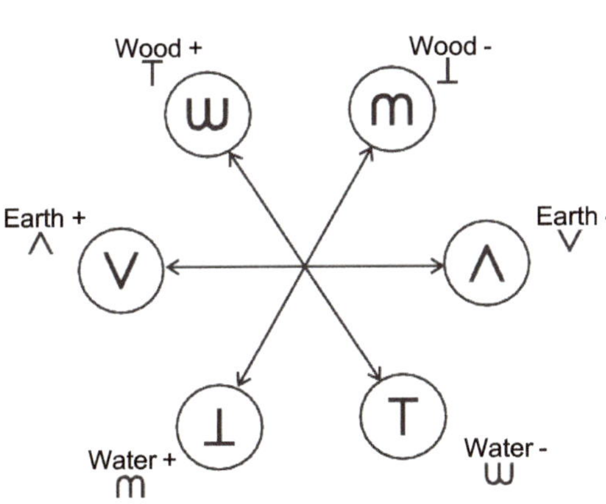

Husband & Wife Cycle

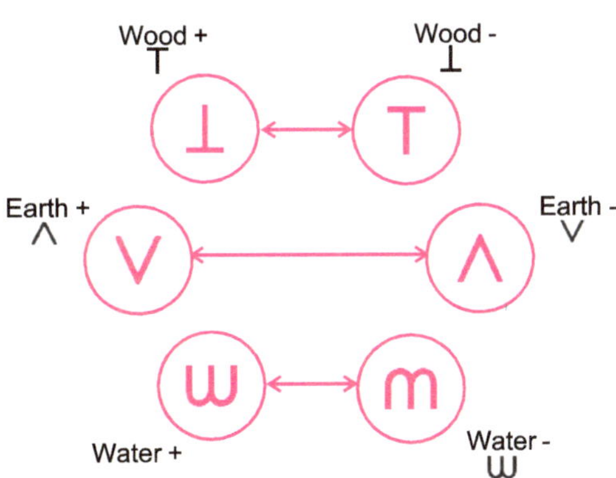

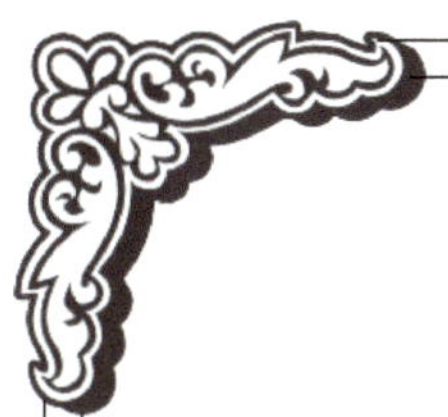
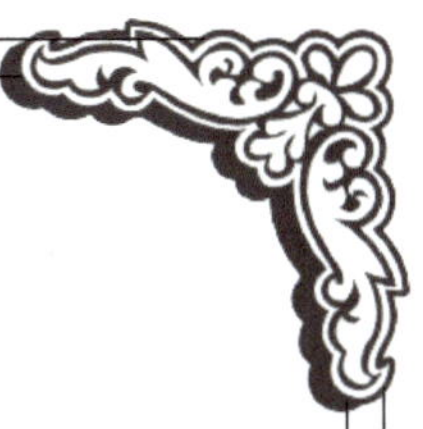

Part Ten

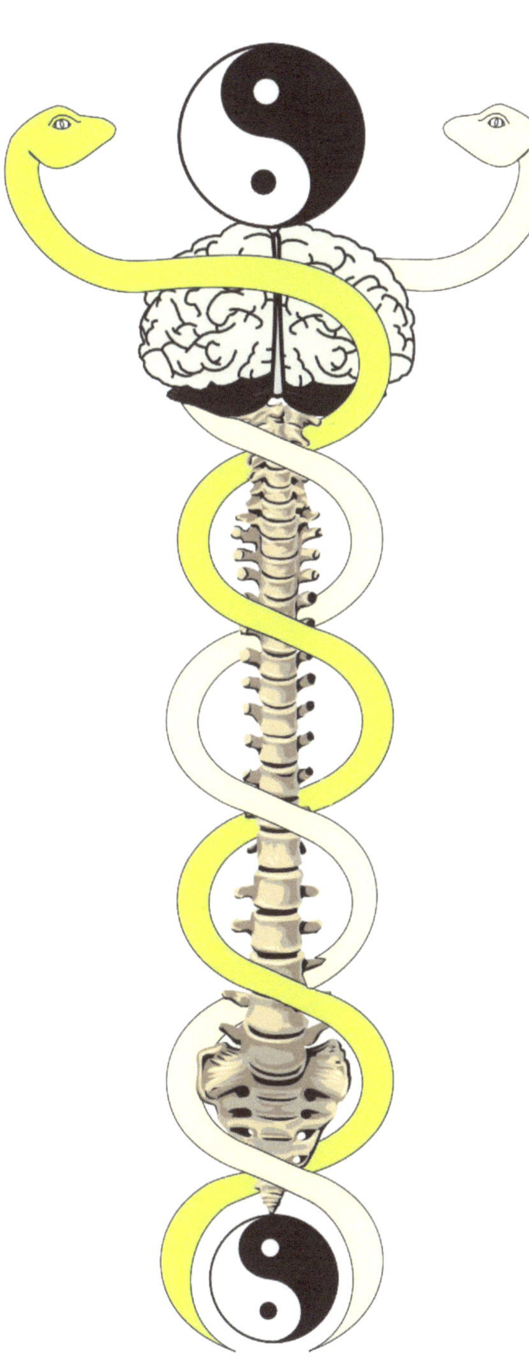

EXPANSION OF SIX ELEMENTS ENERGY CYCLING

GROWTH-GROWTH&SURVIVAL-SURVIVAL

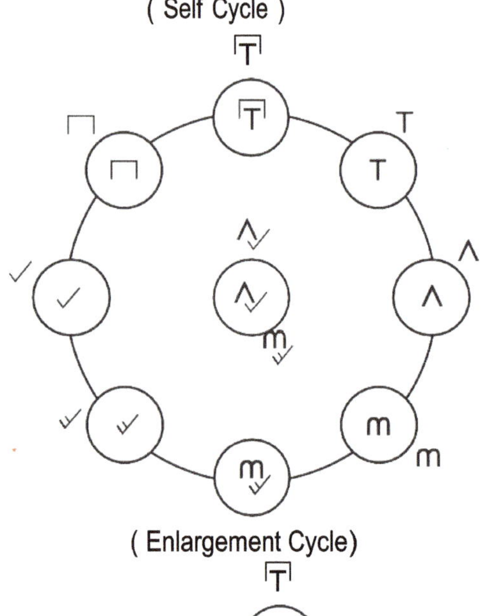

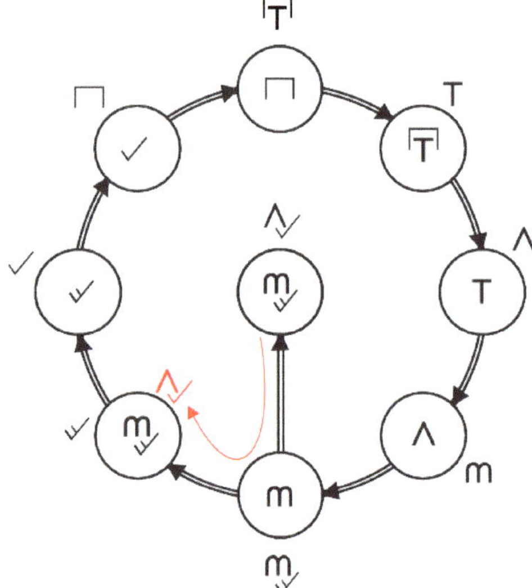

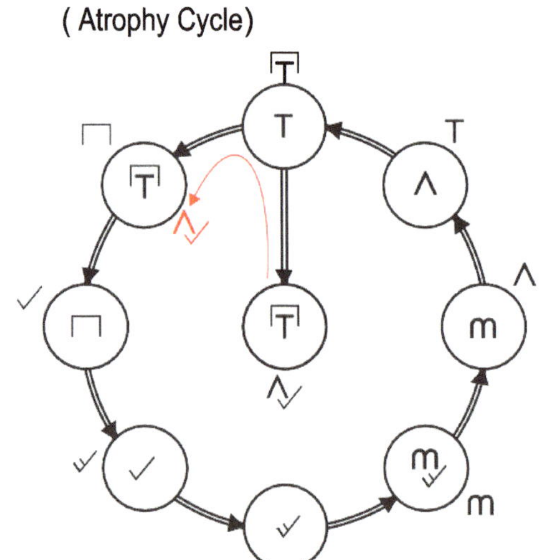

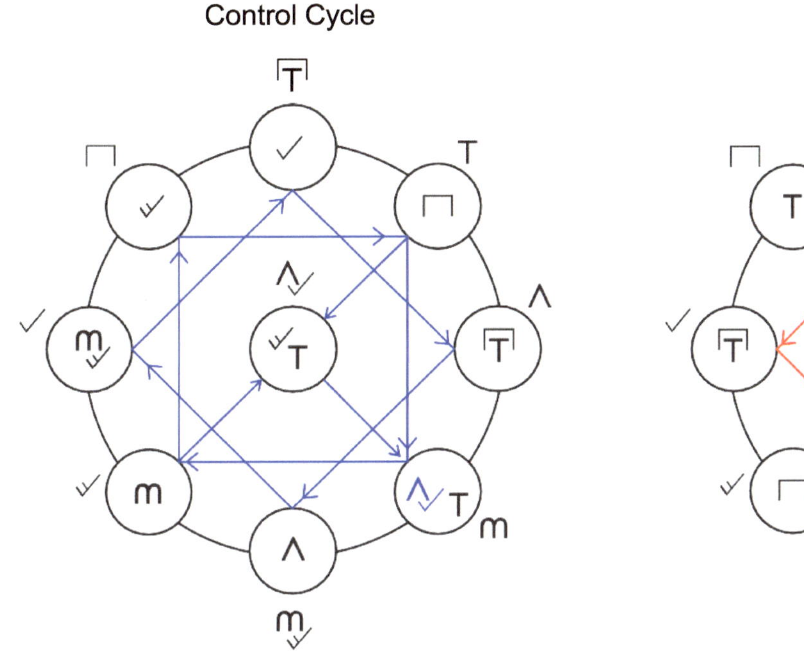
Control Cycle

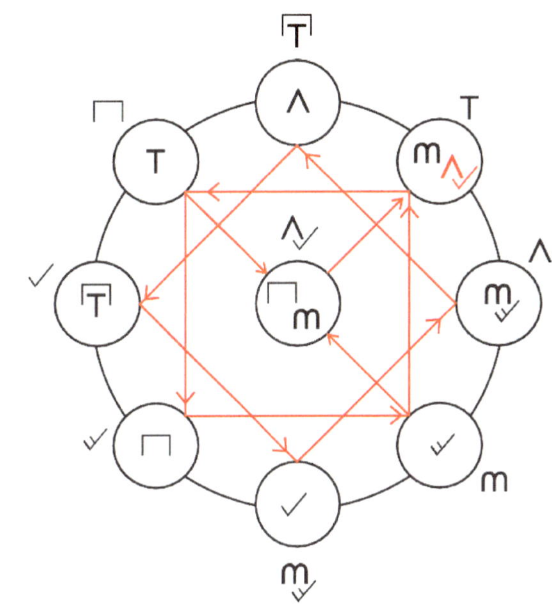
Suck Cycle

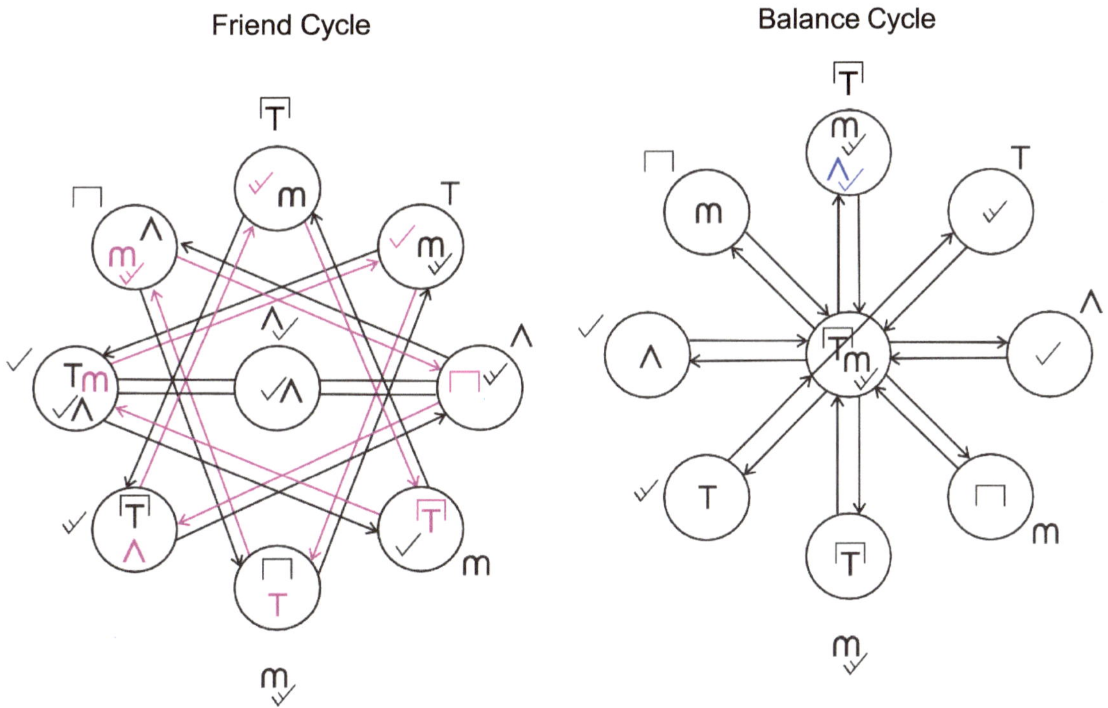
Friend Cycle
Balance Cycle

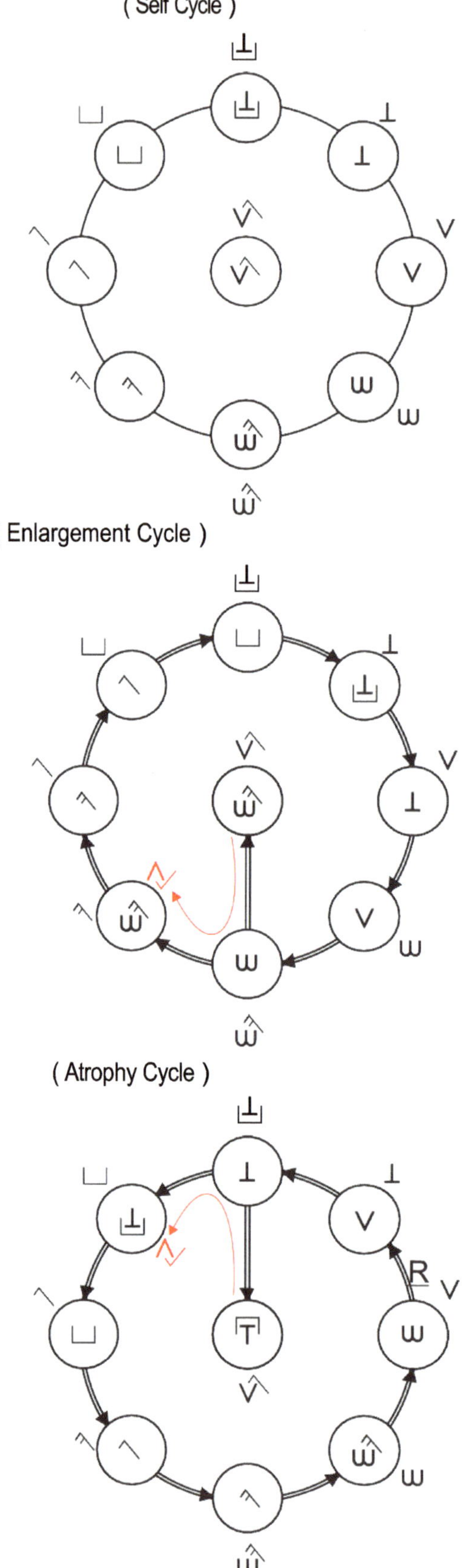
(Self Cycle)
(Enlargement Cycle)
(Atrophy Cycle)
R

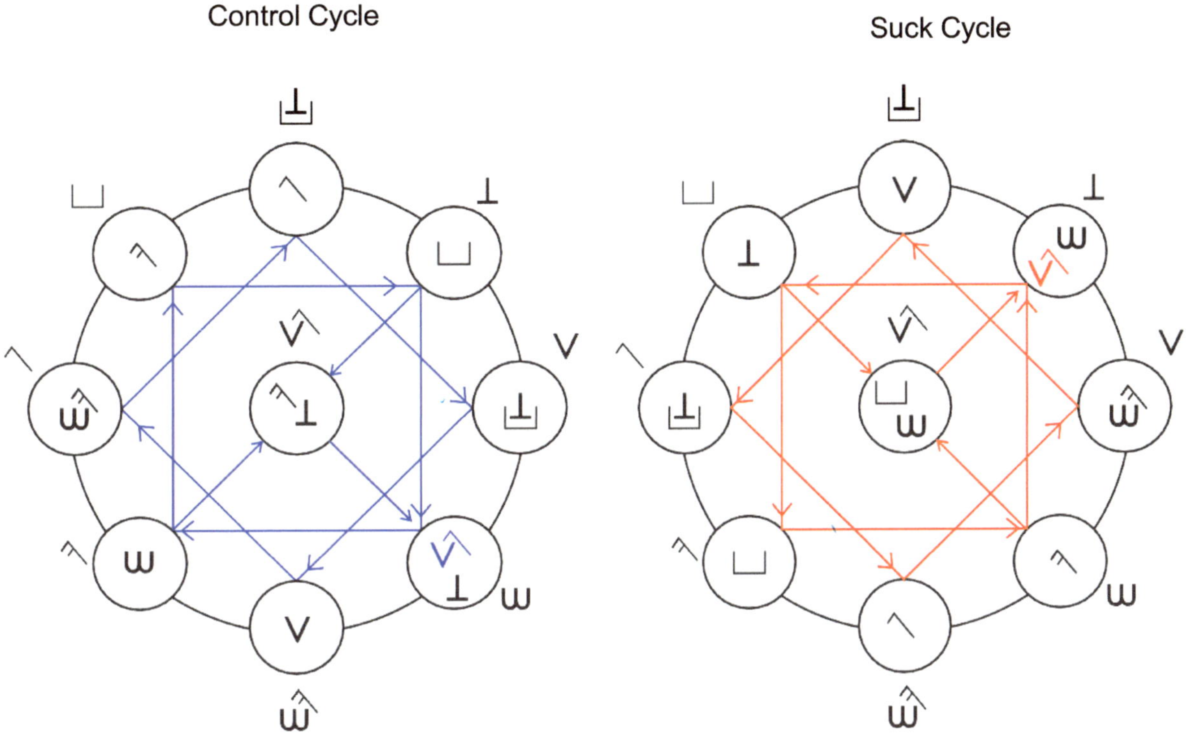
Control Cycle
Suck Cycle

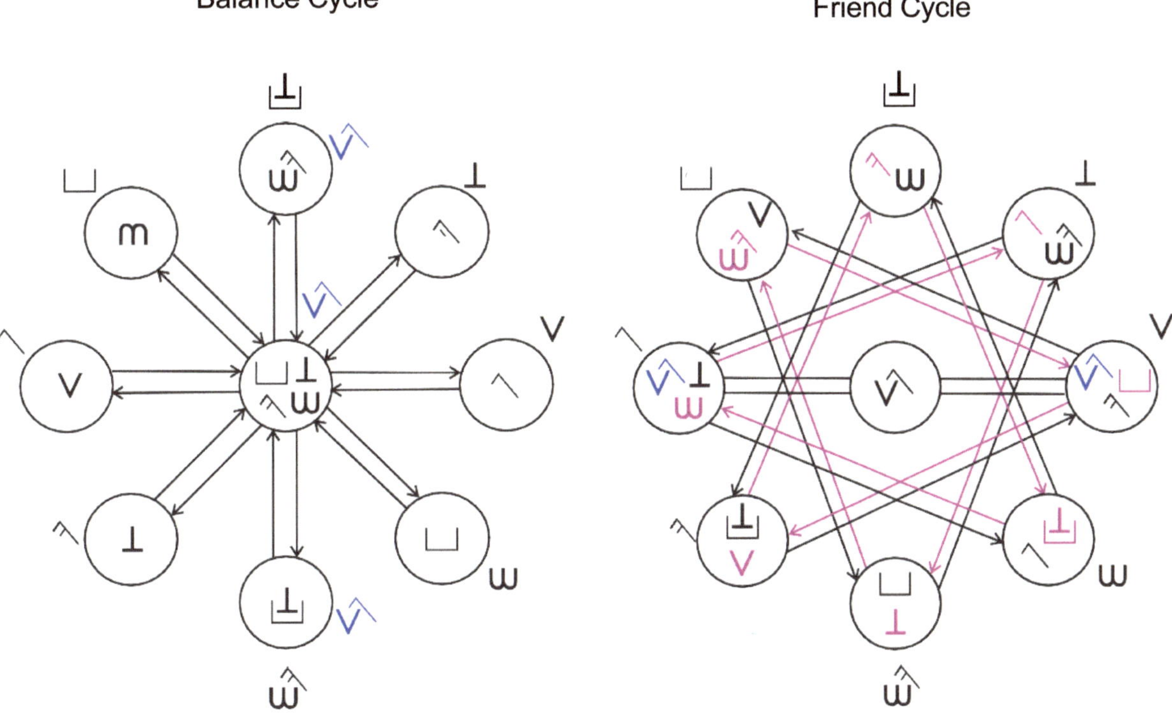
Balance Cycle
Friend Cycle

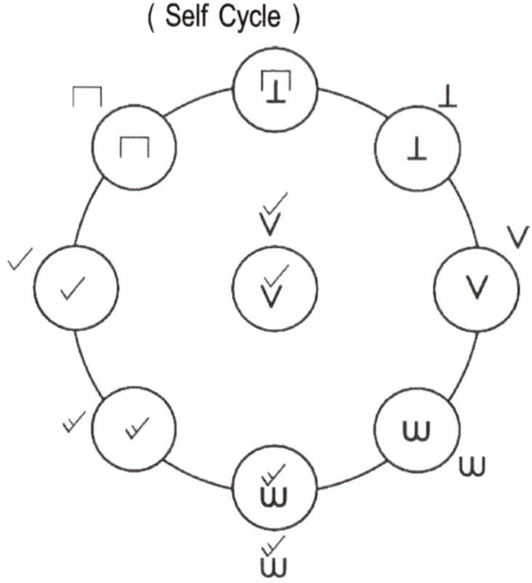
(Self Cycle)

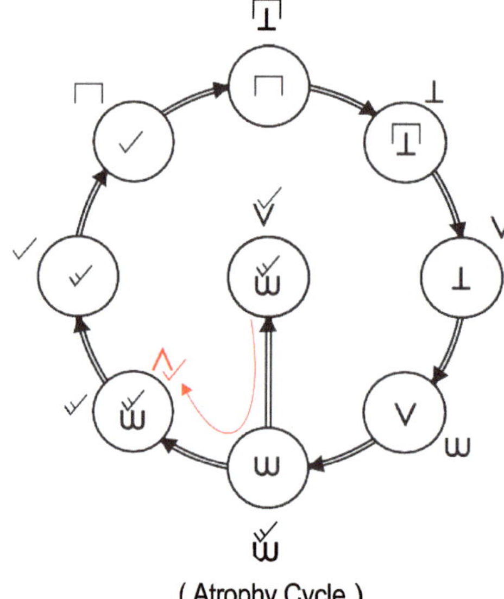
(Enlargement cycle)

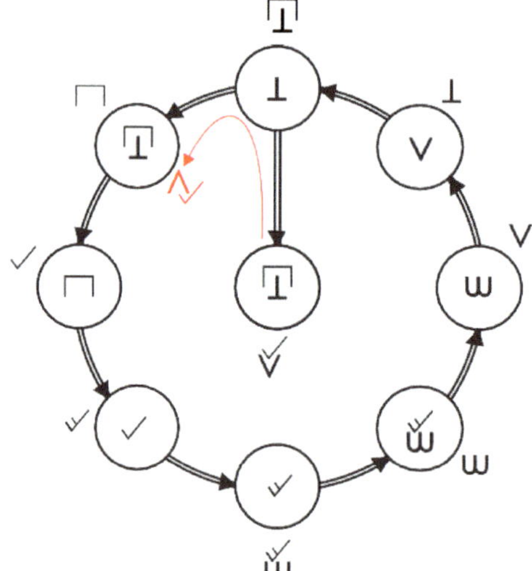
(Atrophy Cycle)

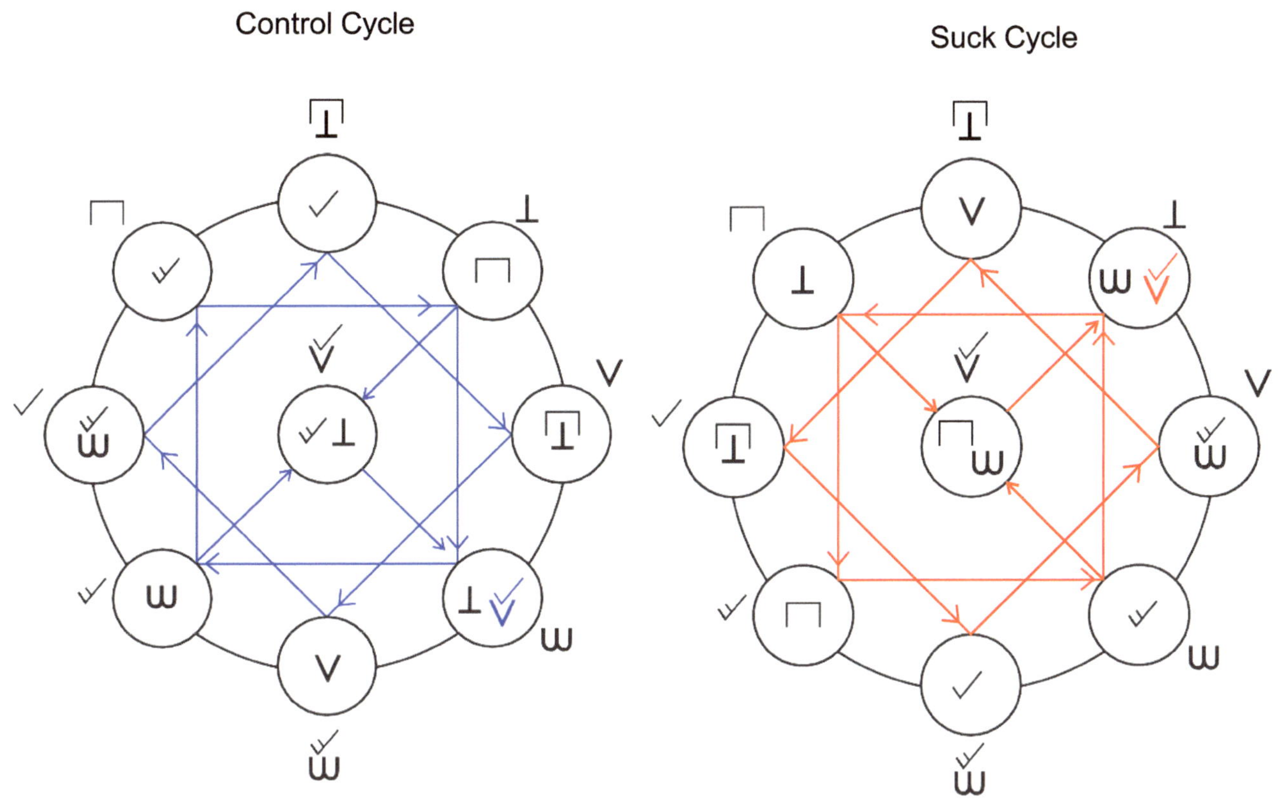

Balance Cycle

Friend Cycle

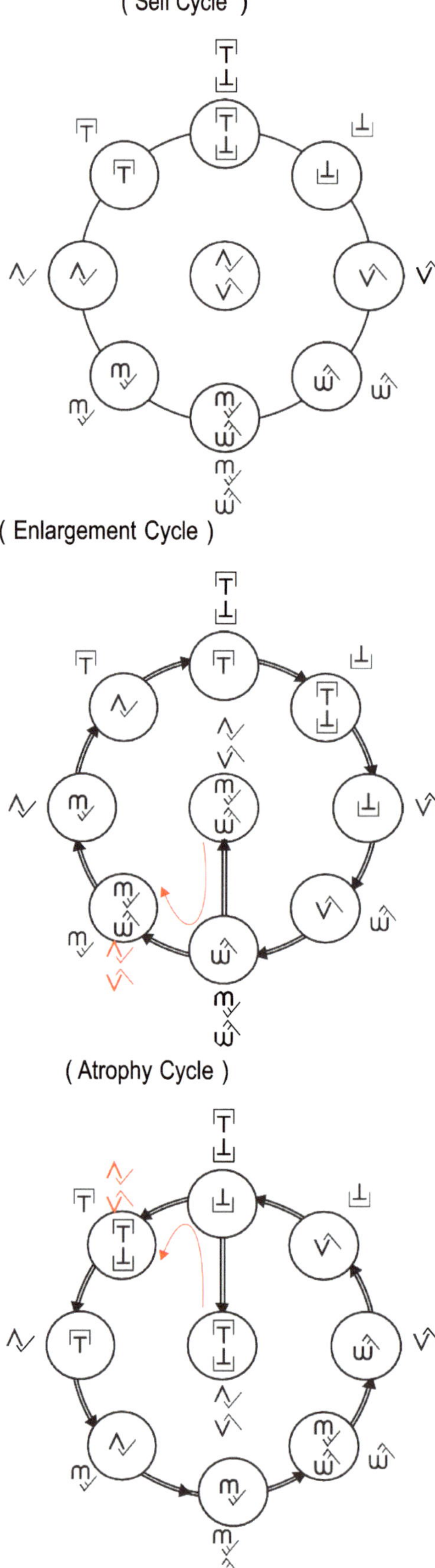
(Self Cycle)
(Enlargement Cycle)
(Atrophy Cycle)

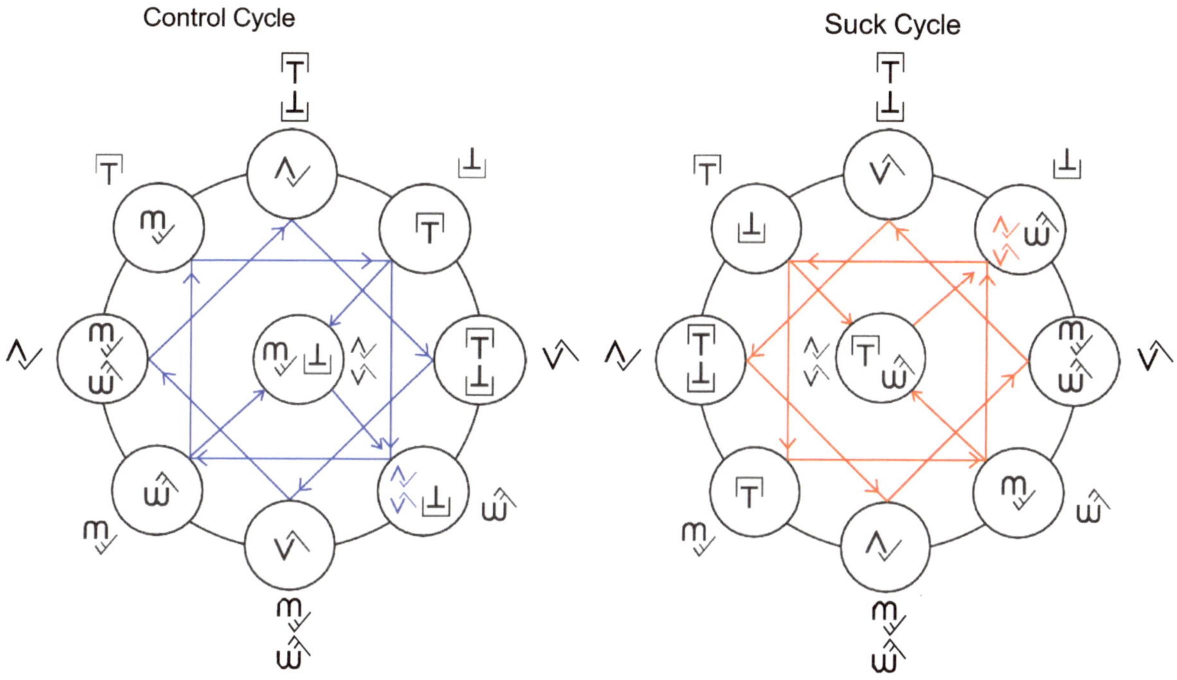
Control Cycle
Suck Cycle

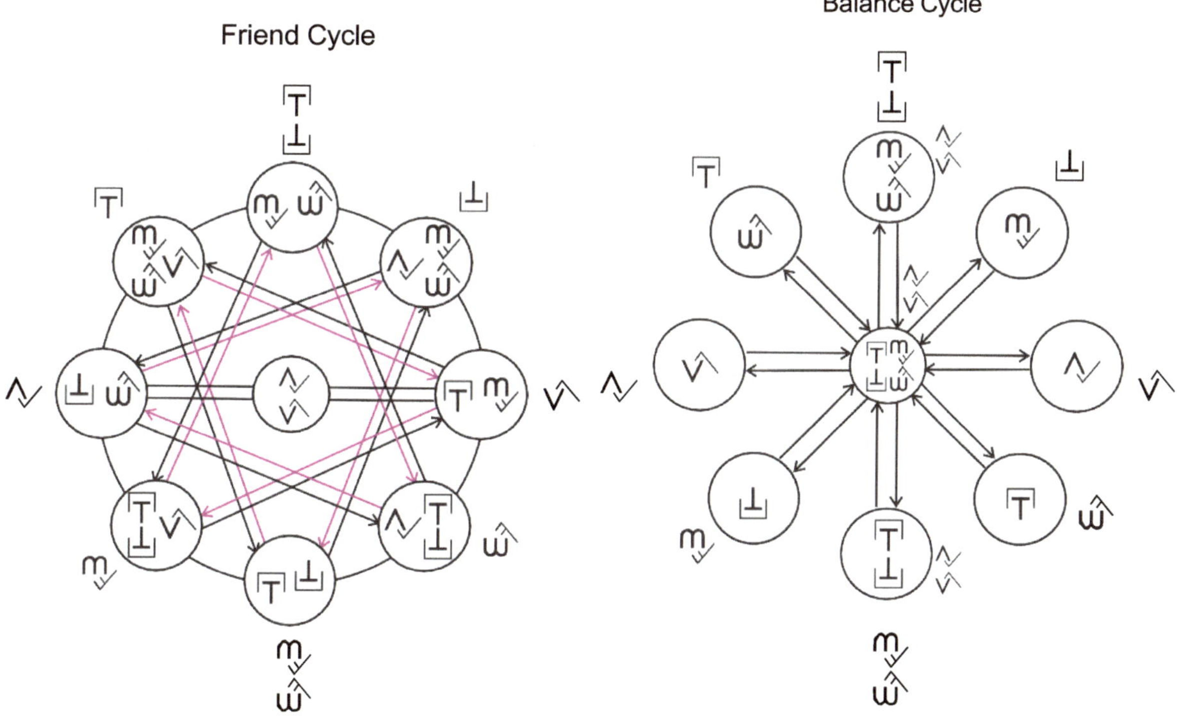
Friend Cycle
Balance Cycle

(Self Cycle)

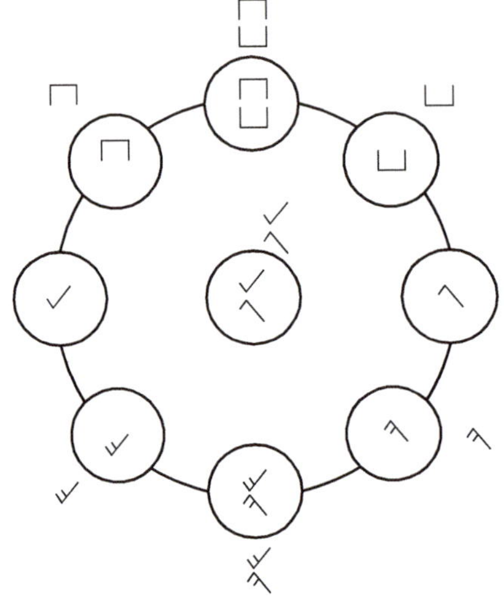

(Enlargement Cycle)

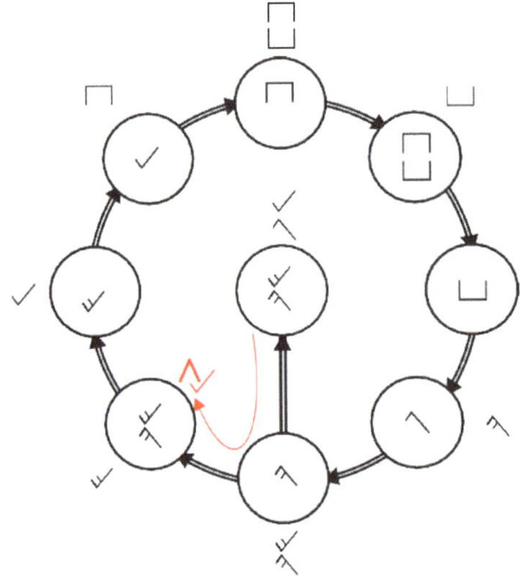

(Atrophy Cycle)

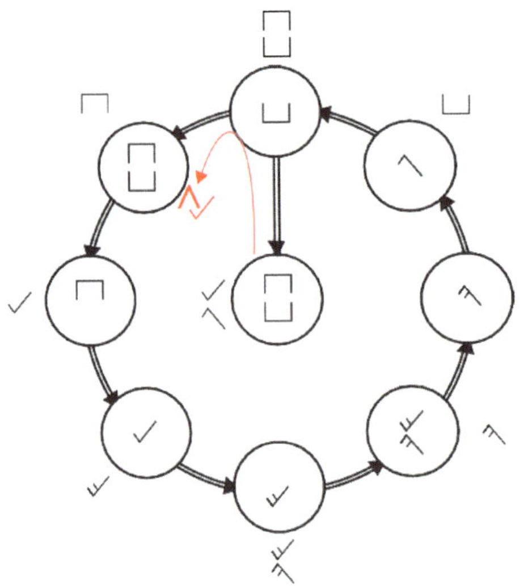

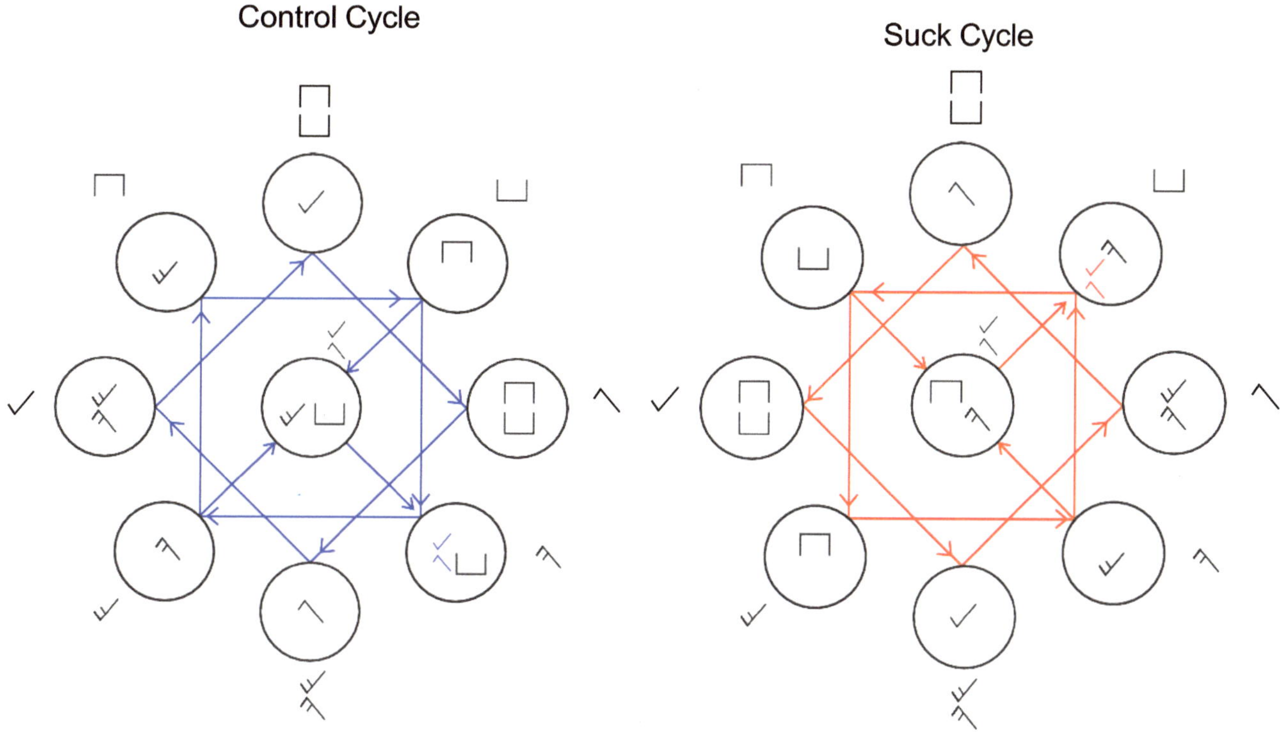
Control Cycle
Suck Cycle

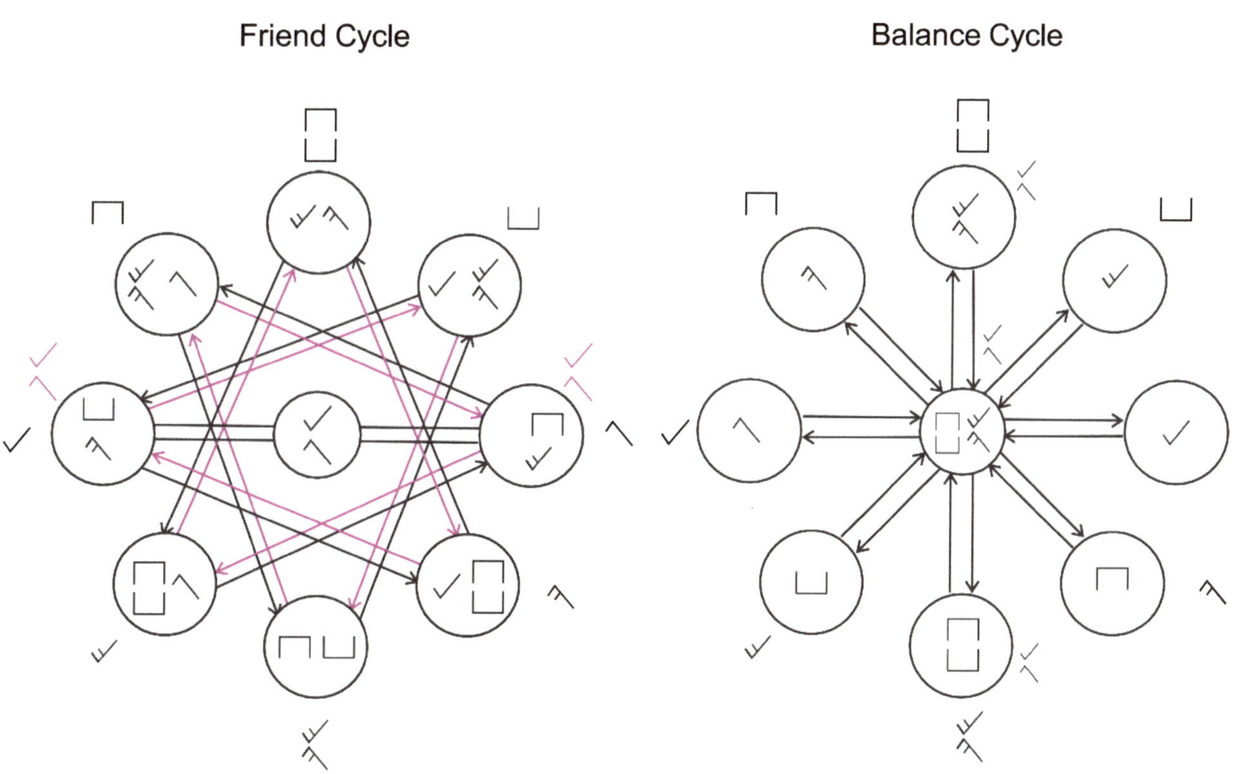
Friend Cycle
Balance Cycle

(Self Cycle)

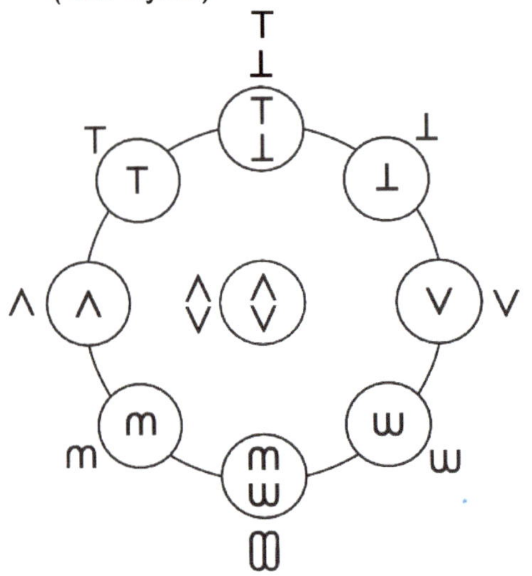

(Enlargement Cycle)

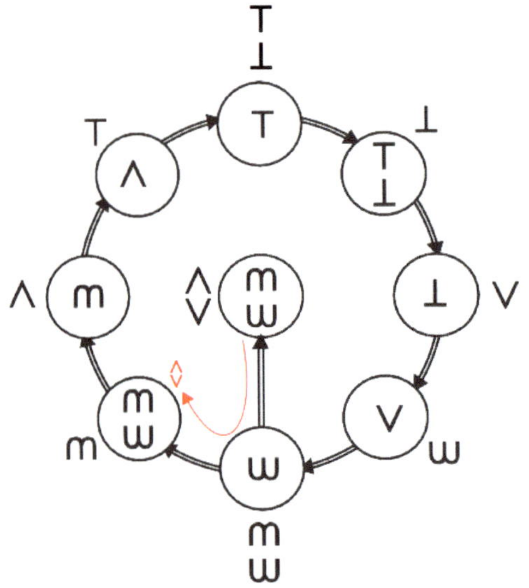

(Atrophy Cycle)

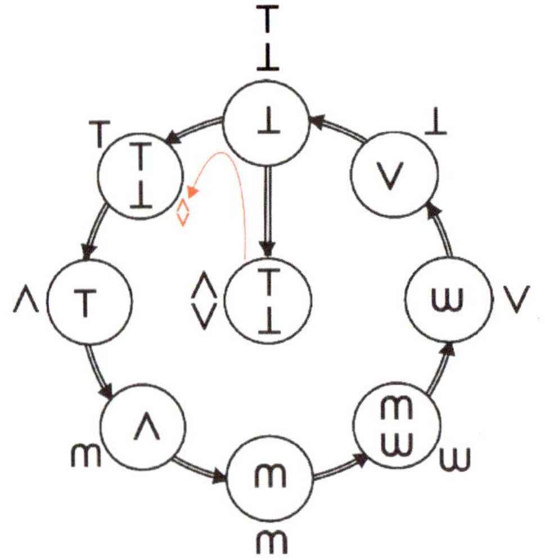

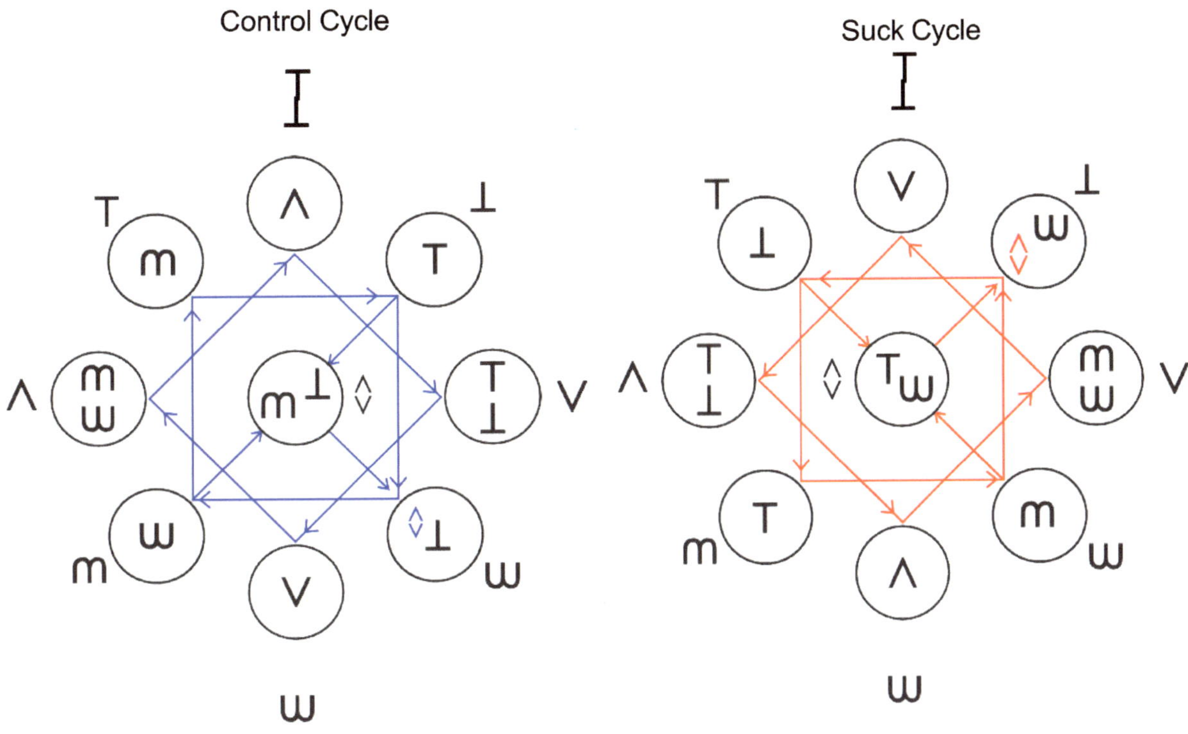
Control Cycle
Suck Cycle

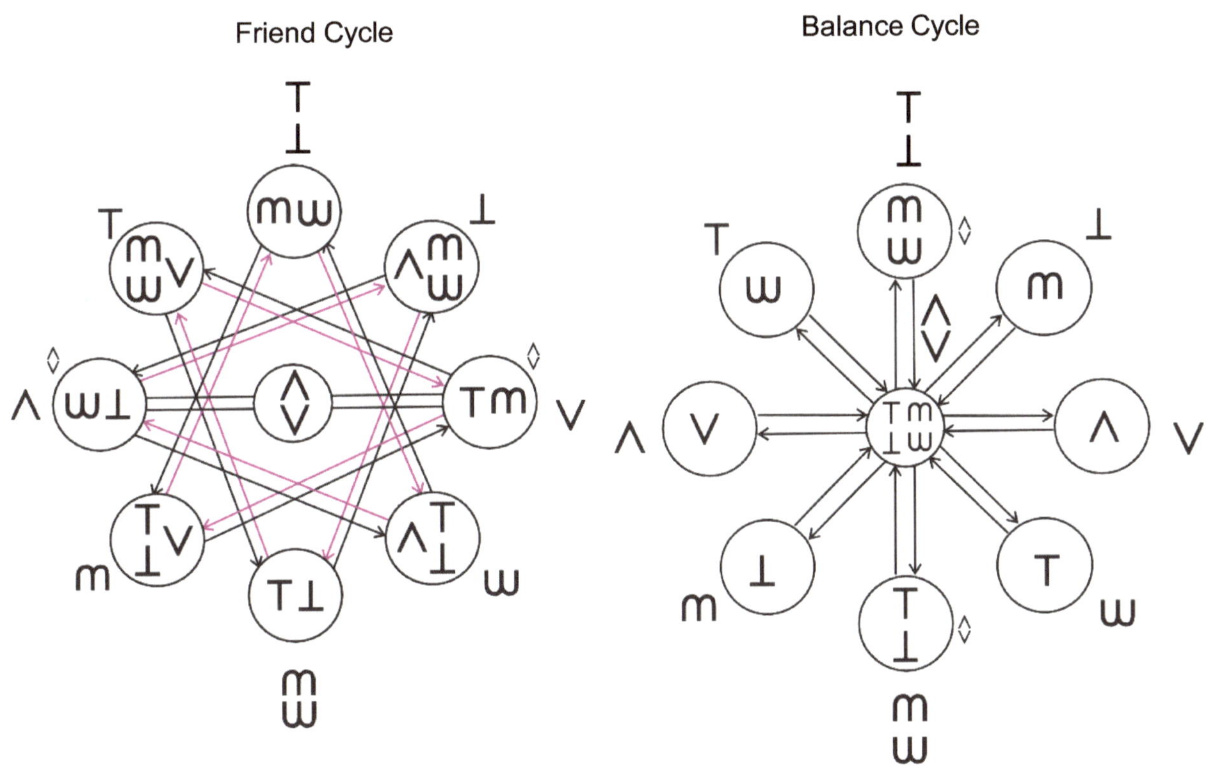
Friend Cycle
Balance Cycle

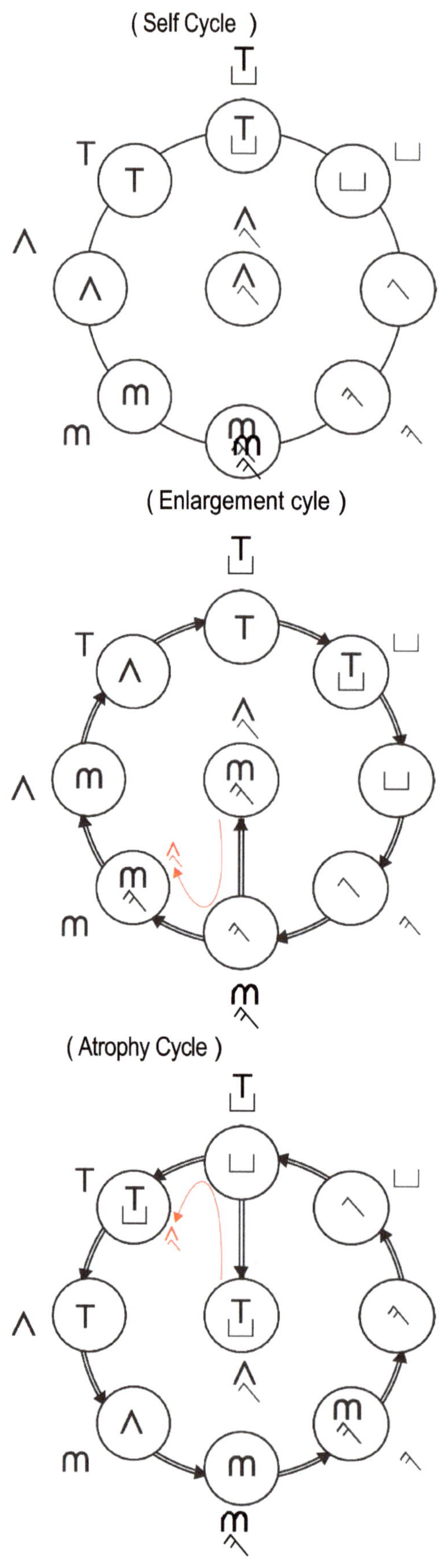
(Self Cycle)
(Enlargement cyle)
(Atrophy Cycle)

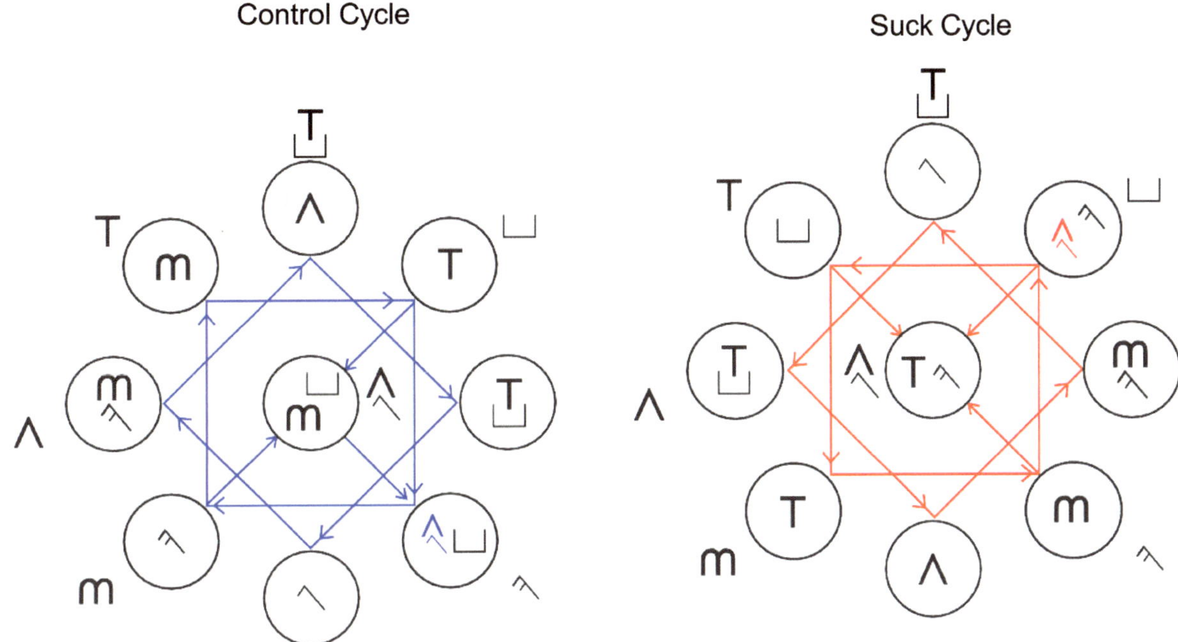
Control Cycle
Suck Cycle

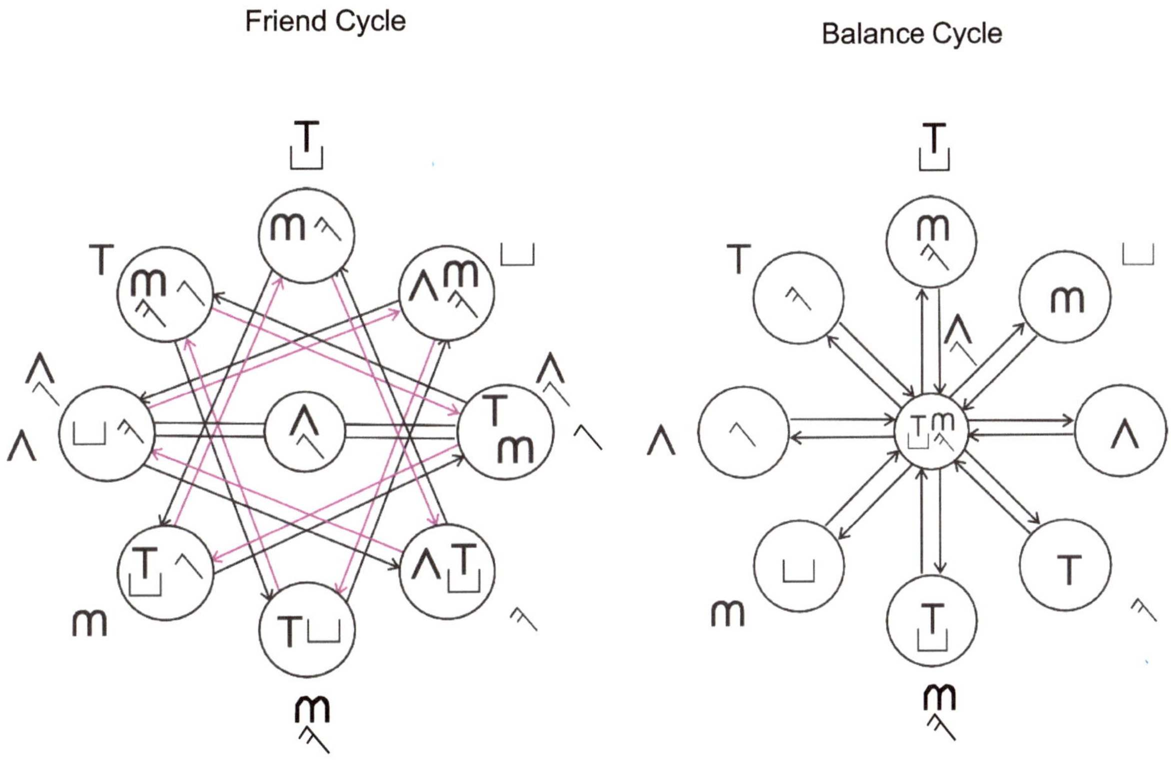
Friend Cycle
Balance Cycle

GROWTH CYCLING IN GROWTH

(GAS-GAS&SOLID-SOLID)

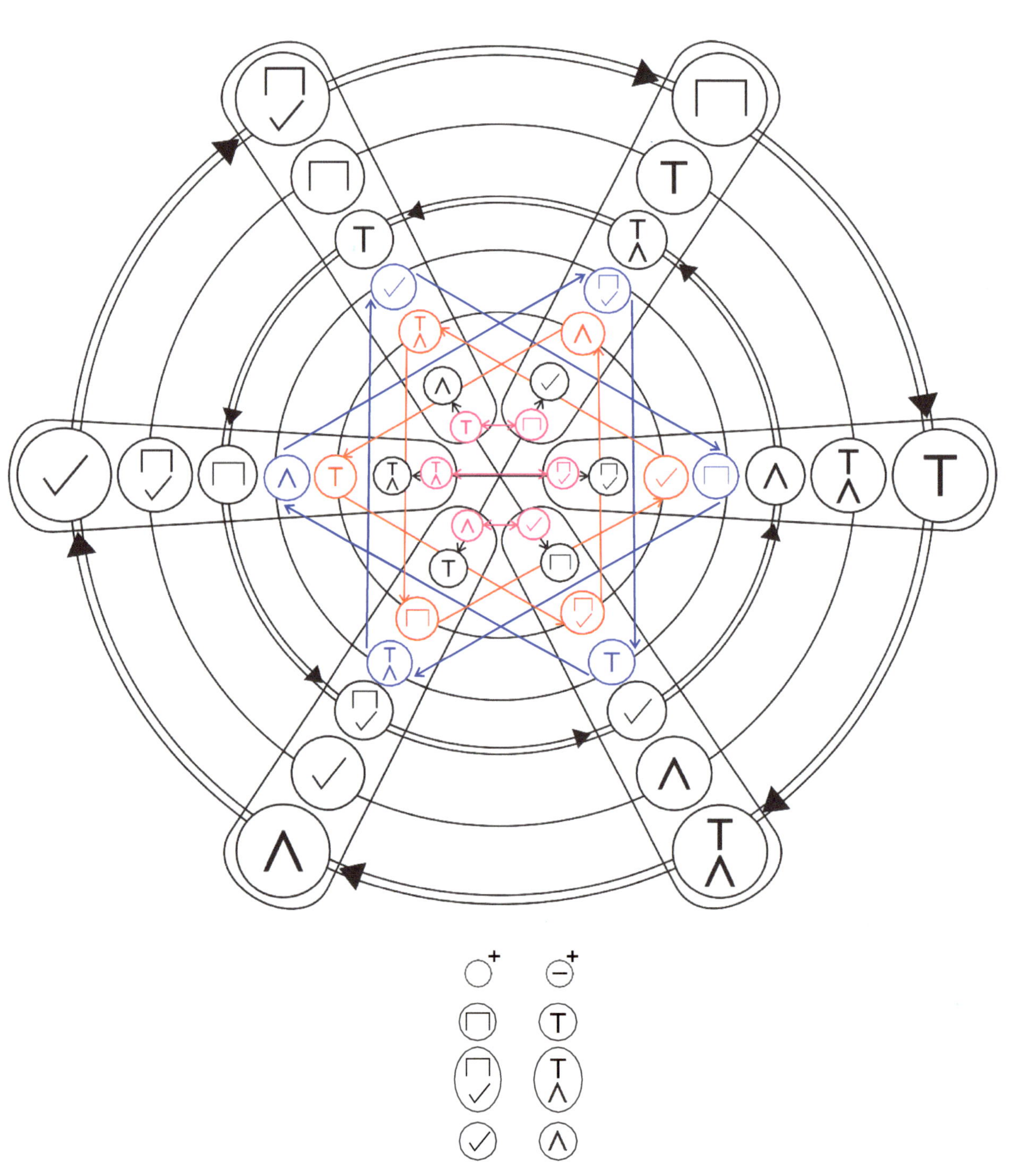

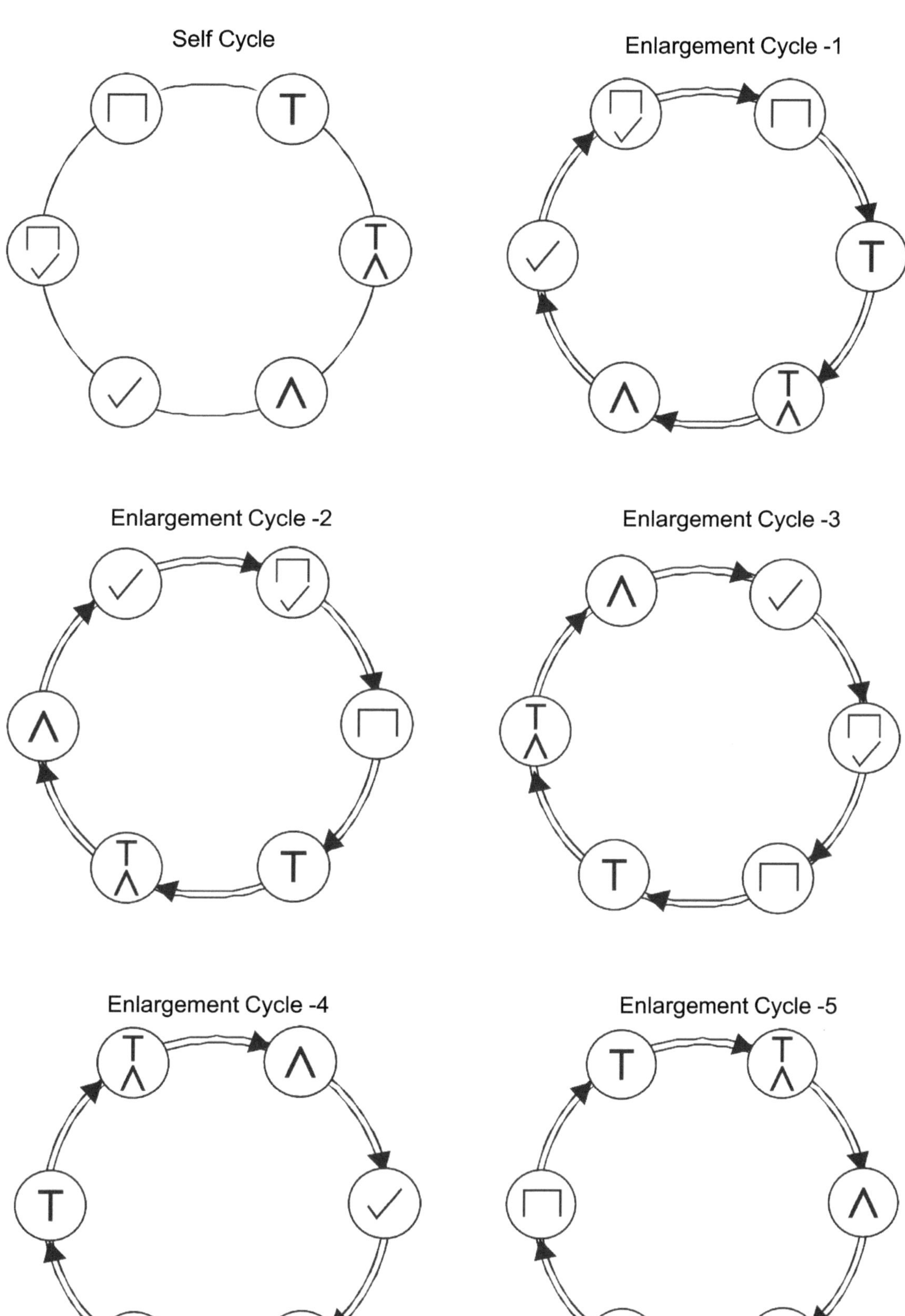
Self Cycle
Enlargement Cycle -1
Enlargement Cycle -2
Enlargement Cycle -3
Enlargement Cycle -4
Enlargement Cycle -5

Atrophy Cycle -1

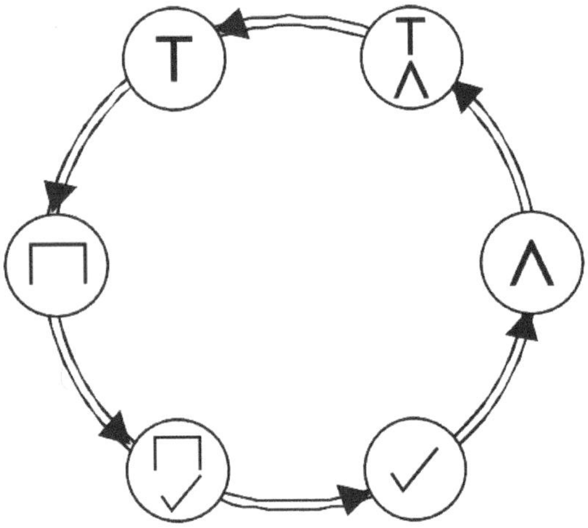

Atrophy Cycle -2

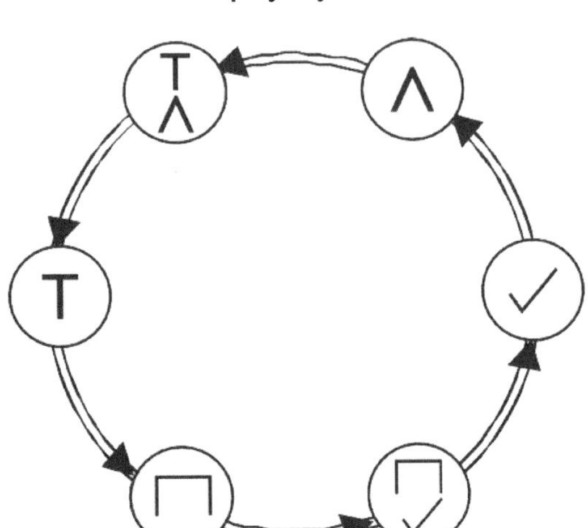

Atrophy Cycle -3

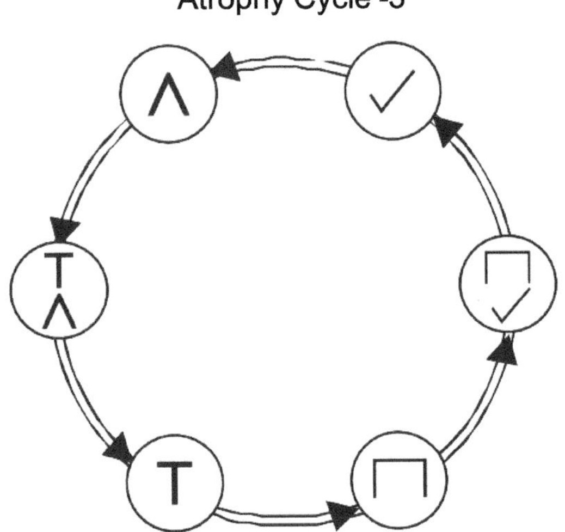

Atrophy Cycle -4

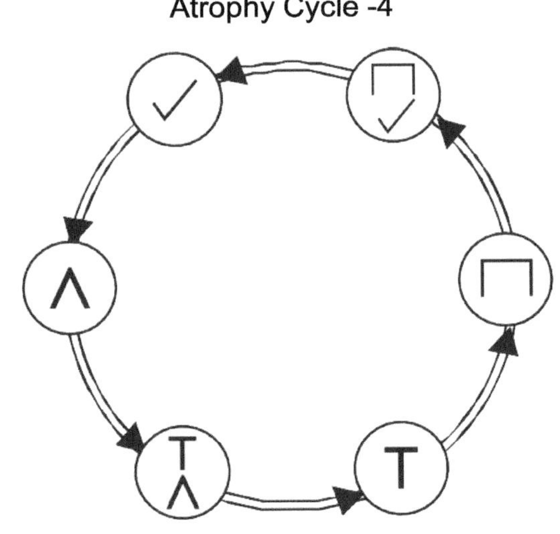

Atrophy Cycle -5

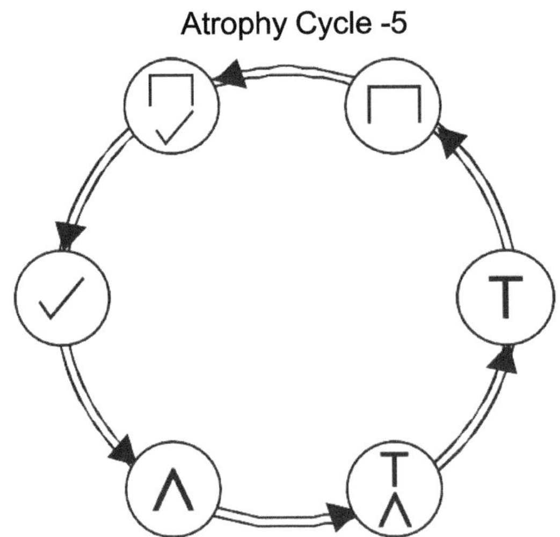

Control Cycle

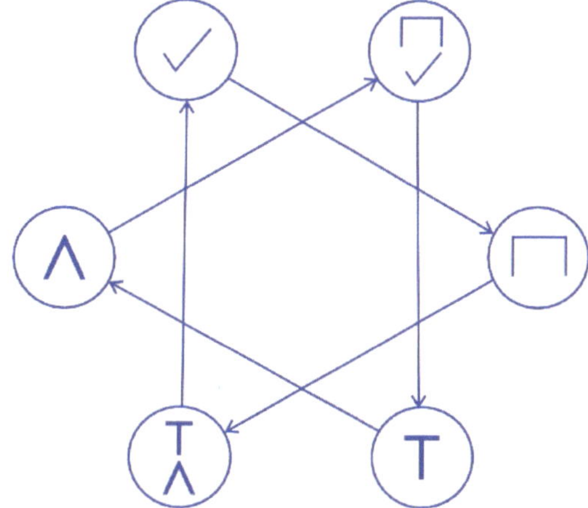

Suck Cycle

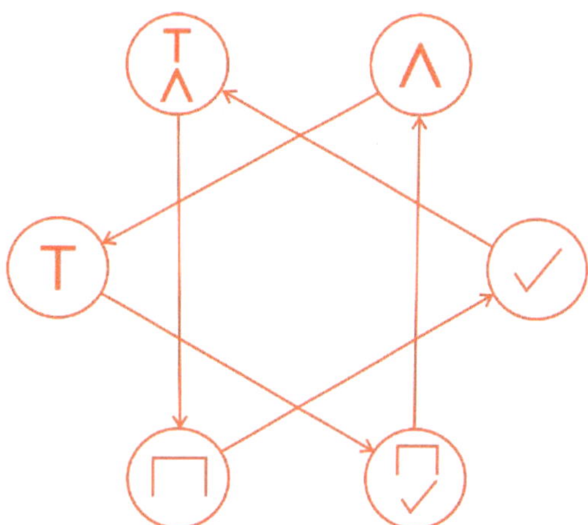

Balance Cycle

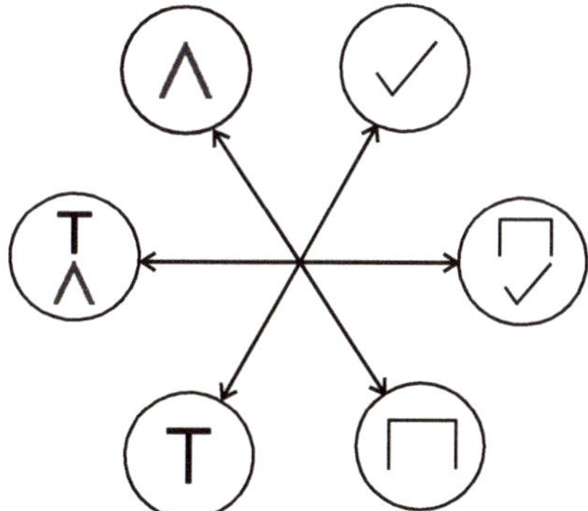

Husband & Wife Cycle

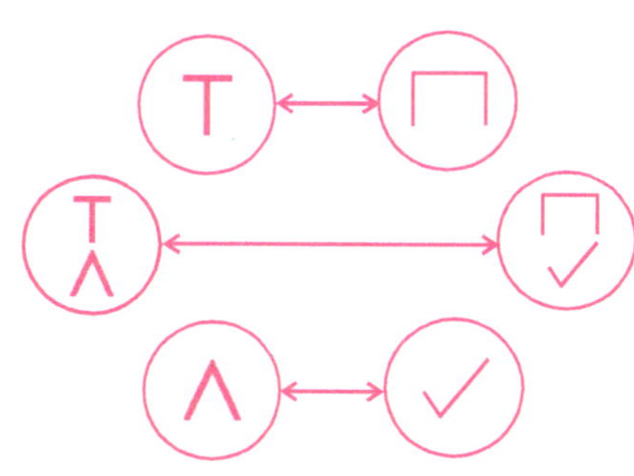

SURVIVAL CYCLING IN SURVIVAL

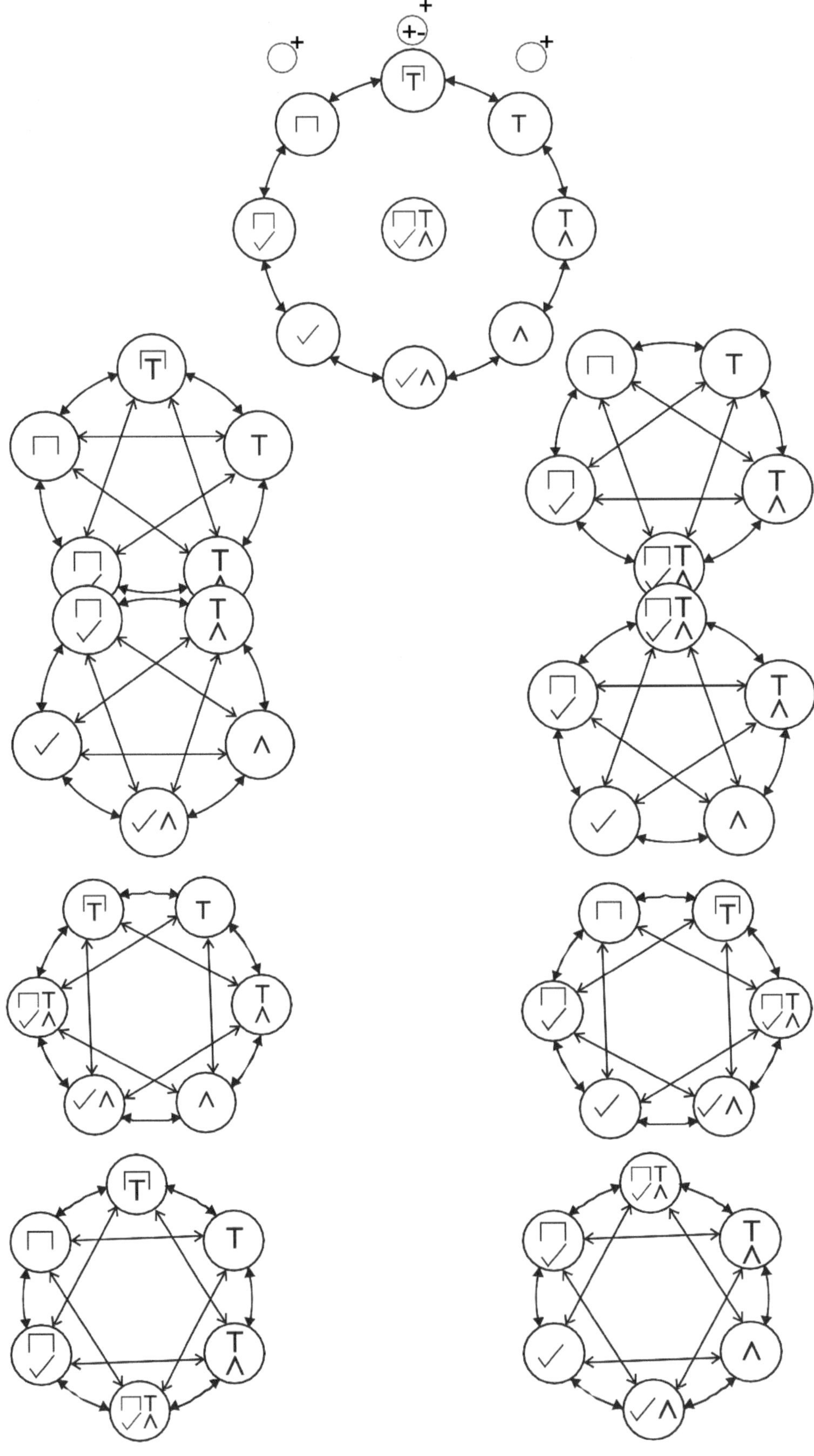

SURVIVAL CYCLING IN SURVIVAL

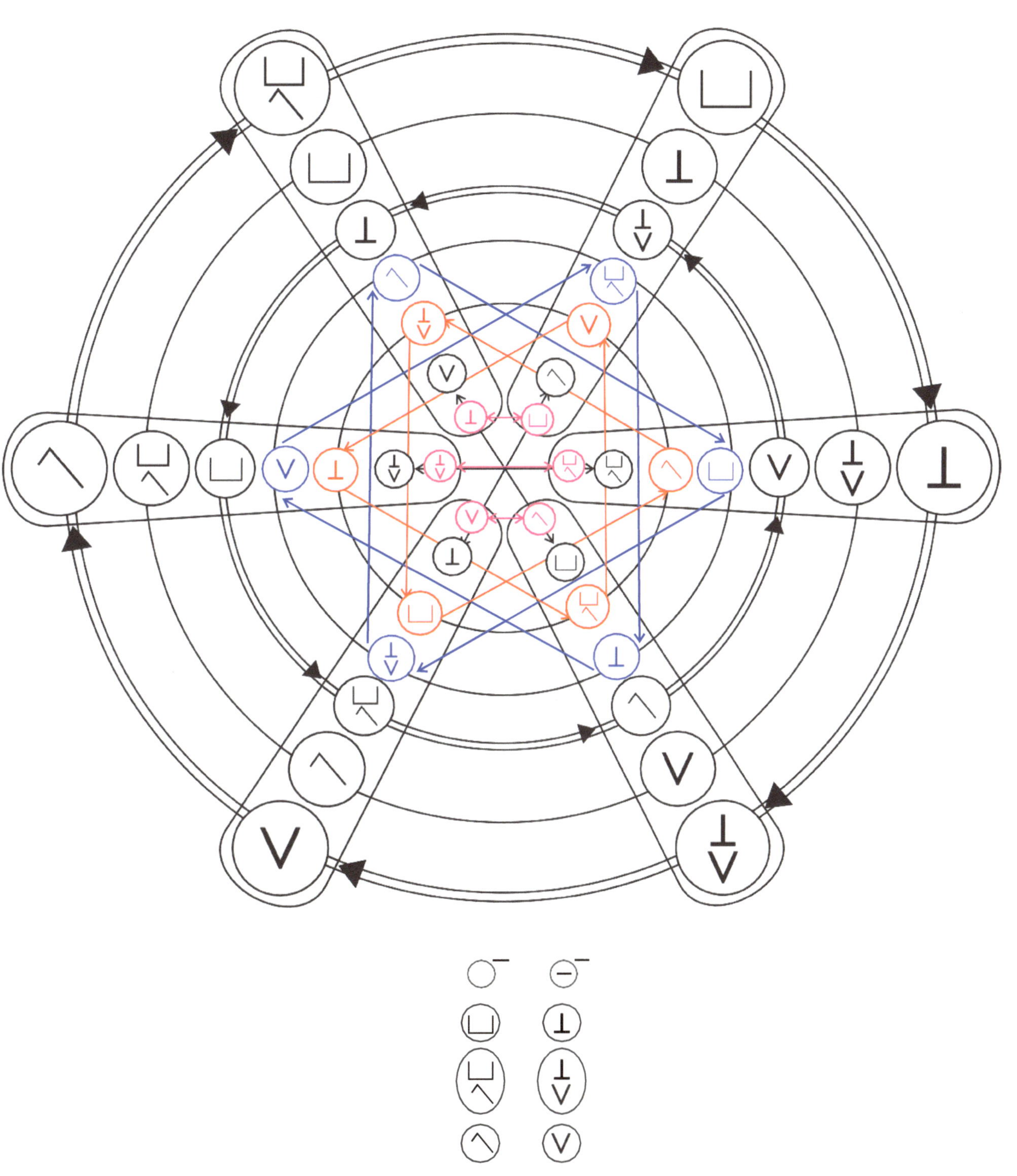

Self Cycle

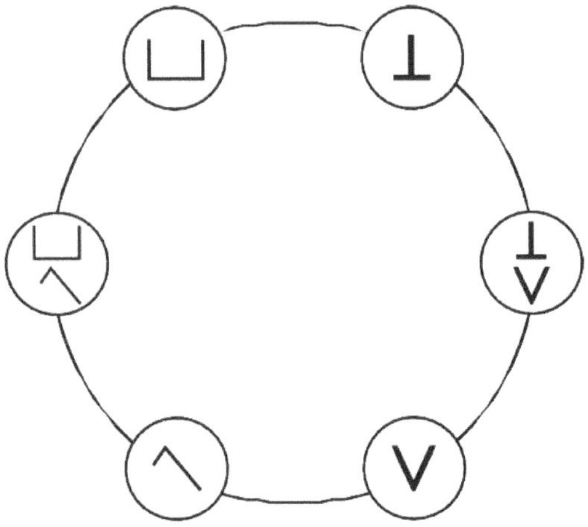

Enlargement Cycle -1

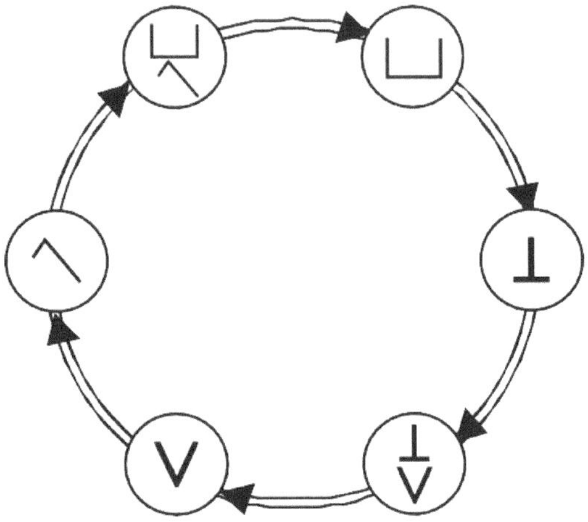

Enlargement Cycle -2

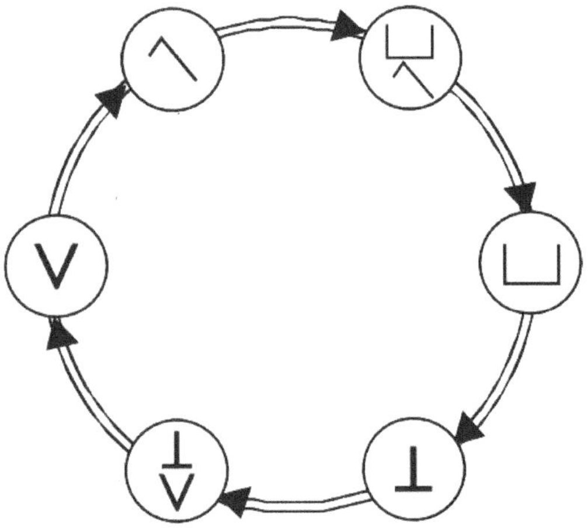

Enlargement Cycle -3

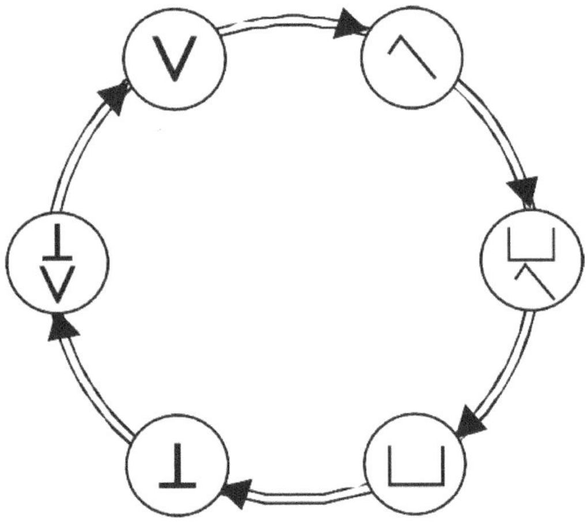

Enlargement Cycle -4

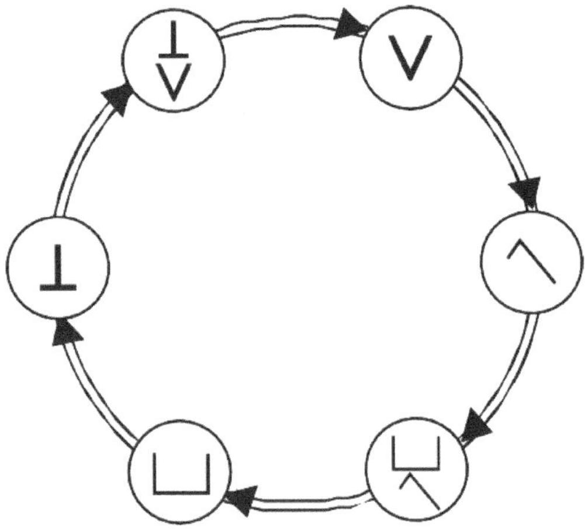

Enlargement Cycle -5

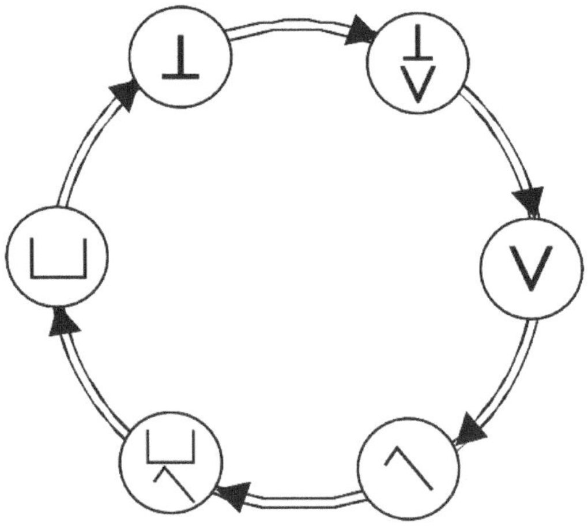

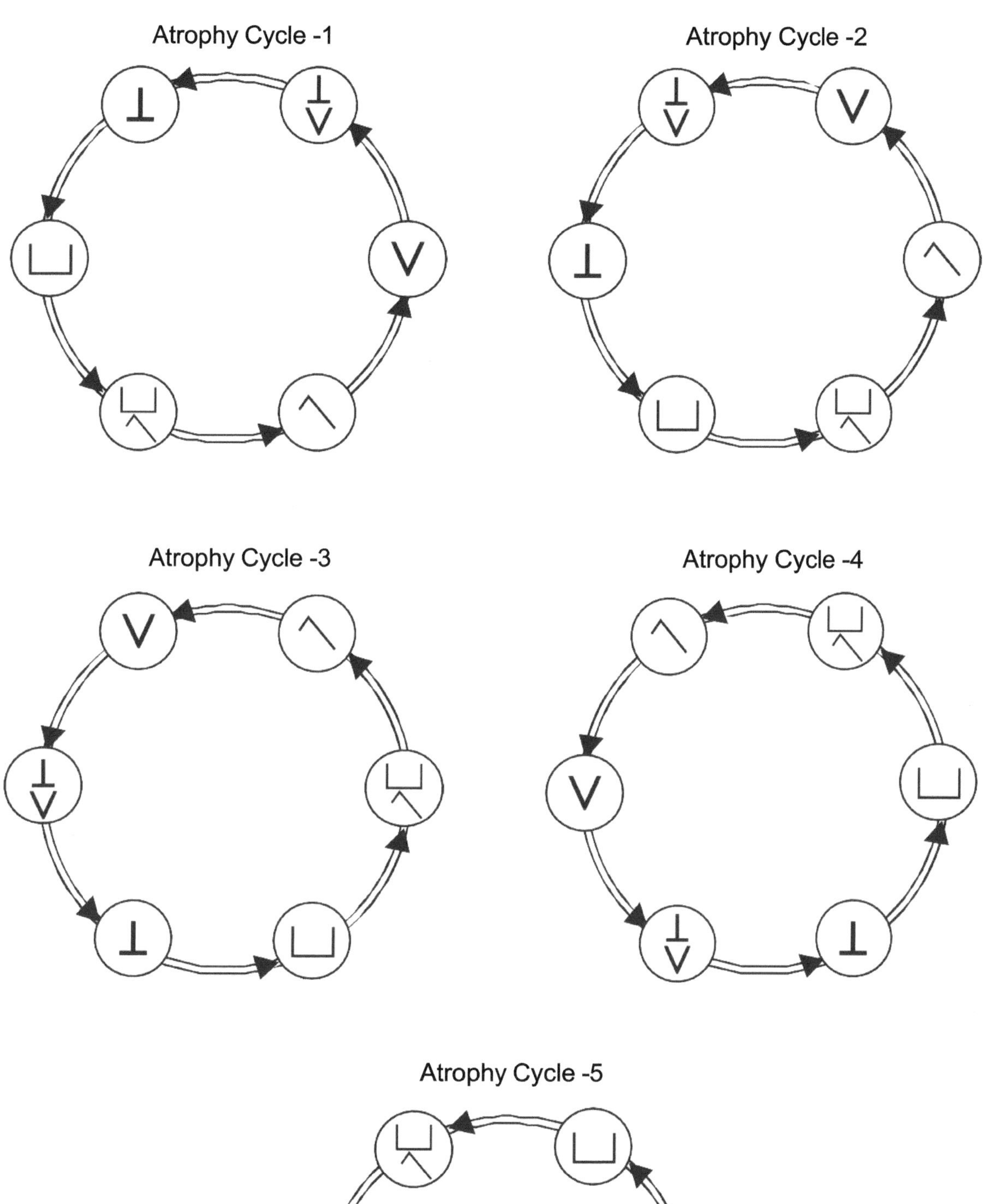
Atrophy Cycle -1
Atrophy Cycle -2
Atrophy Cycle -3
Atrophy Cycle -4
Atrophy Cycle -5

Control Cycle

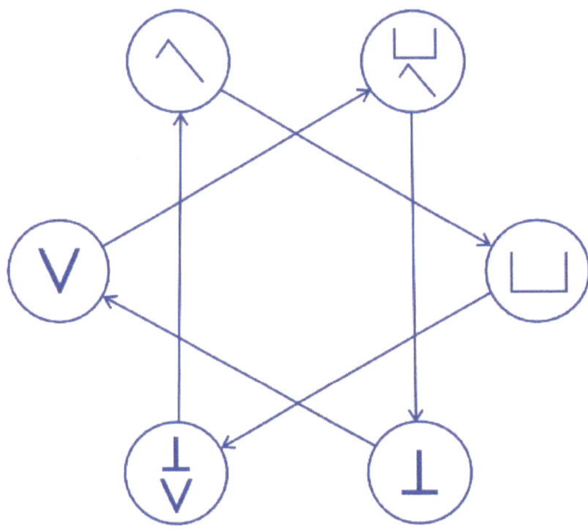

Suck Cycle

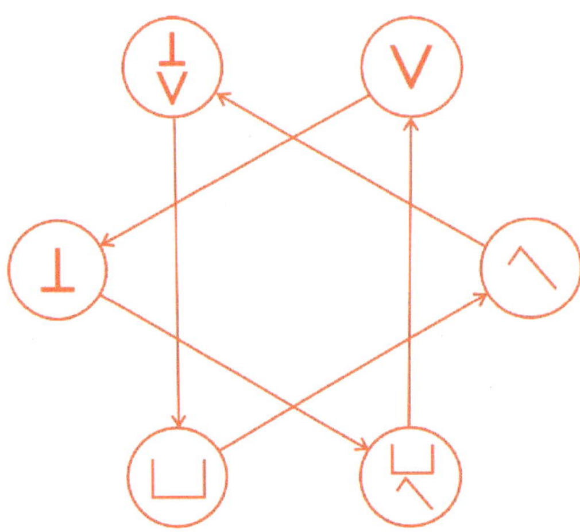

Balance Cycle

Husband & Wife Cycle

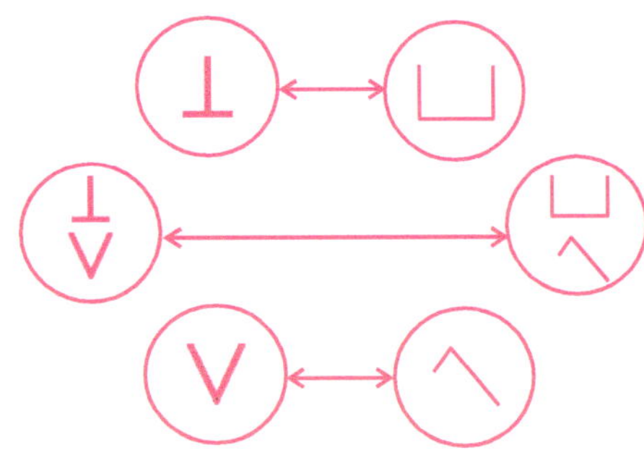

SURVIVAL CYCLING IN SURVIVAL

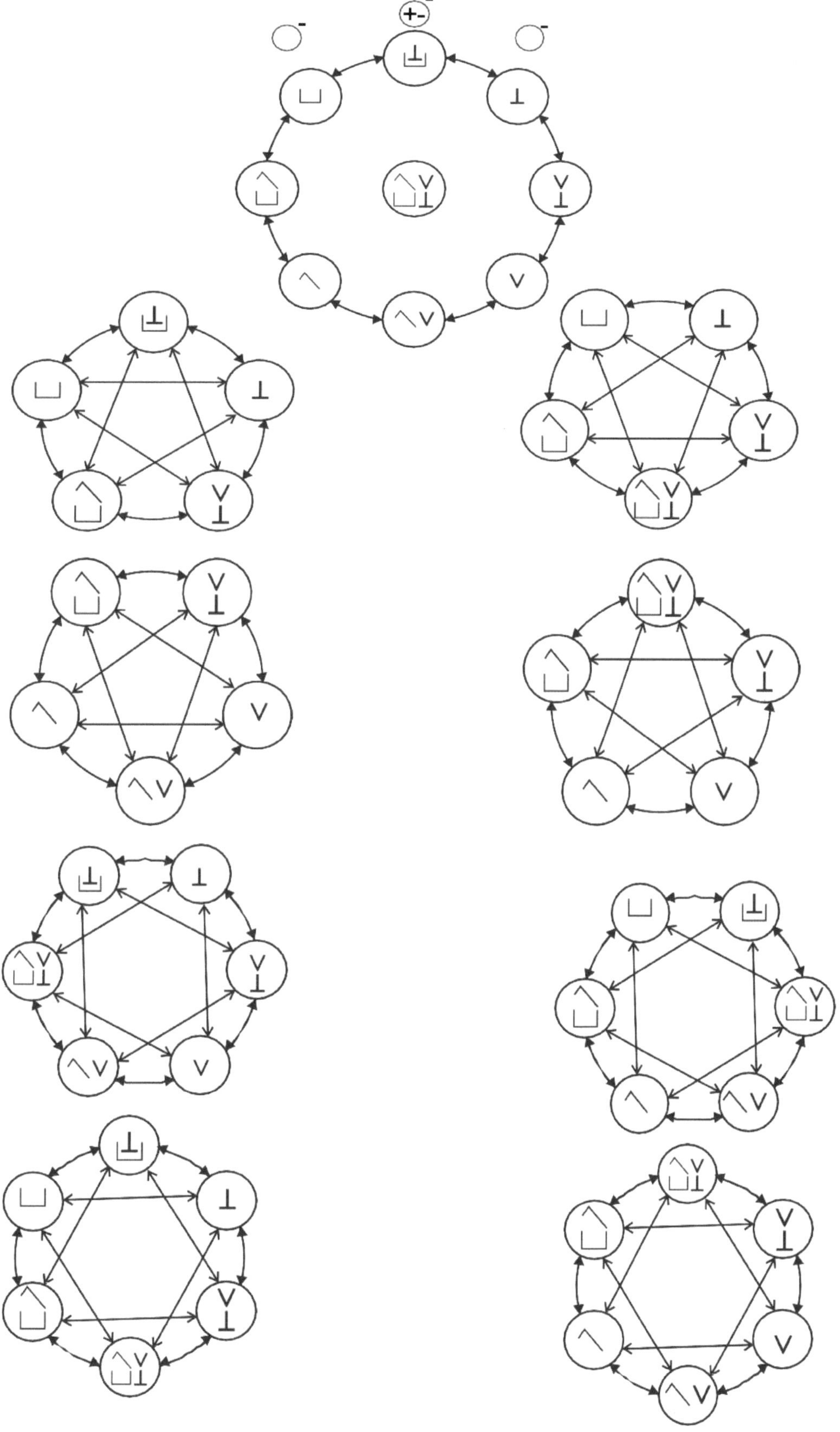

Part Eleven

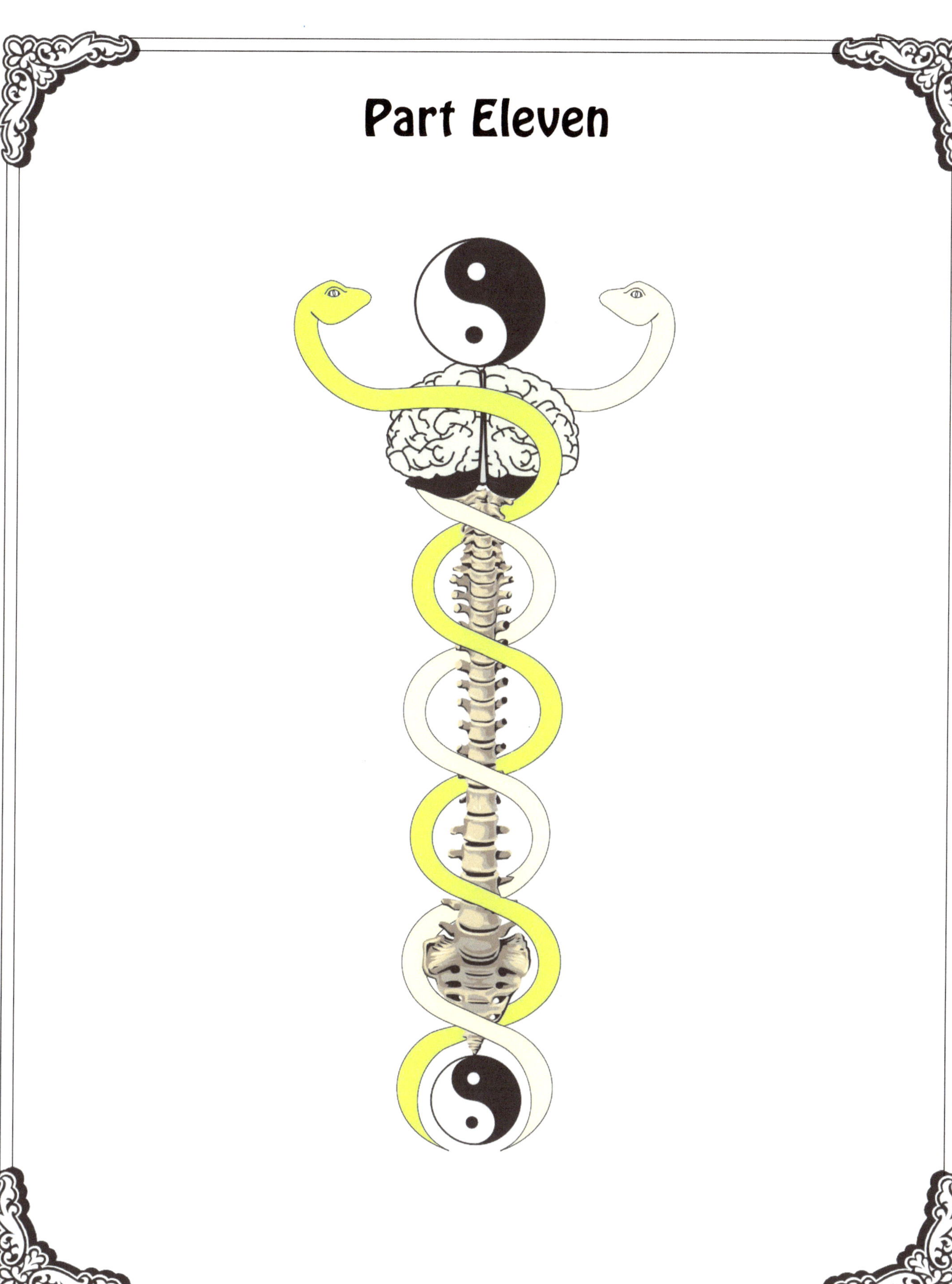

Method of Selecting the Five Elements Points Based on the Law of Five Elements (Six Elements)

11.1. Explanation of How to Diagnose the Five Elements Pulse Through Sensing Them.

11.2 Fire Big

11.3 Fire Small

11.4 Earth

11.5 Metal

11.6 Water

11.7 Wood

11.8 Case Studies

11.9 Conclusion

11.1 Explanation of How to Diagnose the Five Elements' Pulse Through Sensing Them.

Five Elements	Related organs	Symbols	Sensation
Fire big	Heart	(✓)	It is a sense where it feels as if the sharp edge of a pin is rubbing on one's fingers.
Fire small	Pericardium	(✓)	Though the same as Fire big, this pulse goes up and down.
Earth	Spleen	(/)	Piercing sense from the elbow towards the wrist.
Metal	Lungs	(\)	The sense of touching a thin metal wire, it runs from the wrist to the elbow.
Water	Kidneys	(—)	Feels like water passing through one's fingers when we touch it while it passes through the pipe. This runs from the elbow to the wrist.
Wood	Liver	(I)	A small ball or bead-like lump comes upward towards our finger and dashes.

Method of Selecting the Five Elements Points Based on the Law of Five Elements (Six Elements)

11.2 Fire Big

Five element organs	Six element cycles	State of creative, destructive cycles	Point of selection in five elements
Fire big heart	Self-energy Cycle Excess	Destructive Cycle	H4 (or) H3 (or)
		Creative Cycle	H9 (or) H7 (or) H.7.5 (or)
Fire small, small intestine	Self-energy Cycle Excess	Destructive Cycle	S11 (or) S12 (or)
		Creative Cycle	S13 (or) S18 (or)
Fire big Heart	Enlargement Energy Cycle Excess	Destructive Cycle	H4 (or) H3 (or)
		Creative Cycle	H7 (or) H8 (or) H.7.5
Fire small, small intestine	Enlargement Energy Cycle Excess	Destructive Cycle	S11 (or) S12 (or)
		Creative Cycle	S14(or) S15 (or) S18
Fire big Heart	Atrophy Energy Cycle Excess	Destructive Cycle	H4 (or) H3 (or)
		Creative Cycle	H9(or) H8 (or) H.7.5
Fire small, Small intestine	Atrophy Energy Cycle Excess	Destructive Cycle	S11 (or) S12 (or)
		Creative Cycle	S14 (or) S15 (or) S11
Fire big Heart	Atrophy Energy Cycle Excess	Destructive Cycle	H4 (or) H3 (or)
		Creative Cycle	H9(or) H8 (or) H.7.5
Fire small, Small intestine	Atrophy Energy Cycle Excess	Destructive Cycle	S11 (or) S12 (or)
		Creative Cycle	S14 (or) S15 (or) S11
Fire big Heart	Control Energy Cycle Excess	Destructive Cycle	H4
		Creative Cycle	H9, (or) H8 (or) H.7.5 (or) H7 (or)
Fire big small intestine	Control Energy Cycle Excess	Destructive Cycle	S11
		Creative Cycle	S14 (or) S15 (or) S18 (or) S13 (or)
Fire big Heart	Suck Energy Cycle Excess	Destructive Cycle	H3
		Creative Cycle	H9 (or) H8 (or) H.7.5(or) H7
Fire big small intestine	Suck Energy Cycle Excess	Destructive Cycle	S12
		Creative Cycle	S14(or) S15 (or) S18 (or) S13(or)

11.3 Fire Samll

Five element organs	Six element cycles	State of creative, destructive cycles	Point of selection in five elements
Fire small Pericardium	Self-cycle Energy Excess	Destructive Cycle	P3, (or) P5 (or)
		Creative Cycle	P9 (or) P7 (or) P.7.5(or)
Fire Small Triple warmer	Self-cycle Energy Excess	Destructive Cycle	Tw1 (or) TW2 (or)
		Creative Cycle	TW3 (or) TW10 (or)
Fire small Pericardium	Enlargement Cycle Energy Excess	Destructive Cycle	P3 (or) P5 (or)
		Creative Cycle	P7 (or) P8 (or) H.7.5 (or)
Fire small Triple warmer	Enlargement Cycle Energy Excess	Destructive Cycle	TW1 (or) TW2
		Creative Cycle	TW4 (or) TW6(or) TW10
Fire small Pericardium	Atrophy Cycle Energy Excess	Destructive Cycle	P5(or) P3 (or)
		Creative Cycle	P9(or) P8 (or) P.7.5(or)
Fire small Triple warmer	Atrophy Cycle Energy Excess	Destructive Cycle	TW1 (or) TW2 (or)
		Creative Cycle	TW4 (or) TW6 (or) TW3 (or)
Fire Small Pericardium	Control Energy Cycle Excess	Destructive Cycle	P5
		Creative Cycle	P9(or) P8 (or) P7 (or) P.7.5 (or)
Fire Small Triple warmer	Control Energy Cycle Excess	Destructive Cycle	TW1
		Creative Cycle	TW4 (or) TW6(or) TW3 (or)TW10 (or)
Fire Small Pericardium	Suck Energy Cycle Excess	Destructive Cycle	P3
		Creative Cycle	P9 (or) P7 (or) P8 (or) P.7.5 (or)
Fire Small Triple Warmer	Suck Energy Cycle Excess	Destructive Cycle	TW2
		Creative Cycle	TW4 (or) TW6 (or) TW10 (or) TW3

11.4 Earth

Five element organs	Six element cycles	State of creative, destructive cycles	Point of selection in five elements
Earth Spleen Excess	Self-cycle Energy	Destructive Cycle	SP1(or)SP9
		Creative Cycle	SP1.5(or)SP2(or)SP5
Earth Stomach	Self-cycle Energy Excess	Destructive Cycle	ST43(or)ST44
		Creative Cycle	ST45(or)ST42
Earth Spleen	Enlargement Cycle Energy Excess	Destructive Cycle	SP1(or)SP9
		Creative Cycle	SP1(or)SP5(or)SP3
Earth Stomach	Enlargement Cycle Energy Excess	Destructive Cycle	ST43(or)ST44
		Creative Cycle	ST36(or)ST45
Earth Spleen	Atrophy Cycle	Destructive Cycle	SP1(or)SP5
		Creative Cycle	SP1(or)SP1.5(or)SP2
Earth Stomach	Atrophy Cycle	Destructive Cycle	ST43(or)ST44
		Creative Cycle	ST36(or)ST41(or)ST42
Earth Spleen	Self-cycle Energy Excess	Destructive Cycle	SP9
		Creative Cycle	SP1(or)SP1.5(or) SP2(or) SP3(or)SP5
Earth Stomach	Self-cycle Energy Excess	Destructive Cycle	ST44
		Creative Cycle	ST36(or)ST41(or)ST42 (or)ST45
Earth Spleen	Enlargement Cycle Energy Excess	Destructive Cycle	SP1
		Creative Cycle	SP1.5(or)SP2(or)SP3(or) SP5
Earth Stomach	Enlargement Cycle Energy Excess	Destructive Cycle	ST43
		Creative Cycle	ST(36)ST41(or) ST42(or) ST45

11.5 Metal

Five element organs	Six element cycles	State of creative, destructive cycles	Point of selection in five elements
Metal, Lungs	Self-cycle Energy Excess	Destructive Cycle	LU10(or)LU9.5(or)LU11
		Creative Cycle	LU9(or)LU5
Metal, Large Intestine	Self-cycle Energy Excess	Destructive Cycle	LI4(or)LI5(or)LI3
		Creative Cycle	LI2(or)LI11
Metal, Lungs	Enlargement Cycle Energy Excess	Destructive Cycle	LU10(or)LU9.5(or)LU11
		Creative Cycle	LU8(or)LU5
Metal, Large Intestine	Enlargement Cycle Energy Excess	Destructive Cycle	LI4(or)LI5(or)LI3
		Creative Cycle	LI2(or)LI1
Metal, Lungs	Atrophy Cycle	Destructive Cycle	LU10(or)LU9.5(or)LU11
		Creative Cycle	LU8(or)LU9
Metal, Large Intestine	Atrophy Cycle	Destructive Cycle	LI4(or)LI5(or)LI3
		Creative Cycle	LI11(or)LI1
Metal, Lungs	Self-cycle Energy Excess	Destructive Cycle	LU11
		Creative Cycle	LU5(or)LU8(or)LU9
Metal, Large Intestine	Self-cycle Energy Excess	Destructive Cycle	LI3
		Creative Cycle	LI2(or)LI1(or)LI11
Metal, Lungs	Enlargement Cycle Energy Excess	Destructive Cycle	LU10(or)LU9.5
		Creative Cycle	LU8(or)LU5(or)LU9
Metal, Large Intestine	Enlargement Cycle Energy Excess	Destructive Cycle	LI4(or)LI5
		Creative Cycle	LI2(or)LI1(or)LI11

11.6 Water

Five element organs	Six element cycles	State of creative, destructive cycles	Point of selection in five elements
Water Kidney	Self-cycle Energy Excess	Destructive Cycle	K2(or)K3(or)k6
		Creative Cycle	K1(or)K7
Water Urinary Bladder	Self-cycle Energy Excess	Destructive Cycle	UB54(or)UB62(or)UB60
		Creative Cycle	UB65(or)UB67
Water Kidney	Enlargement Cycle Energy Excess	Destructive Cycle	K2(or)K3(or)K6
		Creative Cycle	K1(or)K10
Water Urinary Bladder	Enlargement Cycle Energy Excess	Destructive Cycle	UB54(or)UB62(or)UB60
		Creative Cycle	UB65(or)UB66
Water Kidney	Atrophy Cycle	Destructive Cycle	K2(or)K3(or)K6
		Creative Cycle	K10(or)K7
Water Urinary Bladder	Atrophy Cycle	Destructive Cycle	UB54(or)UB62(or)UB60
		Creative Cycle	UB66(or)UB67
Water Kidney	Self-cycle Energy Excess	Destructive Cycle	K2(or)K3
		Creative Cycle	K1(or)K10(or)K7
Water Urinary Bladder	Self-cycle Energy Excess	Destructive Cycle	UB62(or)UB60
		Creative Cycle	UB65(or)UB66(or)UB67
Water Kidney	Enlargement Cycle Energy Excess	Destructive Cycle	K6
		Creative Cycle	K1(or)K10(or)K7
Water Urinary Bladder	Enlargement Cycle Energy Excess	Destructive Cycle	UB54
		Creative Cycle	UB65(or)UB66(or)UB67

11.7 Wood

Five element organs	Six element cycles	State of creative, destructive cycles	Point of selection in five elements
Wood Liver	Self-cycle Energy Excess	Destructive Cycle	Liv4(or)Liv3(or)
		Creative Cycle	Liv8(or)Liv1.5(or)Liv2
Wood Gallbladder	Self-cycle Energy Excess	Destructive Cycle	GB44(or)GB34(or)
		Creative Cycle	GB43(or)GB40(or)GB38
Wood Liver	Enlargement Cycle Energy Excess	Destructive Cycle	Liv4(or)Liv3
		Creative Cycle	Liv1.5(or)Liv2()Liv1
Wood Gallbladder	Enlargement Cycle Energy Excess	Destructive Cycle	G44(or)GB34
		Creative Cycle	GB40(or)GB38(or)GB41
Wood Liver	Atrophy Cycle	Destructive Cycle	Liv4(or)Liv3
		Creative Cycle	Liv8()Liv1
Wood Gallbladder	Atrophy Cycle	Destructive Cycle	GB44()GB34
		Creative Cycle	GB44()GB41
Wood Liver	Self-cycle Energy Excess	Destructive Cycle	Liv3
		Creative Cycle	Liv1()Liv8()Liv1.5()Liv2
Wood Gallbladder	Self-cycle Energy Excess	Destructive Cycle	GB34
		Creative Cycle	GB43()GB41()GB40() GB38
Wood Liver	Enlargement Cycle Energy Excess	Destructive Cycle	Liv4
		Creative Cycle	Liv1.5()Liv2()Liv1()Liv8
Wood Gallbladder	Enlargement Cycle Energy Excess	Destructive Cycle	GB44
		Creative Cycle	GB43()GB40()GB38() GB41

The author discussed the five different cycles of the five elements, their functions along with the creative and destructive cycles and the method of selecting the point for treatment when these cycles become an excess. When these energies become excessive in ***yin***, then the points of treatment must be tonified. By the tonification method, if these energies are less in *yin*, then the selected points for treatment should be sedated (by sedating method).

Whereas, if these energies become excess in *yang*, it indicates that these energies are spent excessively. So, the points selected for treatment must be sedated. If these energies are less in *yang*, then all the selected points for treatment should be tonified.

Hence, irrelevant of the symptoms and the laboratory reports, one can diagnose the patient's *Panchaboodha* energy level through his/her pulse and diagnose the stagnant or lost energy, its channel and the relevant, affected organs, the relevant element which is affected, etc. Through this ***Panchaboodha*** pulse diagnosis and treatment method, the root causes of the symptoms are thoroughly diagnosed and the point of treatment is selected and treated. Hence, all the diseases and symptoms of the patient will be cured totally.

11. 8 Case Studies

Name: Akila

Age:32

Address: Salem-5

Patient's statement

She attained puberty at the age of 13. She had a 25-day menstrual cycle. She has been married for 10 years. Till three years after her marriage, her menstrual cycle was regular. Then she was under medication for fertility. Since then, the menstruation became irregular and she had her periods only once a year. At present, it occurs only after administering an injection or medicines. The last period occurred a year before. Her limbs hurt (like drilling). She experiences no sound and good sleep. She gets headaches often and has no appetite.

Doctor's Diagnosis Using Six Elements Pulse Diagnosis Method.

R)

M(↘)	E(↗)	IIF(✓)
—	|	—

L)

IF(✓)	Wo(I)	Wa(−)
—	|	|

The wood and water elements are in excess.

The liver and the kidneys are working excessively because of the liver. The spleen is affected

Since the spleen is related to the lymphatic system, it is also affected. Since the kidneys affect the heart, the water quantity in the blood will be in excess which causes headaches and menstrual problems.

All these problems occur because of the less functioning of the heart and spleen and excessive functioning of the liver and the kidneys.

Hence, we must reduce the excessive functioning and kindle the less functioning organs by balancing between the organs to give a complete cure to the patient.

First Phase of Treatment

Wood (Wo) and Water elements (Wa) are excess.

R (12 Organ Pulses)

M	E	IIF
—	|	—
—	|	—

L

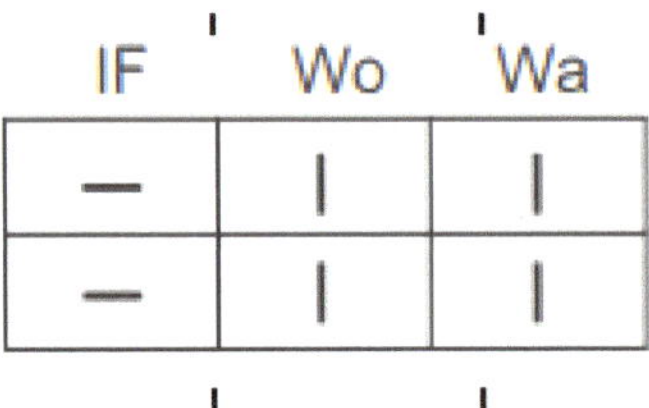

IF	Wo	Wa
—	|	|
—	|	|

Liv 1—the wood point related to the liver organ

SP 1—the wood point related to the spleen organ

Liv 1 and SP1points are selected on the right side tracks of the spleen and the liver.

One of the points has been selected to reduce the liver's function and the other has been selected to balance the spleen and reduce the link between the spleen and the liver. After this, to enhance the functioning of the spleen, the earth point of the spleen on the left side of the spleen track has been applied, which will develop the self-cycle of the spleen.

The basic reason to treat these two organs is that the liver and the kidneys are working excessively. Because of this, the patient's heart and spleen functions are reduced. Apart from these problems, the kidneys' function was not controlled by the spleen since the spleen has been affected. Hence, the liver and the spleen organs' six elements' points were selected.

After the functions of these two organs were checked and confirmed (that the required changes had occurred), the K3 earth point related to the spleen organ has been applied to control the kidney function. After this, the patient was sent back.

Second Phase of Treatment

Statement of the Patient

Headaches were reduced by 50% and sleep improved by 50%. Leg pain had completely stopped. Menstruation did not start.

Doctors' Diagnosis of the Problem Based on the Six Element Pulse Diagnosis Method.

R

M(↘)	E(↗)	IIF(✓)
↘	↗	✓

L

IF(✓)	Wo(I)	Wa(–)
✓	I	–

The water (Wa) element was working excessively.

The link between the lungs and the kidneys became excessive. There was no connection between the lungs and the liver by which the lungs should have been controlled.

The points selected to treat the patient during the second phase.

LU5—the water point in the lung organ

LU4—the metal point in the lung organ

Liv4—metal point in the liver.

The LU5 was selected to reduce the connection between the kidneys and the lungs.

The LU4 was selected to increase the function of the lungs since it increases the function of the lungs' self-cycle.

Liv4 was selected to control the function of the liver. After ensuring the desired functioning of all the above points, the patient was sent home.

LU5 was administered on the right hand, LU4 was administered on the left hand and Liv4 was administered on the left leg.

Third Phase of Treatment

Statement of the Patient

The headaches were completely cured, had sound sleep, a very good appetite, no leg pain and menstruation had not started yet.

Doctor's Diagnosis Based on the Six Element Pulse Diagnosis Method.

R

M(\)	E(/)	IIF(✓)
\	/	✓

L

IF(✓)	Wo(I)	Wa(−)
✓	I	−

The water element was in excess.

There was no connection between the kidneys, the heart and the pericardium.

The points selected for the third phase treatment.

K2—first fire point in the kidney organ

K3—second fire point in the kidney organ

UB60—first fire point in the urinary bladder organ

H9—wood point in the heart organ

Si3—wood point in the small intestine organ

P9—wood point in the pericardium organ

Tw3—wood point in the triple warmer organ

The heart and the pericardium points related to the kidney organ point had been selected because the heat energies in the kidney were not working properly. Moreover, when one kindles the heat energies of the urinary bladder, all the stagnant waste energies, which had to be eliminated would get eliminated.

Except for UB60, all the other points (K2, K3, H9, Si3, P9, Tw3) were applied on the left side of their respective tracks and the UB60 was applied on its right side track.

After ensuring all the energies were working properly the patient was sent home.

The statement of the Patient.

All the problems were completely cured. Menstruation had started on its own.

Doctor's Diagnosis Based on the Six Element Pulse Diagnosis Method.

R

M(\\)	E(/)	IIF(✓✓)
\\	/	✓✓

L

IF(✓)	Wo(I)	Wa(—)
✓	I	—

The water element pulse was functioning perfectly.

The patient had declared that all her problems and symptoms were cured completely. So, the doctor asked her to come back for a review after three months.

R

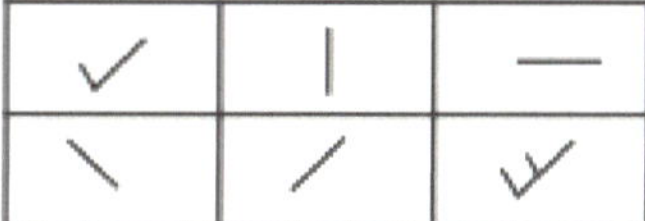

✓	I	—
\\	/	✓✓

L

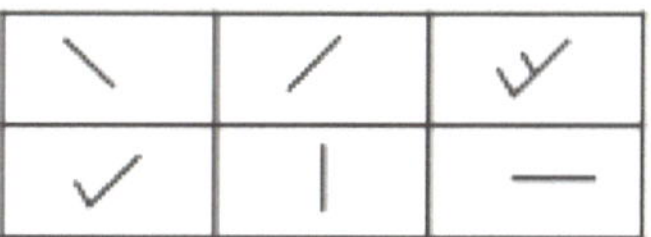

\\	/	✓✓
✓	I	—

Patient 2

Name : R. Rani

Age : 25

Address: Salem

Statement of the patient

Menstruation problems started at the onset of the menstrual cycle. The first menstruation occurred at the age of 10 years. White discharge is present. For the past 13 years, she has had headaches which affect the whole head and it hurts more at the back side of the head. Once or twice, every six months, along with the headache, the temperature would go high. She had a history of wheezing during the rainy season. There was occasional shortness of breath. Continuous nausea was present. She experienced itching in the elbow folds of both arms. She had lower abdomen pain and lumbar pain. She had constipation-related problems. Every time, after sexual intercourse, she would have hip pain, a burning sensation in the vagina and dark yellow urination. After two days of this, she would have the feeling of having a milky secretion. If she indulged in sexual intercourse the next day, then she would feel like passing stools during the act.

Doctor's Diagnosis Based on the Six Element Diagnosis Method

R

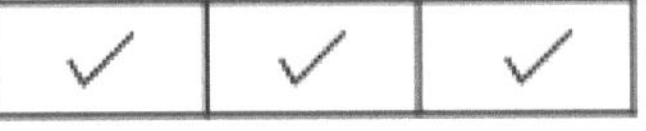

L

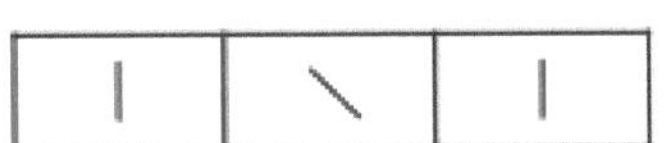

Through the Six Pulse Diagnosis method, it was diagnosed that the IF (first fire) element was working excessively.

First Phase of the Treatment

It was made sure by the Six Pulse Diagnosis method that because of the excessive function of the element, first fire, the first fire organs, namely, the heart and the small intestine were working excessively. The second fire element, which is linked with the first fire and its organs, namely, the pericardium and triple warmer were affected. Apart from this, the element metal (M) which must be controlled/or destroyed, had been affected. Hence, the metal organs, the lungs and the large intestines were also affected.

Next, the son element of fire, the earth was created excessively and the first fire function in the earth was also excessive. Because of this the water element which would get affected by the earth was completely destroyed and the water element's function shrunk.

All the above pulse and organ functions were diagnosed through the Six Element Pulse Diagnosis method. It was made sure that the patient had described the ailments related to the abovementioned affected organs.

It was also diagnosed whether the disease was chronic or acute, the state of the problems, the affected organs, etc.

Since the water element was destroyed, it was not enough to control the first fire element. So, it was decided to atrophy the first fire element and the first fire was made atrophy.

H7—the earth point in the heart organ

Sp3—the wood point in the spleen organ

R)

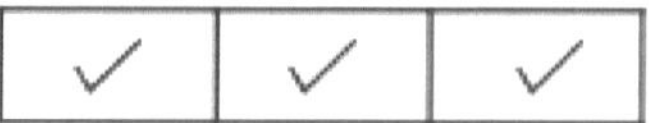

Lu9—the earth point in the lungs organ

L)

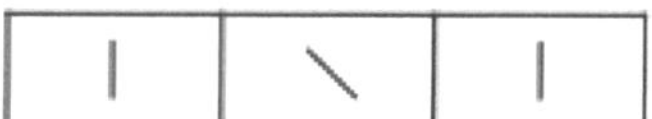

The H7, Sp3 and LU9 points were applied to the respective organs' energy tracks of the left hand and left leg.

H9—wood element point related to the heart organ

LU10—fire element point related to the lung organ

Sp2—fire element point related to the spleen organ

Si3—fire element point related to the small intestine organ

Li5—fire element point related to the large intestine organ

St41—fire element point related to the stomach organ.

All the above points were applied on the respective right side organs' energy tracks of the patient.

As soon as the treatment was over, the patient felt relieved of her problems. It was made sure that all the points were working as desired and the patient was sent home.

Second Phase of Treatment

Statement of the Patient

After the first phase of treatment, menstruation occurred. Nausea had stopped completely. The white discharge had reduced. Headaches, wheezing, lower abdomen pain and lumbar pain had reduced to a moderate level. All the problems that occurred after sexual intercourse had reduced to a moderate level. The feeling of passing stools during the second day of sexual intercourse and the feeling of secret in milk from the breasts had not reduced.

The water and the wood element energies were very less.

R)

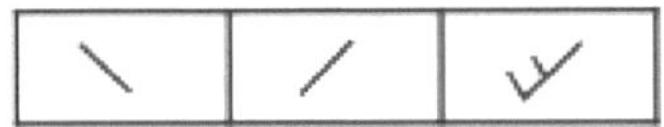

L)

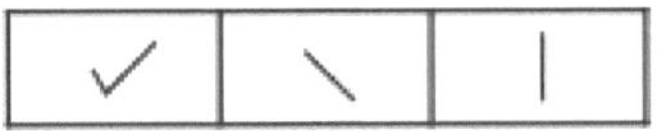

Since the water and wood elements' energies were very less, it was diagnosed through the pulse that there was no link between the fire and water elements and there was no link between the wood and earth elements. The above diagnosis was made sure by the statement of the patient. It was also diagnosed that the link between the lungs and the kidneys was not properly developed.

The Details of the Points Selected During the Second Phase of Treatment

K7—metal point related to the organ, the lungs

K10—water point related to the organ, the lungs

H3—water point related to the organ, the heart

P3—water point related to the pericardium

Liv8—water point related to the liver

All the above points were administered on the left side of the respective energy tracks.

K3—earth point related to the organ, the kidneys

K1—water point related to the organ, the kidneys

Liv4—metal point related to the organ, the liver

Ub54—earth point related to the organ, the kidneys

All the above points were administered on the right side of the respective energy tracks.

After the treatment, the pulse pattern of the patient was checked immediately and ensured that the desired results were gained by the patient. The patient also said that all her symptoms had reduced. She was sent back home.

Third Phase of Treatment

Statement of the Patient

After 10 days from the second phase of treatment, menstruation started with lower abdominal pain. A white-coloured cyst had got discharged during menstruation. The menstrual cycle lasted for five days. During this cycle, there was no abdominal pain or back pain. The white discharge had almost stopped and if it occurred, it was very mild. All the problems that occurred after sexual intercourse had vanished. Headaches stopped. The feeling of passing stools during the second day of sexual intercourse had minimised. The feeling of secreting milk from the breasts stopped. The itching in the inner elbow had minimised.

Doctor's Diagnosis Based on the Six Element Pulse Diagnosis Method.

R

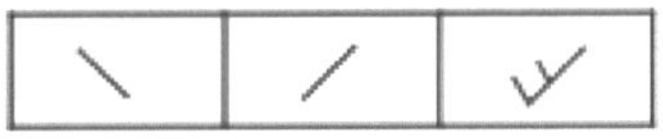

╲	╱	✓╱

L

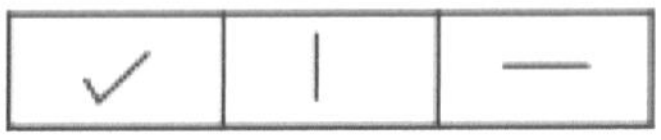

✓	|	—

Six Element Pulse Diagnosis

R

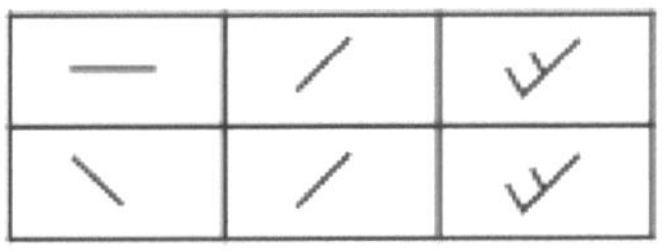

—	╱	✓╱
╲	╱	✓╱

L

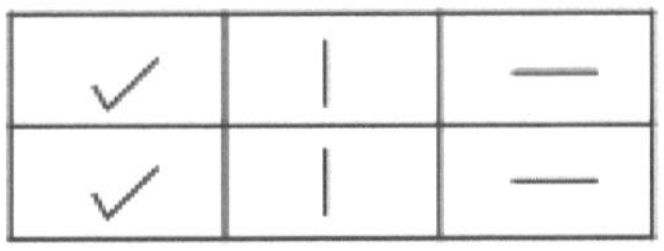

✓	|	—
✓	|	—

(12 organs pulse)

It was diagnosed that the water element and wood element were working less.

There was no link between the earth and wood elements because the wood and water elements were less working.

Points Selected for the Treatment

L12—Large intestine-related water point

UB67—kidney-related metal point

These two points were applied on the right side of the patient on the respective tracks.

ST43—stomach-related wood point

GB34—gallbladder-related earth point

Tw2—triplewarmer-related water point

UB61—urinary bladder-related second fire point

LI5—large intestine-related first fire point

Si1—small intestine-related metal point

All these points were applied on the left side in their respective energy tracks.

After ensuring that all the above-mentioned right side and left side pulses were working as desired, the patient was sent back.

Fourth Phase Treatment

Statement of the Patient

The headache had relapsed. The white discharge had started. Itching and pain in the elbow had started. If she indulge in sexual intercourse for two days continuously, the feeling of passing stools was still there.

Doctor's Diagnosis Based on the Six Element Pulse Diagnosis Method.

Though the treated pulses were working, the first fire was still working excessively, as it was on the first day.

R

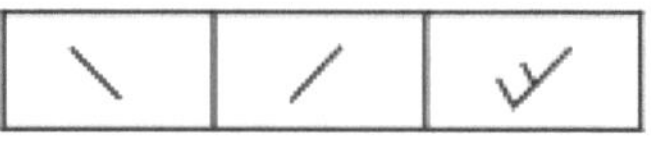

L

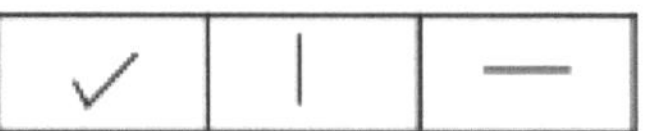

Six Element Pulse Diagnosis

R

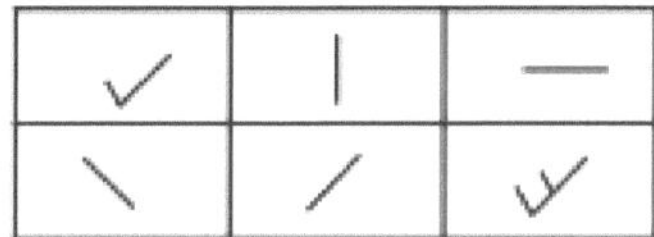

L

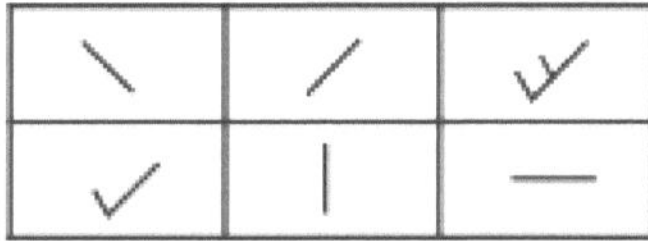

(12 organs)

Since the first fire element was working excessively, it consumed the wood element indirectly. Apart from this, the link between the water and fire had become very less. Hence, we had to connect the heart function with the liver and the kidneys. Also, the pericardium function had to be connected with the liver and the kidneys. The link between the heart and the pericardium had to be reduced.

Points Selected for the Treatment

Liv2.5—Liver-related first fire point

Liv2—Liver-related second fire point

K6—Kidney-related first fire point

K2—Kidney-related second fire point

H8—Pericardium-related second fire point

All the above points were applied on the left side of their respective channels.

P7.5—Pericardium-related first fire point

This point was applied on the right side of its energy channel.

It was verified that all the above pulses were working properly as desired. The patient had declared that the headache and itching with pain in the elbow had reduced to the maximum extent.

She was asked to come after three months for a follow-up.

Patient 3

Name : Manivannan

Age : 36

Address : Hasthampatti, Salem-7

Statement of the Patient

History of cold and phlegm from 1990, yearly thrice, the patient was affected by this problem. It would start either with the itching of the nose, throat irritation or bronchitis. The patient had chest pain on the left side for the past 10 days and constipation. There was a burning sensation in the area where it hurt (the chest). All the tests had been done to check the heart's function in the allopathy hospital and the results were negative.

Doctor's Diagnosis Based on the Six Elements Pulse Diagnosis Method

R

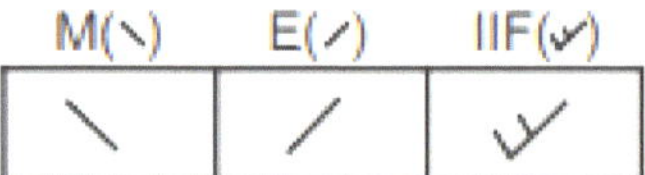

L

IF(✓)	Wo(I)	Wa(–)
✓	|	—

The water and the metal elements were working excessively

Based on the Pulse Diagnosis Method, it was diagnosed that the patient's lungs and kidneys were working excessively. The liver function has been affected because of the excessive function of the lungs and the heart. The pericardium was affected because of the excessive function of the kidneys. Apart from this, it was diagnosed that heat energy had accumulated in the liver and the spleen. Because of all these reasons, the patient was often affected by cold and pain, along with a burning sensation in the heart, etc.

There were three different angles, which were the starting symptoms of the patient's cold.

The cold would start after the itching sensation in the nose. This indicates that the element wood (Wo) is in excess in the kidneys.

The cold would start after the blocking feeling in the throat. This indicates that the element wood is in excess in the lungs.

The cold would start after the chest congestion. This indicates that the water (Wa) element is in excess in the heart and the pericardium.

(12 organ pulse)

R

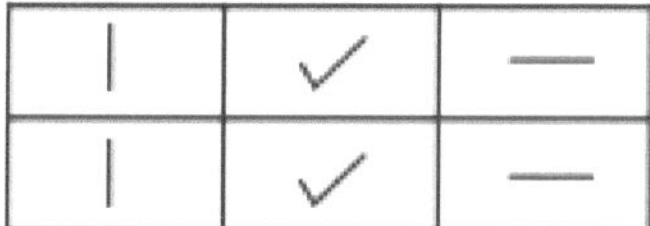

L

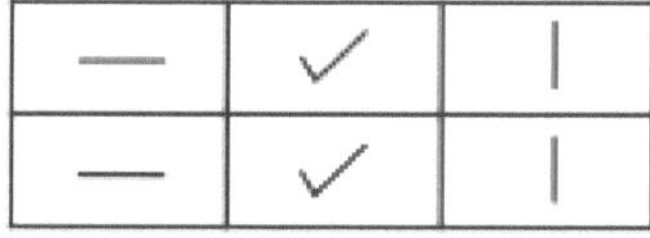

Details on the first day's treatment

LU 11—Lungs-related wood point

Li 3—Large intestine-related wood point

K 1—Kidney-related wood point

These five element points were selected on his right hand and leg. After the treatment, the pulse was checked for the desired actions and after ensuring the improvement of the patient by the Pulse Diagnosis Method, he was asked to go for that day.

Second Phase of the Treatment

(12 organ pulse)

R

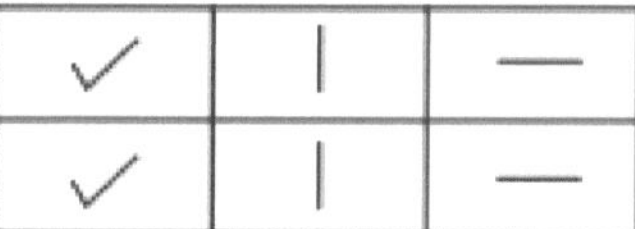

L

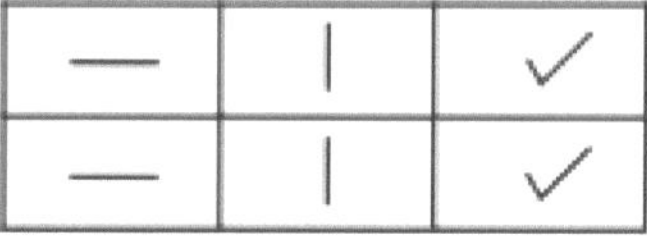

Statement of the Patient

The patient did not get affected by the cold. There was no constipation. There was no pain in the left chest but there was a heaviness in the left chest.

The Doctor's Diagnosis Based on the Six Elements Pulse Diagnosis Method

R

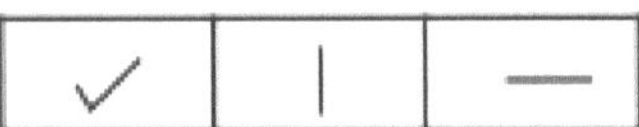

L

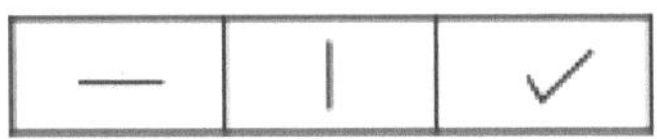

(Six Elements Pulse Diagnosis Method)

It was diagnosed that the water element (Wa) was working excessively.

The details on the point of selection during the second phase of treatment

H3—Heart-related water point

P3—Pericardium-related water point

K2—Kidneys-related second fire point

K6—Kidneys-related first fire point

The heart and the pericardium-related kidney water points were selected.

H3 and P3 were pointed on the right side.

In the same way, the kidney-related heart and pericardium fire points were selected. K2 and K6 were pointed on the left side.

After diagnosing the patient with the Pulse Diagnosis Method, and checking whether his pulses were working in the desired way, he was sent home.

Third Phase of Treatment

Constipation had occurred again. Instead of the pain, he had a heavy feeling in his chest.

R

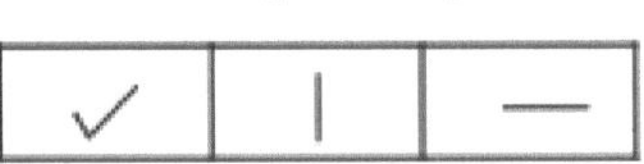

L

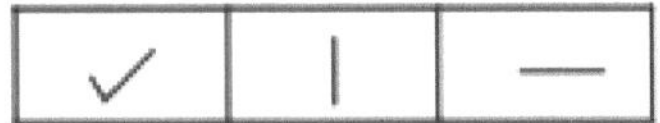

Six Elements Pulse Diagnosis Method

Based on the Six Element Pulse Diagnosis Method, it was diagnosed that all the energies were properly present in their respective places.

R

✓	|	—
✓	|	—

L

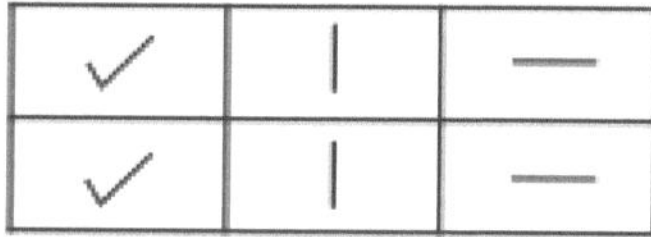

(12 Organs' Pulse)

The 12 Organ Pulse Diagnosis Method also ensured that all the energies were present in their places along with their opposite energies.

Since both the pulse diagnosis methods were indicating that the patient was completely cured, he was asked to come after three months for a review.

(Since the five elements' functional cycles are linked with the four seasons and their cycles, I requested the patient to come after three months.)

R

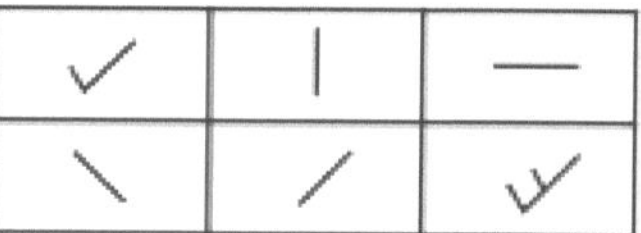

L

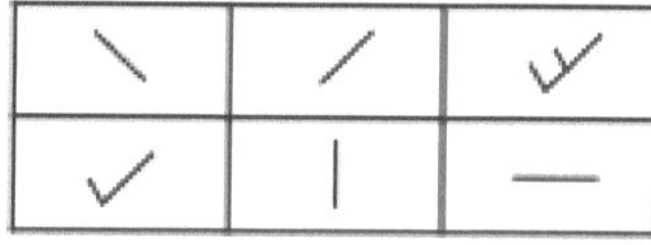

Patient 4

Name : Ashwin

Age : 12

Address : Salem

Statement of the Patient

H/O headache, cold, cough and fever from the first standard, had allopathy and homoeopathy medicines for the above-mentioned problems. While studying in the third standard, all the above-mentioned problems worsened, along with vomiting. After this, the cough never stopped but continued for three to four months. If he ate legumes, such as beans or red beans with their outer skin after cooking them, the patient would vomit after a while. When vomit occurred, only the skin would come out but no food eaten along with the legume's skin would come out with the vomit. If he had a cough, it would continue for three to four hours till he became totally tired and fainted. Then the cough would stop. The patient had gone to all the schools of medicine but could not get a permanent remedy. He was not eating properly.

Doctor's Diagnosis Based on the Six Element Pulse Diagnosis Method

Six Elements Pulse Diagnosis Method

R

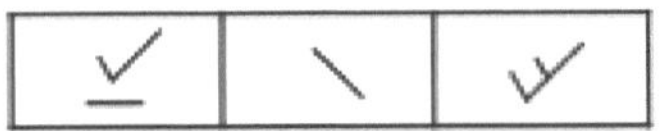

L

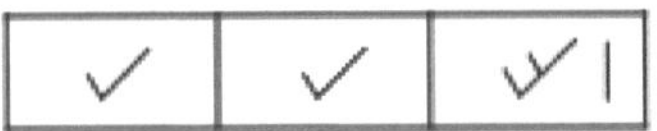

It was diagnosed that the first fire (I) and the second fire ()were in excess.

When this boy was brought to me, he was very sick and was in a serious condition. The function of his liver, spleen, lungs and kidneys was severely damaged. Because of this, he did not have proper immunity, proper breathing energy or proper life energy. It took four years to cure this boy and his parents brought him without breaking down. During these four years, his condition became fatal because of his continuous cough for hours.

It was diagnosed that the heart, the small intestine, the pericardium and the triple warmer were working excessively. Because of this, the boy was affected by hot and cold diseases. The disease also worsened because of the psychosomatic state of the boy. Hence, the disease was worsening or sober, based on his mind.

The details on the points selected for the first phase of treatment:

LU10—I fire ( ) **lungs-related fire point**

K6—II fire ( ) **kidneys-related fire point**

These two points were applied on the respective energy channels of the right side.

H8—I fire ( ) **heart-related fire point**

P8—II fire ( ) **pericardium-related second fire point**

These two points were also applied on the right side of the respective channels.

Apart from these, it was diagnosed that there was no energy link between the heart and pericardium of the patient. This state had affected the earth element and the related organs, the stomach and the spleen. Because of this, the patient could not tolerate any food and the food was creating problems. All the above-mentioned problems of the patient were diagnosed through the Six Element Pulse Diagnosis Method.

Second Phase of Treatment

Statement of the Patient

The fever had become normal. Coughing and vomiting had reduced. Eating habits had not changed.

Doctor's Diagnosis Based on the Six Elements Pulse Diagnosis Method.

R

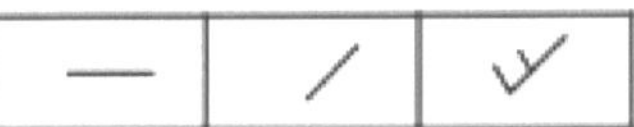

L

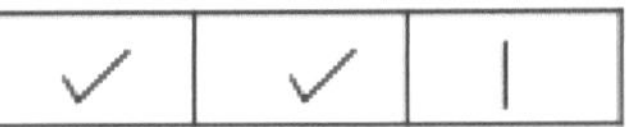

(Six Pulse Element Diagnosis Method)

R

—	/	✓
—	/	✓

L

✓	✓	|
✓	✓	|

(Twelve Organ Pulse Diagnosis Method)

It was diagnosed that the first and second fire elements were working excessively.

First, the link between the heart and the pericardium was created.

The points selected for the second phase of treatment were:

H8—II fire, Heart-related fire point

P7.5—I fire, Pericardium-related fire point

Both these points were selected on the left side of the respective energy channels.

A link between the heart, the pericardium, the spleen and the stomach was created. All these points were applied on the left side of the respective energy channels.

Sp1—I fire ( ) spleen-related fire point

Sp2—II fire ( ) spleen-related fire point

H7—Earth ( ) heart-related earth point

P7—Earth ( ) pericardium-related earth point

S741—I fire ( ) stomach-related fire point

S742—II fire ( ) stomach-related second fire point

All these points were applied and checked. After the desired functioning of these points, the patient was sent.

Third Phase of Treatment

Statement of the patient: Fever affects one at intervals. Coughing and vomiting occur rarely and food intake has improved. The patient had body pain.

Doctor's Diagnosis Based on the Six Element Pulse Diagnosis Method

R

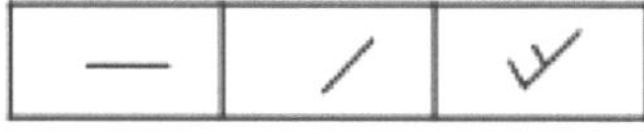

L

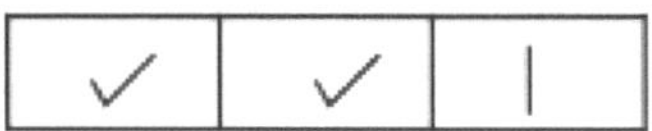

(Six Elements Pulse Diagnosis Method)

R

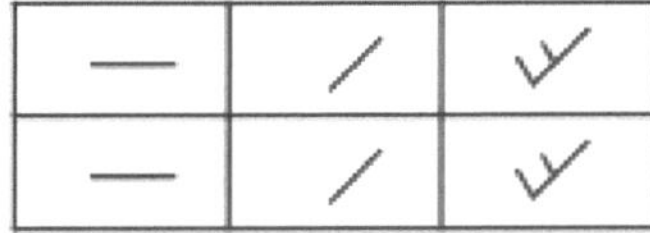

L

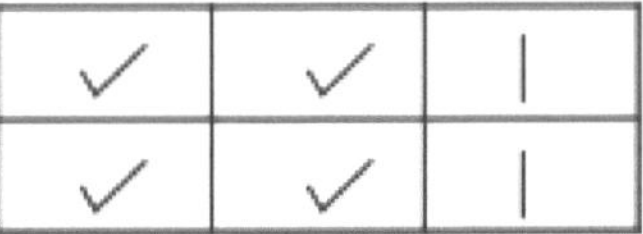

(12 Organs Pulse)

It was diagnosed that the functions of the heart, the pericardium and the spleen had improved. But there was no improvement in the functions of the lungs, the kidneys and the liver.

Details on the points selected for treatment

Lu9—Earth ( ) lungs-related earth point

Lu8—Metal ( ) lungs-related metal point

K7—Metal ( ) Kidneys-related metal point

K10—Water ( ) Kidneys-related water point

To connect the energies between the liver and the pericardium, two more points were selected.

Liv2—II fire ( ) Liver-related second fire point

P9—wood ( ) Pericardium-related wood point

All these points were selected on the left side of the patient in their respective energy channels.

All these points were checked and ensured that they were working as desired and the patient was sent.

Fourth Phase of Treatment

Statement of the Patient

The fever occurred only once. The cough occurred only twice and existed only for a few minutes. Cold was on and off. Food intake has improved. Body pain has reduced.

Doctor's Diagnosis Based on the Six Element Pulse Diagnosis Method

R

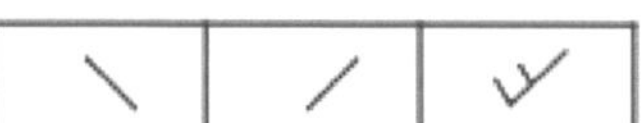

L

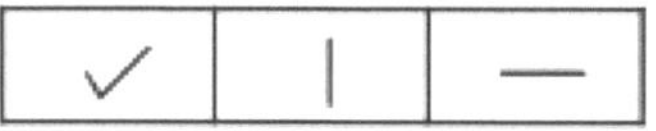

(Six Element Pulse Diagnosis)

R

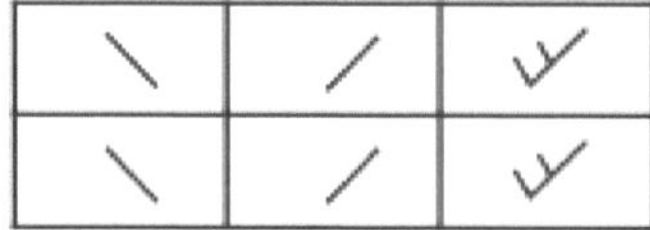

L

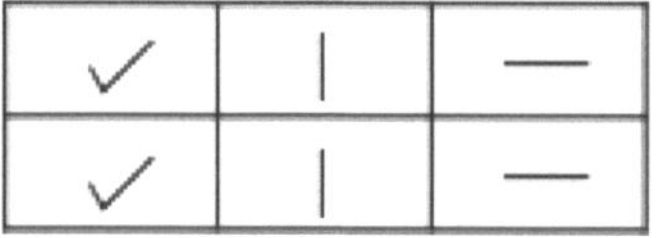

(12 Organs Pulse)

The problems between the liver, the spleen, the gallbladder and the stomach were diagnosed.

The points selected for the treatment were:

Sp1—spleen-related wood point

Liv3—liver-related earth point

St43—stomach-related wood point

Gb34—Gallbladder-related earth point

All these points were applied on the left side of the patient in their respective energy channels. After ensuring the working of the points, the patient was sent home.

Fifth Phase of Treatment

Statement of the Patient

The fever stopped totally. The cough occurred only once. Body pain and cold affect the patient at intervals.

Doctor's Diagnosis Based on the Six Element Pulse Diagnosis Method

R

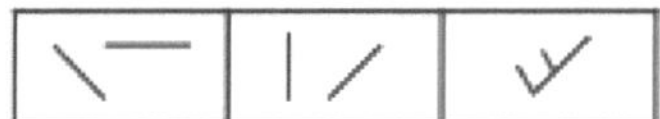

L

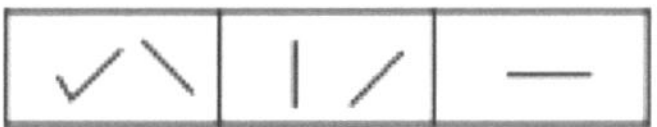

(Six Element Pulse Diagnosis)

R

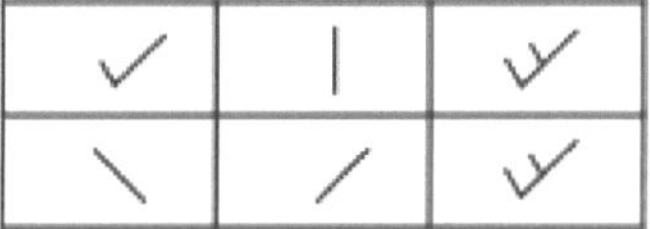

L

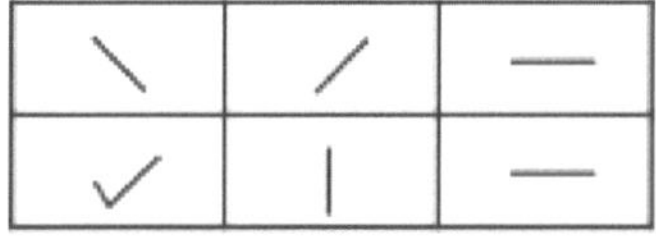

(12 Organs Pulse)

It was diagnosed that there were problems between the spleen and the kidneys, the pericardium and the kidneys.

Points selected to treat the patient were

St44—stomach-related water point

Sp9—spleen-related water point

P3—pericardium-related water point

Tw2—triple warmer-related water point

Ub59—urinary bladder-related water point.

K3—kidney-related water point

Ub61—urinary bladder-related second fire point

K2—kidney-related fire point

All the above points were applied on the left side of the patient in the respective energy channels and their functions were ensured. Later the patient was sent back home.

The treatment had to be continued for this boy, again and again, for the next three years. After that, he was completely cured. He comes for further check-ups once in three to six months.

PATIENT 5

Name : Divya

Age : 20 years

Address : Mettur dam

Statement of the Patient

History of Tuberculosis and other lung-related diseases, H/O epilepsy. Due to these problems, she had a fever and cold often. She was advised to be hospitalised as well as treated and she was told that her conditions are fatal. Suction was advised to implement the removal of phlegm from her lungs. The patient could not stand, walk or talk. She had oedema in her entire body. Her legs and hands were swollen.

Doctor's Diagnosis Based on the Six Element Pulse Diagnosis Method

(Six Element Pulse Diagnosis)

R

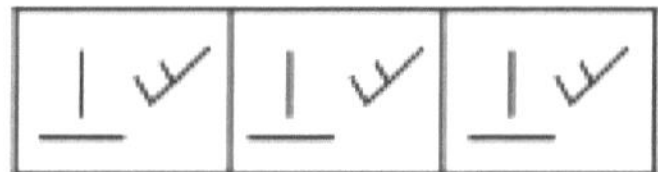

L

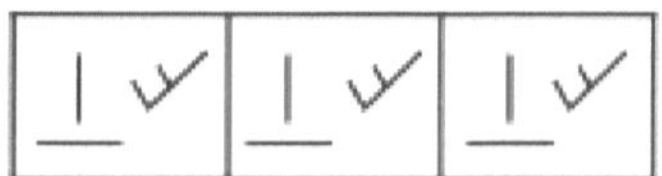

It was diagnosed that throughout the body, wood, water and second fire energies were excessive (all over the body).

This indicated that her kidneys, liver, gallbladder and pericardium functions were very excessive. Because of the excessive function of the liver and the gallbladder, such spleen and stomach-related diseases occurred. Because of the fewer energy levels of the spleen, the lungs could not receive enough energy. This caused lung-related diseases. Since the spleen's energy and function became less, the kidneys and urinary bladder functions became excessive. Because of this, the functions of the heart and the small intestines became less. Apart from this, the function of the parallel organ, the pericardium was working excessively.

It was diagnosed that the wastes of the body, which had to be excreted by the kidneys could not be excreted. Hence, the body started to eliminate them through the lungs as phlegm. Since the lungs also failed to eliminate the wastes, they started to get deposited in the lungs. This caused serious/fatal conditions.

First Phase of Treatment

First, the points which would help the patient to eliminate the wastes from the kidneys and the lungs were selected and applied on the right side of the patient in their respective energy channels.

R

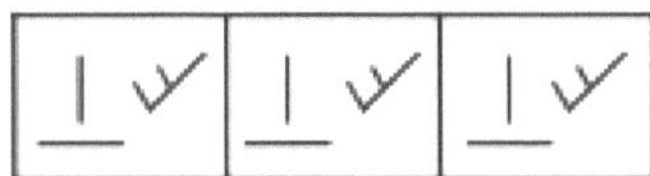

L

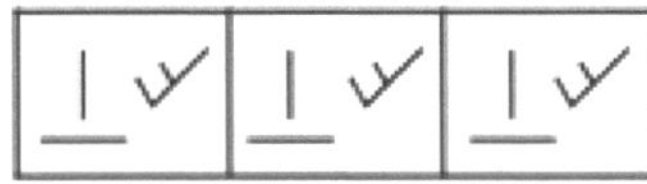

K10—**kidney-related water point**

Ub60—**urinary bladder-related water point**

Lu5—**lung-related water point**

All these three points were applied on the right side of the patient in their respective channels.

After ensuring the working of the applied points through the Six Element Pulse Diagnosis Method, the patient was sent home.

Second Phase of Treatment

Statement of the Patient

Had excessive urine excretion and sputum, after which the oedema was reduced. The patient is now able to stand, walk and talk to some extent.

Doctor's Diagnosis Based on the Six Elements Pulse Diagnosis Method

R

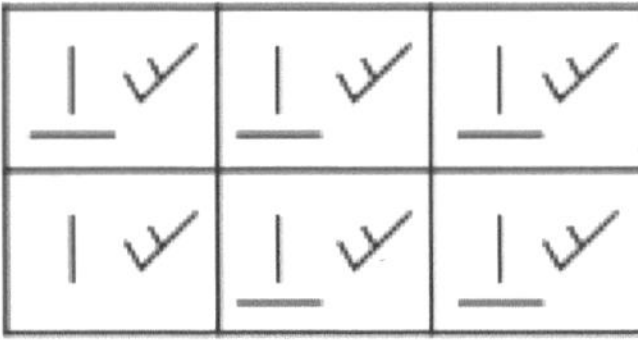

L

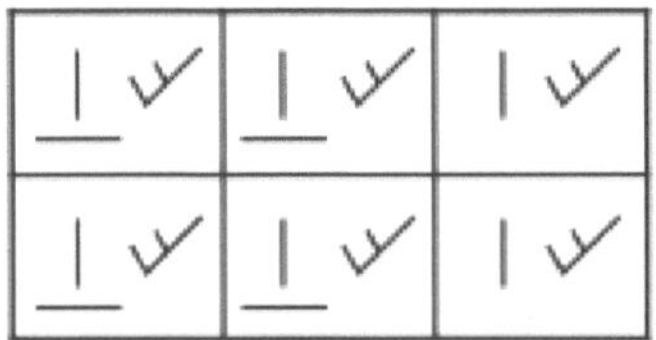

(12 Organs Pulse)

It was diagnosed through the Six Element Pulse Diagnosis Method that the water had been eliminated from the lungs and the kidneys. The previous treatment had brought good results for the patient.

In the second phase of the treatment, the points were selected to eliminate the stagnant water in the large intestine, the stomach and the heart. Also, points were selected to reduce the functions of the triple warmer and the pericardium.

Details on the points selected

Sp9—spleen-related water point

St44—stomach-related water point

Li2—large intestine-related water point

H3—heart-related water point

P3—pericardium-related water point

P8—pericardium-related second fire point

Tw5—triple warmer-related second fire point

All these points were selected and applied on the right side of the patient in their respective energy channels.

Third Phase of Treatment

Statement of the Patient

The patient vomited thrice, which contained mucus, had Diarrhoea six or seven times, which also contained mucus and water, sputum was discharged through the nose too, the oedema of the whole body had vanished and the patient could breathe without difficulties.

Now the hunger feeling had improved and the difficulties in walking and talking had reduced. Fatigue had reduced by 75%.

Doctor's Diagnosis Based on the Six Element Pulse Diagnosis Method

(Six Element Pulse Diagnosis)

R

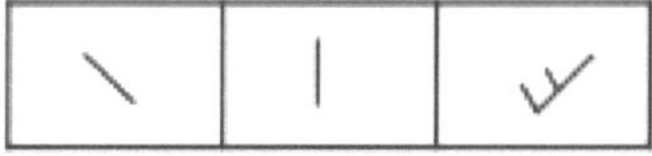

L

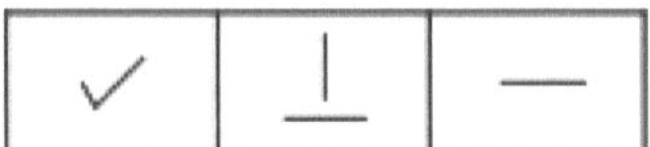

Water and the Wood Pulses Are High (12 Organs Pulse)

R

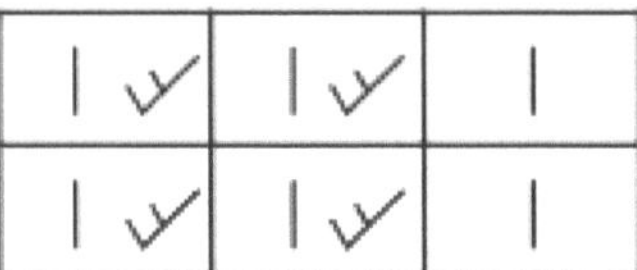

L

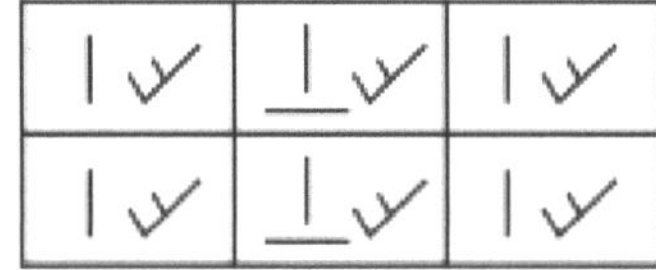

It was diagnosed that water energy was stagnant in the liver and gallbladder organs, and the energies from the kidneys were excessively transferred to the liver.

Details on the Points Selected

K1—kidney-related wood point

Ub65—urinary bladder-related wood point

Sp1—spleen-related wood point

St43—stomach-related wood point

Lu11—lungs-related wood point

Li1—large intestine-related wood point

All the above points were selected and applied on the right side of the patient in their respective energy channels.

Sp3—spleen-related wood point

St36—stomach-related earth point

K3—kidney-related earth point

The above three points were selected and applied on the left side of the patient in their respective energy channels.

All the points were checked through the Six Elements Pulse Diagnosis Method to ensure their proper functioning and after that, the patient was sent home.

Fourth Phase Treatment

Statement of the Patient

The patient could eat normally. She had no problems in standing, walking and talking. She had no problem in breathing. The phlegm had reduced to a maximum level. She neither vomited nor had diarrhoea.

Doctor's Diagnosis Based on the Six Element Pulse Diagnosis Method

R

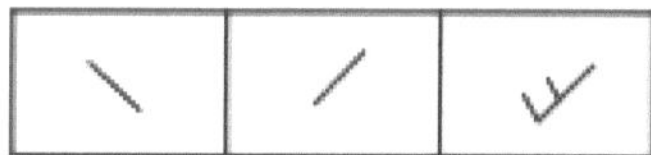

L

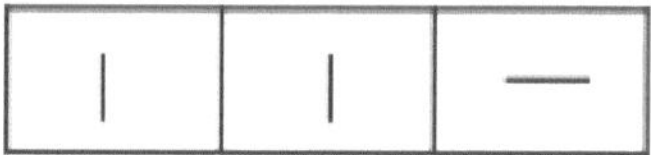

Water and wood pulses were in excess**(12 Organs Pulse)**

R

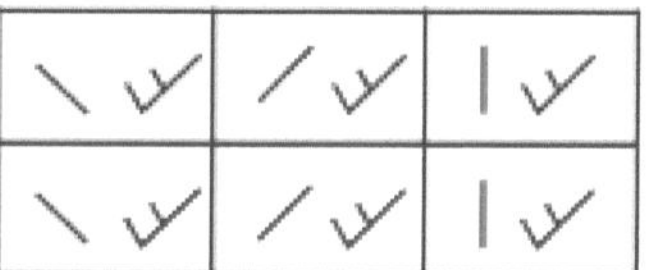

L

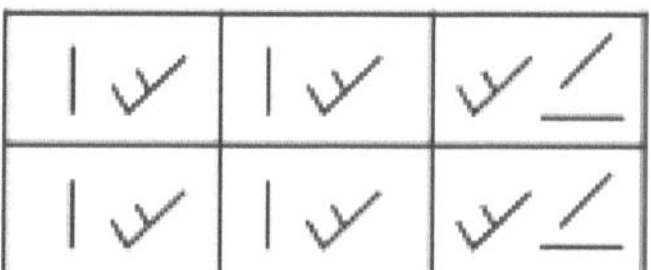

Through the Pulse Diagnosis Method, it was diagnosed clearly that the function of the pericardium was in excess and the energy of the liver was in excess in the heart and the pericardium.

Details on the points selected

H9—heart-related wood point

Si3—small intestine-related wood point

P9—pericardium-related wood point

Tw3—triple warmer-related wood point

K8—kidney-related second fire point

P7.5—pericardium-related first fire point

All the above points were selected and applied on the right side of the patient in their respective energy channels.

H8.5—heart-related first fire point

This point was selected and applied on the left side of the patient in its respective channel.

After ensuring the functions of the applied points towards the desired functions, through the Six Elements Pulse Diagnosis Method, the patient was sent home.

Fifth Phase of Treatment

Statement of the Patient

All the problems which were present on the first day were not there. Sputum was discharged rarely.

R

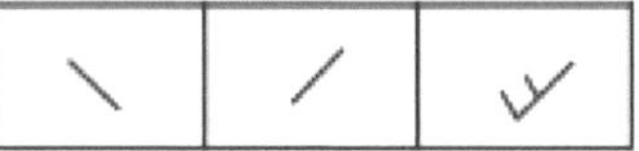

L

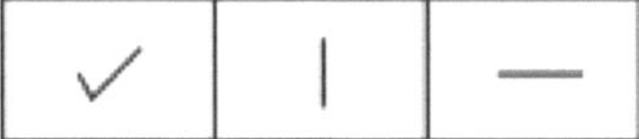

(Six Elements Pulse Diagnosis)

R

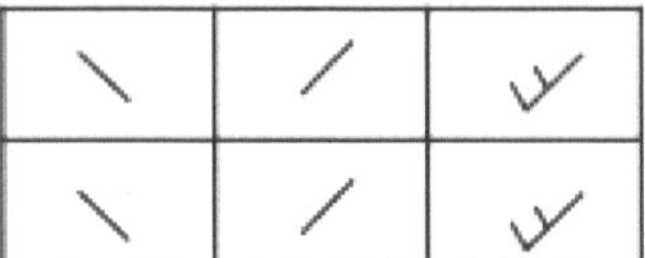

L

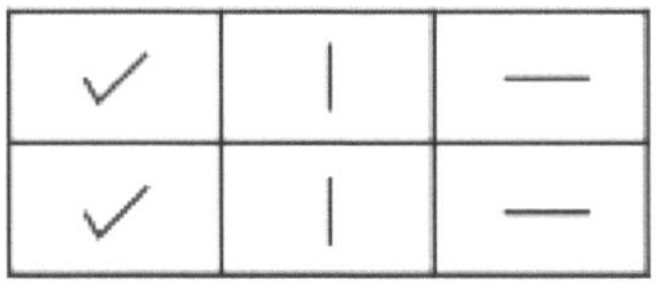

(12 Organ Pulse Diagnosis)

All the pulses and their states of functions were working normally. The control cycle of their energies and their opposite energies were made properly and the patient was sent home.

Details on the points selected

Li5—large intestine-related first fire

Si1—small intestine-related metal point

St43—stomach-related wood point

Gb43—gallbladder-related earth point

Tw2—triple warmer-related water point

Ub61—urinary bladder-related fire point

All the above points were selected and applied on the left side of the patient on the relevant energy channels.

After ensuring the desired functions of the energies, through the Pulse Diagnosis Method, the patient was sent back. The patient was advised to come for a re-check-up after three months.

Patient 6

Name : R. Divya

Age :15

Gender : Female

Address : Tiruchengode

This patient was a type 1 diabetic patient.

Details on the diagnosis through the *Panchaboodha* Treatment
Juvenile Diabetes/type 1 Diabetes

Statement of the Patient

She had H/O Polyuria from childhood. She was diagnosed with diabetes mellitus and excess urea in the blood after fainting in the restroom.

She was using two types of insulin injections for the past eight years. Per day, 45 units of insulin were used. For the past six months, along with insulin injections, she was taking three tablets for diabetes mellitus per day.

She gets headaches and burning of the eyes if the glucose level goes up or down.

She gets stomach pain twice a month.

When the glucose level goes up, she vomits and feels dizzy. She also feels excessively hungry.

When the glucose level goes down, she gets seizures. She was affected like this often.

Doctor's Diagnosis of the Patient Based on the Six Elements Pulse Diagnosis Method

It was diagnosed that the water energy and the lower left energy cycle were working excessively. Her kidneys were affected severely. Because of this, the upper right energy cycle and the metal energy were not working. Hence her disease was not under control and had become worse day by day.

First Phase of Treatment

All the points related to water and the lower side left energies were selected and applied to reduce these energies. After continuous treatment for a month, her glucose level in the blood started to reduce gradually. Her fasting glucose level was 450 mg. This too started to reduce gradually. The insulin intake had been reduced to 25 units per day from 45 units per day.

Second Phase of Treatment

It was diagnosed that the wood element was working excessively. To reduce it, the relevant points on the wood channel and the first fire channel were applied. During this session of 15 days of continuous treatment, her insulin intake was reduced to 15 units from 25 units per day. All the diabetes tablets were stopped as her body was recovering.

Third Phase of Treatment

It was diagnosed through the Six Elements Pulse Diagnosis Method that the wood element, along with the left side upper energy cycle were working excessively. To reduce these energies, the points were selected on the relevant channels. During this phase of the treatment, the insulin intake was reduced to eight units from the fifteen units of injections per day. After fifteen days of treatment, the eight units of insulin were stopped totally and the patient was treated without medicines for diabetes.

Later, she was advised to administer five units of insulin per day. She was advised to continue the treatment for a year.

She was continuing the treatment with only five units of insulin and even after six months, she did not need more medicines than five units of insulin.

She completely got rid of headaches, stomach pain, vomiting, dizziness, seizures and all the symptoms.

Note

The amount of insulin she was taking before treatment was:

Per day : 45 units

Per week : 45x7=315 units

Per month : 1395 units

Per year : 16, 470 units

The amount of insulin after treatment was

Per day : 5 units

Per week : 5x7= 35 units

Per month :5x30=150 units

Per year : 150x12=1800 units

Patient 7

Name : **Balakrishnan**

Age : **32**

Gender : **male**

Marital status : **married**

Occupation : **software engineer**

Address : **Trichy**

Details on the diagnosis through the *Panchaboodha* Treatment

Juvenile Diabetes/type 1 Diabetes

Statement of the Patient

H/O type 1 diabetes mellitus. He was diagnosed with type 1 diabetes mellitus after he met with an accident eight years before, at the age of 24 years. He was advised to take insulin injections immediately after diagnosis.

He was taking twenty-five units of insulin in the morning, fifteen units of insulin in the noon, fifteen units of insulin before dinner and twenty-five units after dinner—a total of eighty units of insulin.

Doctor's Diagnosis Based on the Six Elements Pulse Diagnosis Method

It was diagnosed that the wood and water elements were working excessively in this patient. This indicated that his problems are chronic.

First Phase of Treatment

The patient did not take all eighty units of insulin on the first day of ***Panchaboodha*** treatment. On the first day, before treatment, the glucose level of this patient in the random test was 342 mg, which had been reduced to 234 mg after treatment. A total of 100mg of glucose had reduced after the treatment on the first day. His HBA1C test on the first day of treatment was 266mg before treatment.

Second Phase of Treatment

The patient was taking eighty units of insulin from 6-7-2014 to 11-7-2014. From eighty units, his insulin intake has been reduced to seventy-six units. From that day, every day, five units were reduced per day. Hence, for six days ,thirty units of insulin had been reduced.

When his pulse patterns were diagnosed, it was found that the earth and wood elements of the lower side right and left cycles were working excessively. Accordingly, the treatment was given and his energies were balanced. On 12-7-2014, the total units of insulin intake had been stopped and he was under the ***Panchaboodha*** treatment for the whole day.

Without insulin, his glucose level was reduced from 152 mg to 123 mg.

Third Phase of Treatment

The patient was advised to take only seventy-five units and from that level, he was asked to reduce five units per day from 13-7-2014 to 18-7-2014.

It was diagnosed on 19-7-2014 that the earth and the wood elements were working in excess in the upper right and left side energy cycles.

His intake of insulin was totally stopped on 19-7-2014 and the ***Panchaboodha*** treatment was given for the whole day.(same day)

At the end of the treatment on 19-7-2014, his glucose level had come down from 360mg to 190 mg.

Fourth Phase of Treatment

The patient was asked to reduce the insulin from seventy-five units to sixty units, from 20-7-2014 to 26-7-2014

From that level, he was advised to reduce ten units per day for six days, which gradually decreased the amount of insulin.

On 26-7-2014,a total of 60 units of insulin intake had been completely stopped.

It was diagnosed on 26-7-2014that the wood element was in excess.

He was treated to balance the wood element on that day without insulin.

At the end of the day, his glucose level was reduced to 133mg from 230 mg.

Fifth Phase of Treatment

The patient was advised to take fifty units from 27-7-2014.

He was asked to reduce furthermore 8.3 units from fifty units for another six days till 1-8-2014.

On 2-8-2014, it was diagnosed that the earth element was in excess in his body. To balance this earth element, along with other elements, treatment was given.

On 2-8-2014, the insulin, of fifty units, was totally stopped before giving the ***Panchaboodha*** treatment.

At the end of the day, on 2-8-2014, his glucose level was reduced from 313mg to 180mg.

Sixth Phase of the Treatment

The patient was advised to take only forty-two units of insulin instead of 50, from 3-8-2014.

He was also advised to reduce eight units of insulin per day till 7-8-2014 (for four days). Thus on 7-8-2014, the total intake of insulin was thirty-two units.

On 7-8-2014, the insulin units were reduced to twenty-seven units from thirty-two units.

After the treatment, the patient was advised to take only five units of insulin during the night on 7-8-2014 and 8-8-2014.

On 9-8-2014 the insulin was stopped totally.

On 7-8-2014, the glucose level was reduced to 157mg from 250 mg.

On 8-8-2014, the glucose level was reduced to 152mg from 246 mg.

On 9-8-2014, the glucose level was reduced to 137mg from 244mg.

From 10-8-2014, The patient was advised to take only fifteen units of insulin.

Seventh Phase of Treatment

The patient was taking only fifteen units of insulin from 10-8-2014 to 14-8-2014.

On 15-8-2014, he was advised to take only five units of insulin and had undergone the ***Panchaboodha*** treatment.

His insulin was totally stopped on 16-8-2014.

He was advised to take only ten units of insulin from 17-8-2014 to 28-8-2014.

His insulin intake has been reduced to 300 mg per month(10x30=300) against his previous insulin intake of 2400 mg per month (80x30=2400).

He was advised to come for treatment for three months during which his glucose level would be made normal and his diabetic conditions would be cured.

His glucose levels were maintained steady and low with the ten units of insulin compared to the levels with the previous intake of eighty units of insulin.

He has been advised to maintain records of his food-intake timing and glucose levels after one and a half hours of eating, along with the diet chart.

On 5-7-2014, when the patient came for the treatment, his HBA1C was 9.57%, which is 266 mg on average with eighty units of insulin.

On 15-10-2014, after the *Panchaboodha* treatment, his HBA1C was 8.0%, that is, 192mg on average with ten units of insulin.

Patient 8

Name : **Mrs. Pankajam**

Age : **62 years**

Marital status : **Married**

Occupation :**Retired, from the government's child development department.**

Address : **Salem-7.**

Details on the diagnosis through the *Panchaboodha* Treatment

Diabetic Mellitus and High blood pressure.

History of the Patient

Diabetic for the last 15 years.

Had removed her uterus in the year 2009.

After the surgery, she could not sit on the floor with her legs folded.

Legs felt very soft like foam.

She used to take tablets for diabetes in the morning and at night. From August 2013, for a month, she took twenty-five units of insulin because of the increase in her glucose level. (Human Mixtard—Buphasic Bophane). Along with that, she took tablets thrice a day. (Volix m3, and Trajentamet) She took 20 units of insulin in the evening.

She felt fatigued.

She had H/O high blood pressure and took the tablet, (Eritel) for more than 20 years, in the morning only.

Statement of the Patient on 9-9-2013

She could not stand. She felt dizzy, very weak in her limbs and could not move without help.

She could not eat and had nausea.

All these symptoms were present for one and a half months after starting insulin.

She was advised to continue all the medicines along with insulin.

Doctor's Diagnosis Based on the *Panchaboodha* Pulse Diagnosis Method

It was diagnosed that the element, wood was working excessively. Among the four pulses, the lower right-side pulse alone was working excessively.

First Phase of Treatment

Because the wood element was working excessively, the patient would have excessive stagnation of bile and carbon energies. This had created indigestion and vomiting.

Because of the above-stated problems, the patient experienced dizziness, fatigue, tiredness, could not walk, etc.

Her blood glucose level had high fluctuation.

Since the lower right-side energy cycle alone was working, she could only lie down and this cycling would allow her to neither stand nor walk.

After the treatment on the first day, for about twenty minutes, her glucose level had come down and her high blood pressure was under control. She walked back alone without anybody's support after the treatment.

Improvement status of the patient from 9-9-2013 to 14-9-2013:

On 10-9-2013, five units of insulin dose were reduced. She had only 20 units of insulin. Her blood glucose level on that day was 175 mg before treatment and 146mg after treatment. Her high blood pressure was under control. She had diabetic tablets thrice daily.

On 11-9-2013, the insulin taken by her was fifteen units—ten units of insulin had been reduced. Her blood glucose level was 126mg. Her B.P. was under control. She had diabetic tablets thrice daily.

On 12-9-2013, she had only five units of insulin. On 12-9-2013, a total of twenty units of insulin was reduced. Her blood glucose level was 152mg before treatment and got reduced to 119mg after treatment. Her B.P. was normal. She had taken one tablet for B.P., in the morning and diabetic tablets thrice on that day.

On 13-9-2013, her total insulin intake had been stopped—that is, a total of twenty-five units of insulin had been stopped. Her blood glucose level on that day was 170mg and she had taken one tablet for high blood pressure and diabetic tablets thrice daily.

On 14-9-2013, she stopped taking insulin totally and her blood glucose level on that day was 182mg, which came down to 146mg after treatment. She had taken tablets for high blood pressure in the morning and diabetic tablets thrice daily.

After that, she was advised to reduce her diabetic tablets gradually, such as from three to two, and then from two to one and a half.

In this way, she was under treatment for three months, with tablets gradually reduced at each time of the day, that is, first at night and then, during the day.

She was advised to take her tablets for high blood pressure on alternative days instead of daily. Her blood pressure was monitored and it was made sure that it was under control and normal.

After reducing the diabetic tablets gradually, her diabetic conditions were checked and she was advised to take one tablet in the morning and one at night.

She was also advised to continue the ***Panchaboodha*** treatment for three months and to stop the medicines totally.

PATIENT 9

Name : **Sabari**

Age :**29 years**

Gender : **Female**

Marital status : **married**

Address : **Coimbatore**

Details on the diagnosis through the *Panchaboodha* Treatment
Obesity, Allergic conditions, Asthma, Breathing problems.

Statement of the Patient

- Allergy
- Wheezing
- Obesity

Doctor's Diagnosis Based on the *Panchaboodha* Pulse Diagnosis Method.

It was diagnosed that the patient had an excess of the element, earth. It was also diagnosed that the lower and upper left-side energy cycles were working only. These imbalances created the above-stated symptoms.

First Phase of Treatment

The points were selected to reduce the element, earth. Apart from this, the lower and upper left-side energy points were selected and applied to balance those cycles. She was given treatment continuously for five days and then once a fortnight for three months. Her weight had reduced to 85.5kgs from 89kgs.

Second Phase of Treatment

She was treated for ten days continuously. It was diagnosed that the wood element was linked to the earth element. The points were selected and applied to reduce both the earth and wood elements. Because of this, her weight had reduced to 81 kg.

She was advised to continue the treatment.

PATIENT 10

Name : Dinesh

Age : 29 years

Gender : Male

Occupation : Business

Address : Rasipuram

Details on the diagnosis through the *Panchaboodha* Treatment
Obesity

Statement of the Patient

He was below the normal weight ten years back.

To put on some weight, he had taken homoeopathy treatment.

He had the habit of drinking excessive ice-cool water.

He used to sleep in an air-conditioned room that had the lowest temperature.

After taking the homoeopathy medicines, he put on excessive weight. For the past 10 years, he has endured obesity.

His weight could not be reduced even after following strict diet patterns and exercises.

Doctor's Diagnosis Based on the *Panchaboodha* Pulse Diagnosis Method

It was diagnosed that the water element was working excessively in all the pulses and the lower left side energy cycle was working excessively. These were the reasons for his obesity.

First Phase of Treatment

Points were selected and applied to reduce the water element first.

The water points in the metal and wood elements were treated.

The water points in the earth and fire elements were treated.

He was treated in the morning and evening, twice a day for a week and his weight reduced from 123.5 kg to 116.2 kg within a week.

Second Phase of Treatment

It was diagnosed that the wood element mixed with the water element. The points were selected and applied to reduce these elements.

The treatment continued for a month and his body weight was reduced to 113kg.

In two months, this patient could lose a total of 10.5kgs of weight.

He was advised to reduce consuming the sour-tasting food and chilled food.

He was advised to continue the treatment for three more months continuously.

PATIENT 11

Name : **Sangeetha**

Age : **37 years**

Gender : **female**

Marital status : **married**

Address : **Coimbatore-26**

Details on the diagnosis through the *Panchaboodha* Treatment
Obesity, pain in the legs and hands, Menorrhagia.

Statement of the Patient

She had undergone a Caesarean section.

In 2004, she had surgery to rectify the hernia and a mesh has been fixed in the abdomen.

She was taking medicines for three years.

She was affected by the Chikungunya fever and from that, she had pain in the limbs and her whole body.

She was obese.

She experienced fatigue.

She had continuous bleeding during menstruation. It stopped at times if medicine was taken. At times, it never stopped.

Doctor's Diagnosis Based on the *Panchaboodha* Pulse Diagnosis Method.

It was found that the wood and earth elements were working excessively. The lower right-side energies were working excessively. These were the causes of all her health issues.

It was suspected that she was prone to diabetes and advised to take the random glucose test.

As suspected, she had diabetes.

First Phase of Treatment

Points to reduce wood and earth elements were selected and applied. Points to balance the lower right side energy cycle were also applied. After continuous treatment as has been mentioned above, the patient started to get her menstruation regularly and properly. Her weight started to go down and she started to slim down.

Second Phase of Treatment

When the patient came again for the second phase of treatment, she had dizziness, pain in the legs and hands, ulceration on the tongue, constipation, pain in the lower abdomen and boils on the scalp.

It was diagnosed that her gaseous state and the upper side left energy cycle were not working.

To balance those defects, her wood and earth energies were reduced and the points were selected to reduce the right side lower energy cycle. She was treated for a week continuously and all her problems were solved. Her weight started to reduce. From 108 kgs, she lost 12 kgs during this treatment period.

Her diabetes was in control.

Third Phase of Treatment

Her weight and blood glucose levels had fluctuations. Her weight was fluctuating between 95 kgs–100 kgs.

The treatment was going on for this instability and the pain in the limbs as well as the bones.

She was advised to continue treatment for three more months.

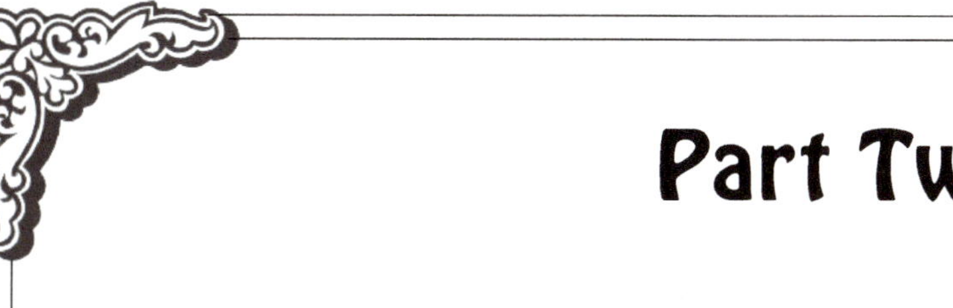

Part Twelve

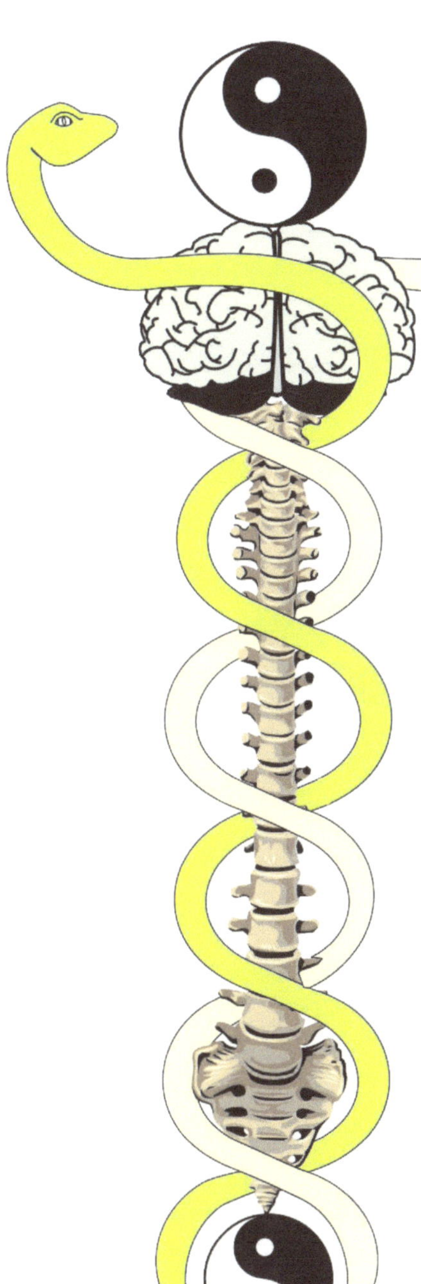

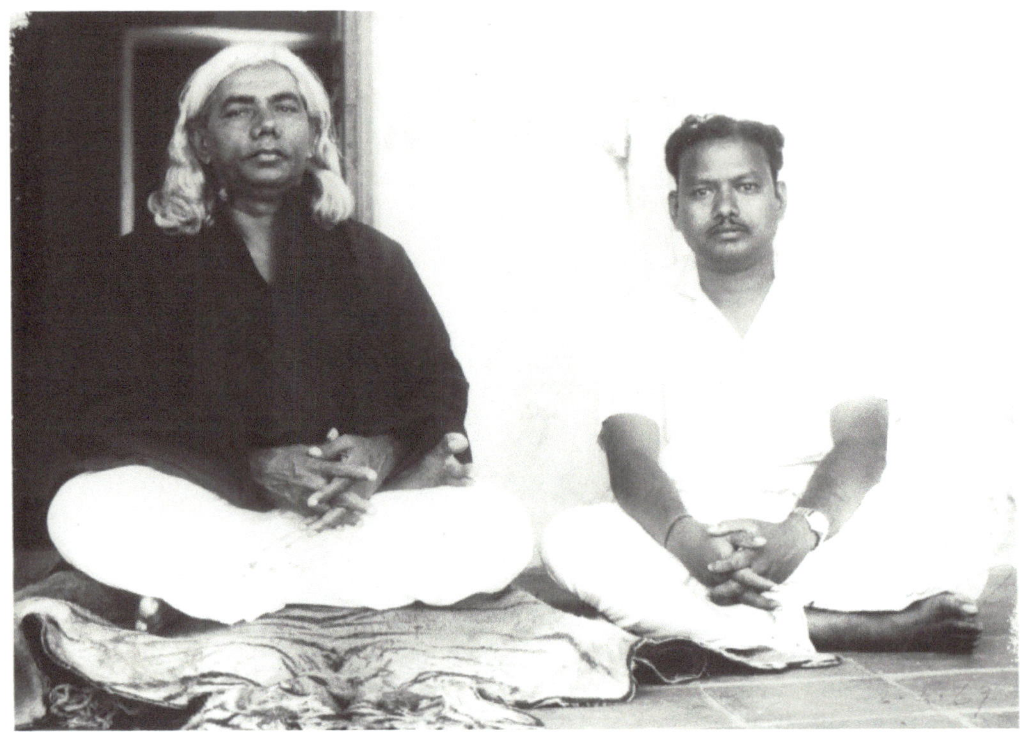

Gnana Vallal Paranjothi Mahan—Guru Gnanaparanjothi

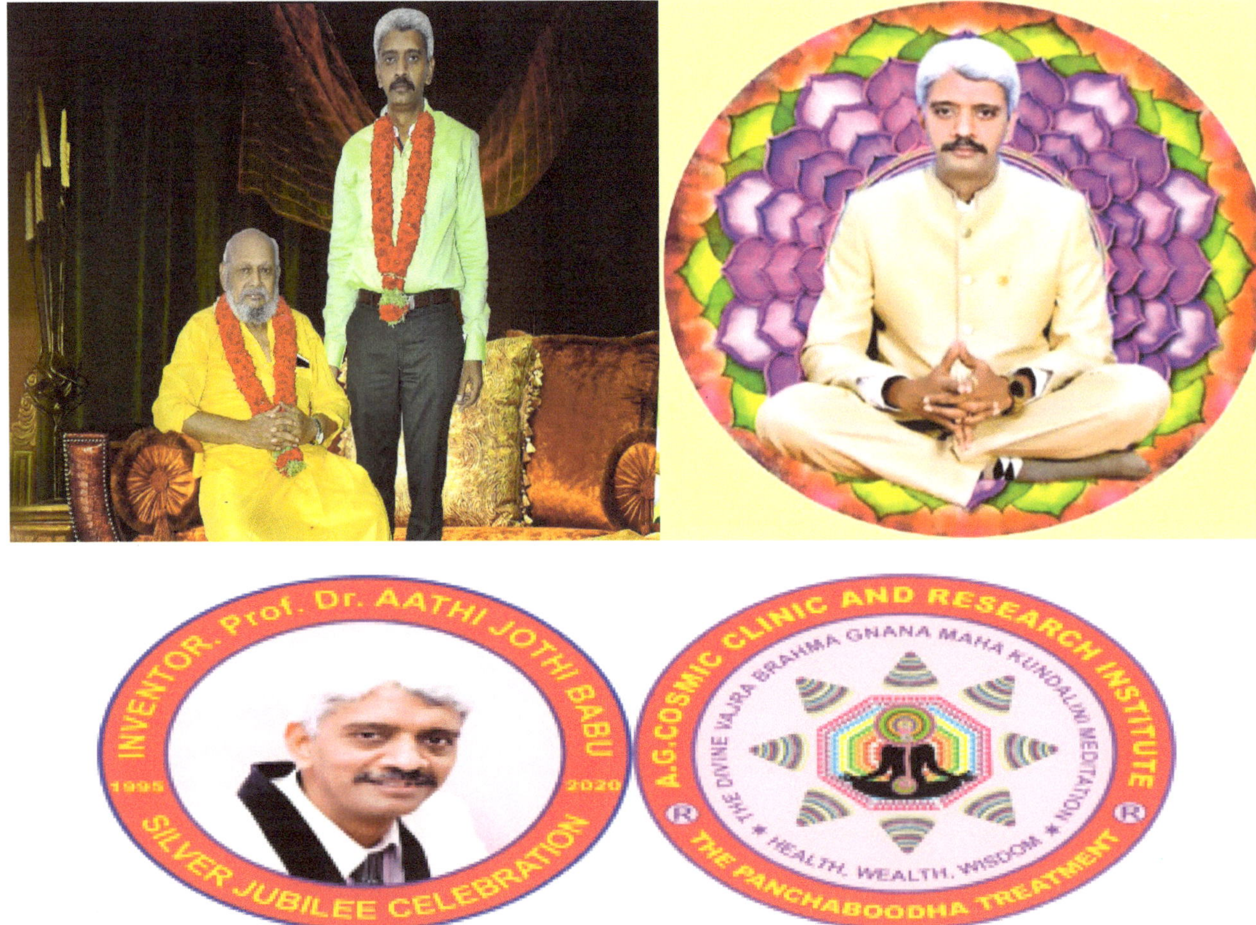

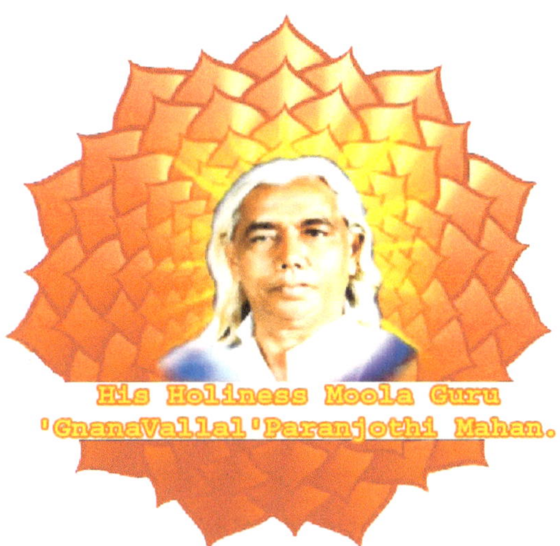

We pray to the incomparable, philosopher and saint of this century, who laid the glorious path and opened it to all, to attain wisdom and eternal happiness—His Holiness Moola *Guru*, ***Gnana Vallal*** Paranjothi Mahan.

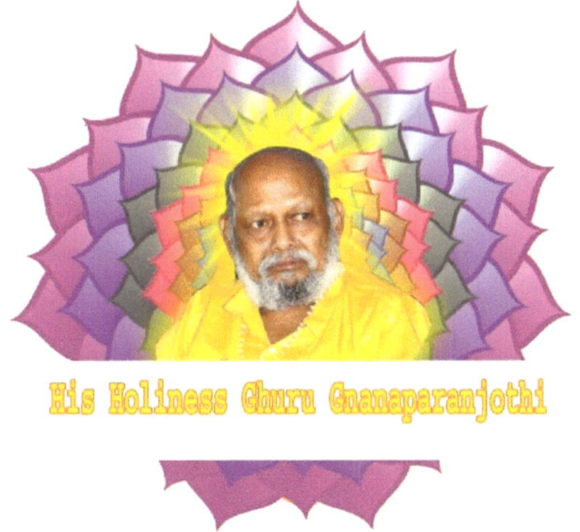

His Holiness *Ghuru* Gnanaparanjothi, with all his divine love for humankind, has created the ***Vasantha Marga*** Meditation. By doing it, people can get a healthy body, peace of mind, happiness, a long life, willpower and wisdom.

His Holiness, Guru Gnanaparanjothi was born to Late Varadhappa Chettiyar and Mrs. Govindammal at Yethapur Village, Salem District, Tamil Nadu, India, on 25th October 1936.

He completed his education in school at Yethapur and Pethanaikkanpalayam villages, near his native village. Then, after successfully completing his diploma in Livestock Inspection course at Madras Veterinary College, he joined the government as a Livestock Inspector in 1958 and rendered his generous services to the villagers till 1994.

Though externally he appeared to be leading a common worldly life, his mind and soul were throbbing with questions about the philosophy of God and the thirst to realise the real ***Truth*** engulfed him. To quench his thirst, he searched for the truth in many ways and means but in vain. Because of his constant search, he met his Guru, the incomparable ***Gnani*** (who had realised the Self and through which he realised the Almighty) of this century, His Holiness Gnanavallal Paranjothi Mahan, on 22.12.1968. He had devised the simplest means, to practice the greatest divine art of meditation, ***Kundalini meditation*** which is the only easiest way to attain wisdom.

After meeting his Guru, he got initiated and started doing the Kundalini Meditation constantly to realise himself and God.

After a year, on 22.12.1969, His Holiness, Gnanavallal Paranjothi Mahan, encouraged our Guru, Gnanaparanjothi to initiate others and spread knowledge about this form of meditation, and from then onwards, he revealed himself and became ***The Guru***.

From that moment onwards, His Holiness, Guru Gnanaparanjothi started his services to lift the world from darkness to divine brightness and has taught this divine art of meditation to all the people from different sectors of the world, for the past 40 years.

To make this Kundalini Meditation feasible, His Holiness, Gnanaparanjothi devised a new simple way of meditation called ***Vasantha Marga*** meditation to make the practice of the Kundalini meditation easier, enable everybody to meditate without the oscillation of the mind and enjoy the essence of the meditation.

When this oscillation of the mind gets arrested, the meditation on one's soul will spontaneously start on its own, to realise wisdom regarding God naturally.

Only by doing this ***Vasantha Marga*** Meditation, one can complete the spiritual journey of ***Sarigai*** (worshipping) ***Girigai*** (chanting ***mantras***) ***Yogam*** (Meditation) and enter the path of wisdom (***Gnana***).

The Three Stages of Initiation

First stage: *Sulimunai*

All human beings have an invisible power—the force of the invisible Almighty in the form of atomic power, called Kundalini, embedded in the place called ***Mooladhara***. This power exists in the semen of the men and the ova of the women. When this power is not realised by the human being because of the darkness of ignorance, it is used only to reproduce the offspring of human nature. This is because the man is covered with a blanket of lust.

When the Guru, with all his kindness and spiritual powers, wakes the ***Kundalini*** from ***Mooladhara***, by lighting the lamp of ***Jeevajyothi***, he links it with the sixth ***chakra*** present at the middle of the eyebrows called the ***Ajna***.(the third eye).

This ***Ajna chakra*** is the first meditating ***chakra***. This exists in our bodies as the third eye (in the middle of the two eyebrows) and the sixth ***chakra*** at the centre of the right and left of the five senses meet. This is the place where the masculine and feminine forces also meet. Since the senses work outwardly and are related to lust and worldliness, this sixth ***chakra***, the third eye, once awakened, directs the senses in the correct path and helps to turn them inwardly towards Divinity.

To uncover the darkness which covers the ***chakra***, the Guru touches it and lights the ***Jeeva jyothi*** (the light with life) in it. When constantly meditating, this ***Jeeva jyothi*** of the sixth ***chakra*** attains the state of cosmic consciousness and the mind becomes neutral—without the oscillations. Because of this neutral state, it conquers the three states i.e., **desire, wavering and worries**. This clarity of consciousness becomes more when constantly meditating and the mind becomes totally concentrated without diversions.

The second stage: Mooladhara

In this stage, the ***Ajna***, the sixth ***chakra***, will be united with the Mooladhara, the first ***chakra***.

This is achieved by uniting the ***Ajna chakra***, which has become holy and has the power of true consciousness through continuous meditation, with the place of its origin being the first chakra ***Mooladhara***(the last phase of the spinal cord).By doing so, this place which is the cause of our birth and used only to produce our offspring becomes holy.

Because of this holiness, all the sins created by the ***karma*** of our previous births are destroyed and the incarnation of birth and death created by this ***karma*** will be destroyed. Finally, it comes to an end.

This stage also helps to eliminate the side effects of the meditation (Kundalini) and all sorts of diseases caused in the body by the mind.

Third stage: *Sahasrara*

In this stage, the seventh ***chakra*** the ***sahasrara*** (the ***Samadhi chakra***) is united with the ***Mooladhara***. The true consciousness by the continuous meditation, from the ***Ajna*** sent to the ***Mooladhara*** is raised and made to rotate on the top centre of the head, called the ***Sahasrara*** through the spinal cord. This connects the power of consciousness with a concentration on atomic energy along with universal cosmic energy.

Because of this union, the human (***Jeevathma***) is connected to the state of the Almighty i.e., the ***Paramathma.*** This eternal unification causes eternal bliss and the human ego is destroyed, which melts in the universal cosmic energy, the state of the Almighty.

This unification is the realisation of these things. If one becomes learned and gains eternal knowledge, or wisdom, he gains eternal bliss, will power and eternal life without death (that is, when a person is in this state, they would have control over their deaths since they know the secret about birth and death).

In this blissful state, one will realise the secrets about birth and death, mind, fate, intelligence, the purpose of birth, all the secrets of nature, the universe, the soul and God.

When one enters the path of wisdom, the first stage of meditation will get completed, and the false attachments to the material world through the senses will get destroyed. The second stage of meditation on the self will occur spontaneously and the realisation of God will occur naturally. Self-realisation will give us a blissful life, by which we can realise the secrets of nature and the reasons for our births, and get divine peace of mind, happiness, willpower, etc.

To complete the first stage of meditation (*Munnilai* meditation), one must do this *Vasantha Marga* Meditation with ***Bhakti,*** consciousness and surrender themselves to the Lord.

For self-realisation (***Thannilai*** meditation),we must have the realisation of ourselves (our good and bad deeds) and have faith. One must be in the matured state of meditation, do spiritual self-cross-examination, and have the blessings of the ***Guru***.

When meditation is combined with consciousness and prayers, then meditation will not be an act or exercise and shows the path towards wisdom. With this, one gets enlightened and realises the ***Guru.*** Then strong faith will be instilled and one will surrender himself to the feet of the ***Guru***.

With the blessings of the ***Guru***, the mind's negativity will get destroyed and all the evil emotions will vanish. One becomes the ***Gunadidan*** (one without any ***Gunas***—evil emotions).

Then, the worldly attachments created by the five senses will get destroyed then it becomes possible for the one to be in the state of divinity, always.

Vajra Brahma Gnana Maha Kundalini Meditation

Kundalini meditation is the only pathway that everyone can go to realise himself and attain wisdom. In ***Kundalini*** meditation, there is only one way called ***Erupadi.*** In this, the *Kundalini* power will be initiated by the *guru* and raised upwards to the *Ajna Chakra* towards wisdom. The ascending path in *Kundalini* meditation is not an easy one. The reason is that those who choose this route have various qualifications.

They should be devotees, recluses, *paradeshis*, ascetics, renouncers of the world, possessions and worldly life, awakened in meditation without joining the mind, and should have a natural hunger to know oneself and attain enlightenment. If you want so many qualifications, it is only possible for independent people. This is why people do not want to go through this *Kundalini* meditation path. Our founder, His Holiness ***Gnanavallal Paranjyothi Mahan*** invented a new path called ***Irangapadi,*** so that all people can overcome all these obstacles and go for ***Kundalini*** meditation. This ***Irangupadi*** pathway is from ***Ajna*** to ***Mooladara Chakra.***

My ***Guru***, His Holiness Gurubiran Gnanaparanjothi introduced three methods to conquer the mind, namely, ***Thannilai, Munnilai, Irainilai***. My ***Guru*** realised that the mind is an obstacle to going fully into ***Kundalini*** meditation. That is, he realised that only those who are perfect in devotion and free from their inborn defects can attain enlightenment very quickly through ***Kundalini*** meditation.

He said that to overcome the mind, he created the three paths of presence, self-realisation and divine realism. Through this, if the meditation of the real-life state is complete, self-realisation meditation will happen automatically, and the feeling of Godliness will be natural.

The Invention of a Methodology of Kundalini Meditation

Professor Dr. Aathi Jothi Babu invented this method and stated that apart from the back side of the spinal cord, the Kundalini path exists on the front side of the body, parallel to the spine. Also, there is a neutral path between these two.

There are eight sides of the spine—each of the ways helps *Kundalini* energies rise towards *sahasrara* and flow down towards *mooladhara*. They are both surrounded by eight sides of *Kundalini* energies. These two upward and downward paths have a central neutral path which is surrounded by eight sides.

In the head, the Kundalini power from all eight sides joins at the centre of the upward path—at the ***sahasraram*** to open up the portal of wisdom in someone. When all eight sides join, the centre of the downward path at the ***mooladharam*** opens the ***Brahmam.*** Professor Dr. Aathi Jothi Babu has invented the method to evoke all these eight ways of energy and the joining point.

With the blessings of ***Moolaguru*** and his ***Guru***, Professor Dr. Aathi Jothi Babu discovered that one path from the centre of the atom at the root and eight paths from the outer eight corners of the atom lead up to a total of nine paths and connect to the centre of the ***perenu*** located at the top of the head called ***Sahasraram***. For each of these paths, he found three paths, namely, ascending, central and descending. Then, he discovered that one path from the centre of the ***perenu*** located at the top of the head and eight paths from the eight sides of the ***perenu*** lead downwards to join the centre of the atom.

For these nine paths, he discovered the three paths—Ascending, Centring and Descending Paths. He named these two octagonal triangular formations as ***Ajapa Kundalini*** meditation.

In this, he discovered that the upper breath, the lower breath and the balanced breath, combined with the two, can get rid of the three qualities of the mind, i.e., the ***Raja Guna***, ***Sattva Guna*** and the ***Tamo Guna***, and everyone can reach the state of ***Gunadithan***, a characterless and mindless state.

He has discovered 108 paths and 10 steps of its inner centre, including 96 outer paths that directly connect the periphery of the micro atom and the periphery of the macro atom, 12 central paths that connect the centre of the micro atom and the centre of the macro atom to reach enlightenment through the ten steps of ***Kundalini*** meditation.

Professor Dr. Aathi Jothi Babu has named this method of practising meditation ***Vajra Brahma Gnana Maha Kundalini Meditation.***

With this method, practising meditation and attaining wisdom have been made easier for any person who wants to practice it.

PCT

PATENT COOPERATION TREATY PCT/IN2010/000748

ADVANCE E-MAIL

From the INTERNATIONAL BUREAU

PCT

NOTIFICATION OF RECEIPT OF RECORD COPY

(PCT Rule 24.2(a))

To:
DEWAN, Niti
R.K. DEWAN & COMPANY
Trade Mark & Patent Attorneys
Podar Chambers
S.A. Brelvi Road
Fort, Mumbai 400 001
Maharashtra
INDE

Date of mailing (day/month/year) 28 January 2011 (28.01.2011)	IMPORTANT NOTIFICATION
Applicant's or agent's file reference	International application No. PCT/IN2010/000748

The applicant is hereby **notified** that the International Bureau has received the record copy of the international application as detailed below.

Name(s) of the applicant(s) and State(s) for which they are applicants

BAABU, G . D (all designated States)

International filing date: 16 November 2010 (16.11.2010)
Priority date(s) claimed: 26 May 2010 (26.05.2010)
Date of receipt of the record copy by the International Bureau: 04 January 2011 (04.01.2011)
List of designated Offices:

AP: BW, GH, GM, KE, LR, LS, MW, MZ, NA, SD, SL, SZ, TZ, UG, ZM, ZW
EA: AM, AZ, BY, KG, KZ, MD, RU, TJ, TM
EP: AL, AT, BE, BG, CH, CY, CZ, DE, DK, EE, ES, FI, FR, GB, GR, HR, HU, IE, IS, IT, LT, LU, LV, MC, MK, MT, NL, NO, PL, PT, RO, RS, SE, SI, SK, SM, TR
OA: BF, BJ, CF, CG, CI, CM, GA, GN, GQ, GW, ML, MR, NE, SN, TD, TG
National: AE, AG, AL, AM, AO, AT, AU, AZ, BA, BB, BG, BH, BR, BW, BY, BZ, CA, CH, CL, CN, CO, CR, CU, CZ, DE, DK, DM, DO, DZ, EC, EE, EG, ES, FI, GB, GD, GE, GH, GM, GT, HN, HR, HU, ID, IL, IN, IS, JP, KE, KG, KM, KN, KP, KR, KZ, LA, LC, LK, LR, LS, LT, LU, LY, MA, MD, ME, MG, MK, MN, MW, MX, MY, MZ, NA, NG, NI, NO, NZ, OM, PE, PG, PH, PL, PT, RO, RS, RU, SC, SD, SE, SG, SK, SL, SM, ST, SV, SY, TH, TJ, TM, TN, TR, TT, TZ, UA, UG, US, UZ, VC, VN, ZA, ZM, ZW

ATTENTION: The applicant should carefully check the data appearing in this Notification. In case of any discrepancy between these data and the indications in the international application, the applicant should immediately inform the International Bureau. **In addition, the applicant's attention is drawn to:**

- time limits for entry into the national phase (see www.wipo.int/pct/en/texts/time_limits.htmland *PCT Applicant's Guide*, National Phase, especially Chapters 3 and 4)
- requirements regarding priority documents (if applicable) (see *PCT Applicant's Guide*, International Phase, paragraph 5.070)

A copy of this notification is being sent to the receiving Office and to the International Searching Authority.

The International Bureau of WIPO 34, chemin des Colombettes 1211 Geneva 20, Switzerland Facsimile No. +41 22 338 87 40	Authorized officer Olaiz Alicia e-mail pt01.pct@wipo.int Telephone No. +41 22 338 74 01

Form PCT/IB/301 (July 2010) 1/EQUOIXIW0

PATENT - AUSTRALIA

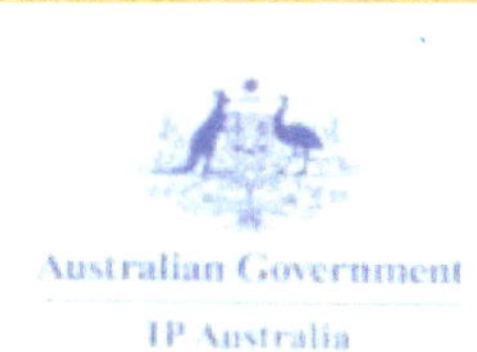

LETTERS PATENT

INNOVATION PATENT

I, Fatima Beattie, the Commissioner of Patents, hereby grant an Innovation Patent

2010101332

to

GD Baabu of 94/C-23 Akashaya Nilayam, 5th Cross, Rajaram Nagar, Salem, Tamil Nadu, 636007, India

for the Innovation Patent titled

A novel system of acupuncture treatment

invented by Baabu, GD

This Innovation Patent is granted for a term of eight years commencing from 29 November 2010.

This Innovation Patent can not be enforced unless and until it has been examined by the Commissioner of Patents and a Certificate of Examination has been issued. See sections 120(1A) and 129A of the Patents Act 1990, set out on the reverse of this document.

Priority Details:

Number	***Date***	***Filed with***
1453/CHE/2010	26 May 2010	IN

Dated this 9th day of December 2010

Fatima Beattie
Commissioner of Patents

PATENTS ACT 1990

PATENT- SOUTH AFRICA

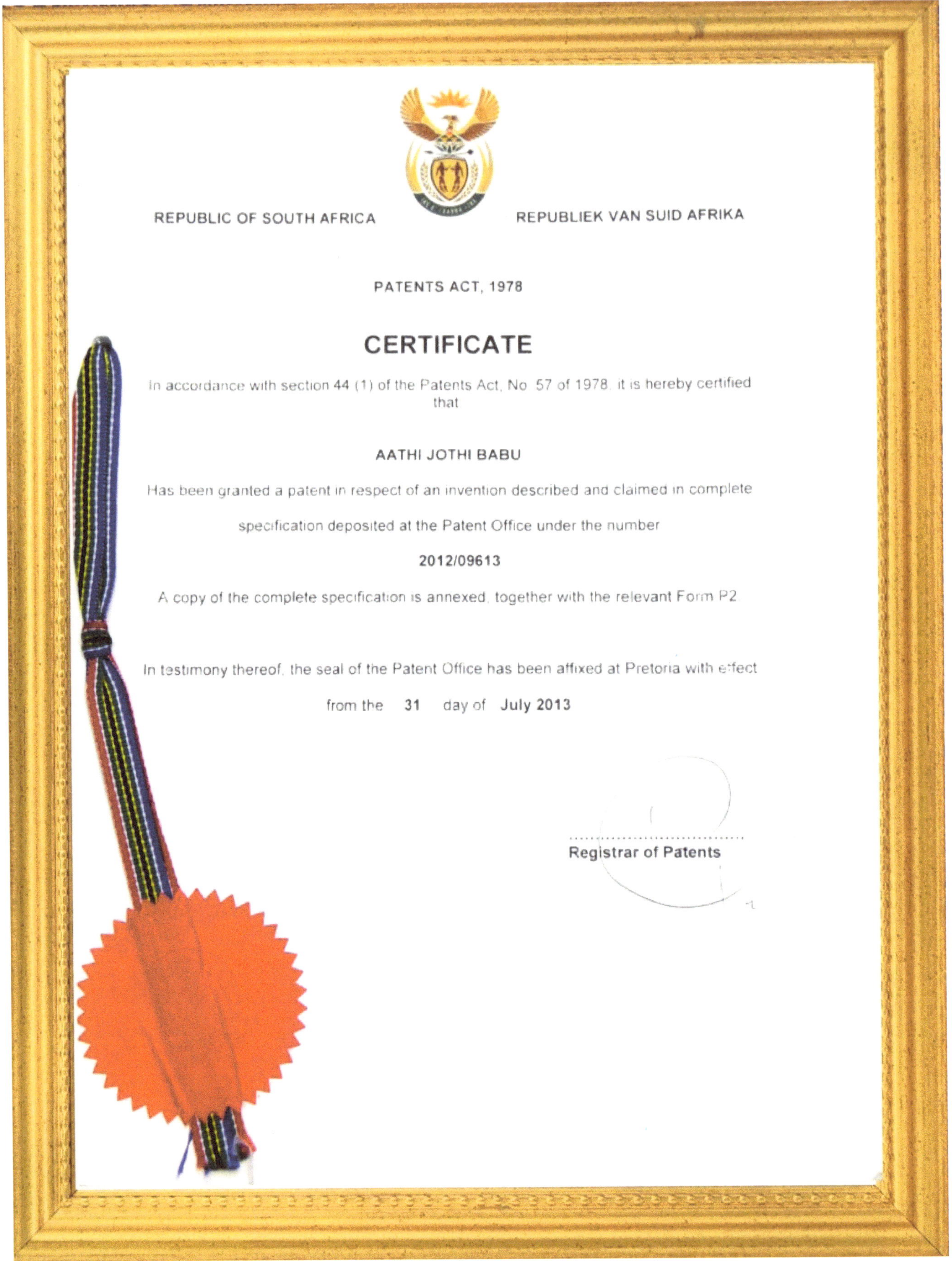

REPUBLIC OF SOUTH AFRICA REPUBLIEK VAN SUID AFRIKA

PATENTS ACT, 1978

CERTIFICATE

In accordance with section 44 (1) of the Patents Act, No 57 of 1978, it is hereby certified that

AATHI JOTHI BABU

Has been granted a patent in respect of an invention described and claimed in complete specification deposited at the Patent Office under the number

2012/09613

A copy of the complete specification is annexed, together with the relevant Form P2

In testimony thereof, the seal of the Patent Office has been affixed at Pretoria with effect from the 31 day of July 2013

Registrar of Patents

PATENT – INDIA

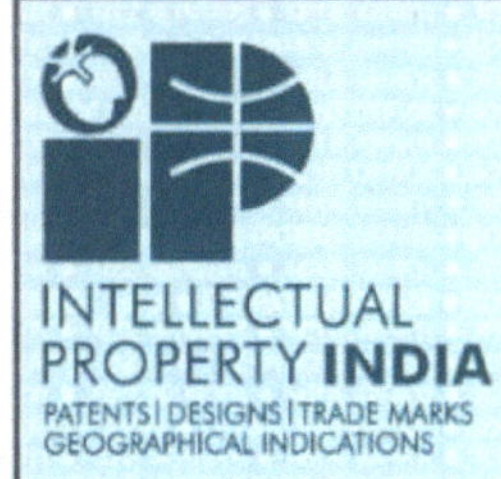

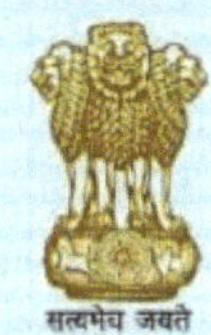

क्रमांक : 044152553
SL No :

भारत सरकार
GOVERNMENT OF INDIA
पेटेंट कार्यालय
THE PATENT OFFICE
पेटेंट प्रमाणपत्र
PATENT CERTIFICATE
(Rule 74 of The Patents Rules)

पेटेंट सं. / Patent No.	:	429282
आवेदन सं. / Application No.	:	1453/CHE/2010
फाइल करने की तारीख / Date of Filing	:	26/05/2010
पेटेंटी / Patentee	:	G.D.BAABU

प्रमाणित किया जाता है कि पेटेंटी को, उपरोक्त आवेदन में यथाप्रकटित A SYSTEM FOR MONITORING FIVE-ELEMENT PULSES नामक आविष्कार के लिए, पेटेंट अधिनियम, 1970 के उपबंधों के अनुसार आज तारीख मई 2010 के छब्बीसवें दिन से बीस वर्ष की अवधि के लिए पेटेंट अनुदत्त किया गया है।

It is hereby certified that a patent has been granted to the patentee for an invention entitled A SYSTEM FOR MONITORING FIVE-ELEMENT PULSES as disclosed in the above mentioned application for the term of 20 years from the 26th day of May 2010 in accordance with the provisions of the Patents Act, 1970.

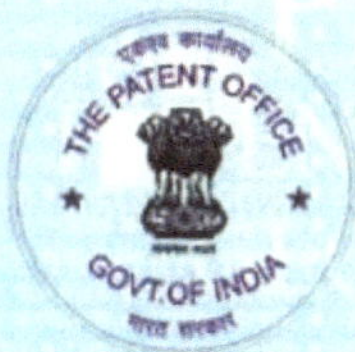

अनुदान की तारीख : 18/04/2023
Date of Grant :

पेटेंट नियंत्रक
Controller of Patent

टिप्पणी - इस पेटेंट के नवीकरण के लिए फीस, यदि इसे बनाए रखा जाना है, मई 2012 के छब्बीसवें दिन को और उसके पश्चात प्रत्येक वर्ष मे उसी दिन देय होगी।

Note. - The fees for renewal of this patent, if it is to be maintained will fall / has fallen due on 26th day of May 2012 and on the same day in every year thereafter.

INDIA DESIGN PATENT: 1

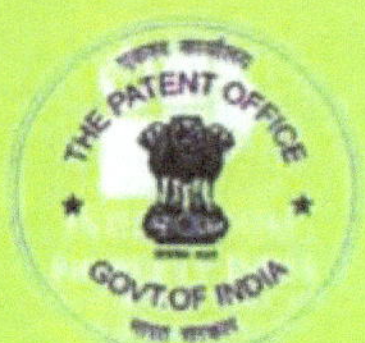

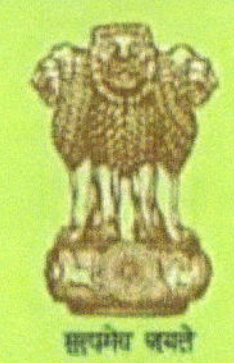

ORIGINAL

मूल/No : 127831

भारत सरकार
GOVERNMENT OF INDIA
पेटेंट कार्यालय
THE PATENT OFFICE
डिजाइन के पंजीकरण का प्रमाणपत्र
CERTIFICATE OF REGISTRATION OF DESIGN

डिजाइन सं. / Design No.	:	356603-001
तारीख / Date	:	12/01/2022
पारस्परिकता तारीख / Reciprocity Date*	:	
देश / Country	:	

प्रमाणित किया जाता है कि संलग्न प्रति में वर्णित डिजाइन जो **MEDITATION ARTICLE** से संबंधित है, का पंजीकरण, श्रेणी **24-99** में Prof Dr.Aathi Jothi Babu के नाम में उपर्युक्त संख्या और तारीख में कर लिया गया है।

Certified that the design of which a copy is annexed hereto has been registered as of the number and date given above in class **24-99** in respect of the application of such design to **MEDITATION ARTICLE** in the name of Prof Dr.Aathi Jothi Babu.

डिजाइन अधिनियम, 2000 तथा डिजाइन नियम, 2001 के अध्यधीन प्रावधानों के अनुसरण में।
In pursuance of and subject to the provisions of the Designs Act, 2000 and the Designs Rules, 2001.

INTELLECTUAL PROPERTY INDIA
PATENTS | DESIGNS | TRADE MARKS
GEOGRAPHICAL INDICATIONS

निर्गमन की तारीख/Date of Issue : 27/01/2023

महानियंत्रक पेटेंट डिजाइन और व्यापार चिह्न
Controller General of Patents, Designs and Trade Marks

पारस्परिकता तारीख (यदि कोई हो) जिसकी अनुमति देश के नाम पर की गई है। डिजाइन का स्वत्वाधिकार पंजीकरण की तारीख से दस वर्षों के लिए होगा जिसका विस्तार, अधिनियम एवं नियम के निबंधनों के अधीन, पाँच वर्षों की अतिरिक्त अवधि के लिए किया जा सकेगा। इस प्रमाण पत्र का उपयोग विधिक कार्यवाहियों अथवा विदेश में पंजीकरण प्राप्त करने के लिए नहीं हो सकता है।

*The reciprocity date (if any) which has been allowed and the name of the country.Copyright in the design will subsist for ten years from the date of Registration, and may under the terms of the Act and Rules, be extended for a further period of five years.This Certificate is not for use in legal proceedings or for obtaining registration abroad.

INDIA DESIGN PATENT: 2

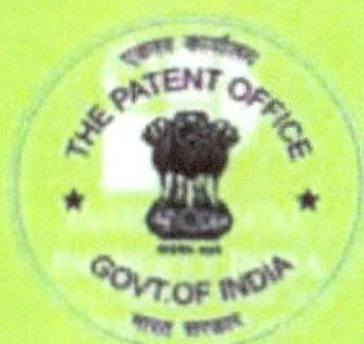

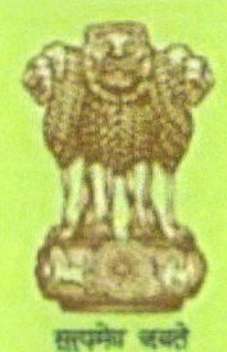

सत्यमेव जयते

ORIGINAL

मूल/No : 127832

भारत सरकार
GOVERNMENT OF INDIA
पेटेंट कार्यालय
THE PATENT OFFICE
डिजाइन के पंजीकरण का प्रमाणपत्र
CERTIFICATE OF REGISTRATION OF DESIGN

डिजाइन सं. / Design No.	:	358411-001
तारीख / Date	:	11/02/2022
पारस्परिकता तारीख / Reciprocity Date*	:	
देश / Country	:	

प्रमाणित किया जाता है कि संलग्न प्रति में वर्णित डिजाइन जो **MEDITATION ARTICLE** से संबंधित है, का पंजीकरण, श्रेणी **24-99** में Prof Dr. Aathi Jothi Babu के नाम में उपर्युक्त संख्या और तारीख में कर लिया गया है।

Certified that the design of which a copy is annexed hereto has been registered as of the number and date given above in class **24-99** in respect of the application of such design to **MEDITATION ARTICLE** in the name of Prof Dr. Aathi Jothi Babu.

डिजाइन अधिनियम, 2000 तथा डिजाइन नियम, 2001 के अध्यधीन प्रावधानों के अनुसरण में।
In pursuance of and subject to the provisions of the Designs Act, 2000 and the Designs Rules, 2001.

INTELLECTUAL PROPERTY INDIA
PATENTS | DESIGNS | TRADE MARKS
GEOGRAPHICAL INDICATIONS

निर्गमन की तारीख/Date of Issue : 27/01/2023

महानियंत्रक पेटेंट डिजाइन और व्यापार चिह्न
Controller General of Patents, Designs and Trade Marks

पारस्परिकता तारीख (यदि कोई हो) जिसकी अनुमति देश के नाम पर की गई है। डिजाइन का सत्वाधिकार पंजीकरण की तारीख से दस वर्षों के लिए होगा जिसका विस्तार, अधिनियम एवं नियम के निबंधनों के अधीन, पाँच वर्षों की अतिरिक्त अवधि के लिए किया जा सकेगा। इस प्रमाण पत्र का उपयोग विधिक कार्यवाहियों अथवा विदेश में पंजीकरण प्राप्त करने के लिए नहीं हो सकता है।

*The reciprocity date (if any) which has been allowed and the name of the country.Copyright in the design will subsist for ten years from the date of Registration, and may under the terms of the Act and Rules, be extended for a further period of five years.This Certificate is not for use in legal proceedings or for obtaining registration abroad.

INDIA DESIGN PATENT: 3

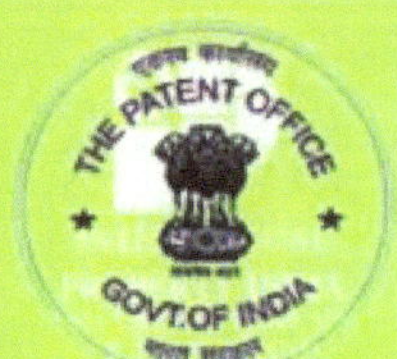

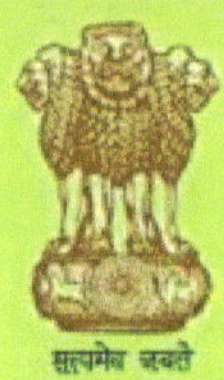

ORIGINAL

मूल/No : 130420

भारत सरकार
GOVERNMENT OF INDIA
पेटेंट कार्यालय
THE PATENT OFFICE
डिजाइन के पंजीकरण का प्रमाणपत्र
CERTIFICATE OF REGISTRATION OF DESIGN

डिजाइन सं. / Design No.	:	357383-001
तारीख / Date	:	27/01/2022
पारस्परिकता तारीख / Reciprocity Date*	:	
देश / Country	:	

प्रमाणित किया जाता है कि संलग्न प्रति में वर्णित डिजाइन जो **MEDITATION ARTICLE** से संबंधित है, का पंजीकरण, श्रेणी **24-99** में Dr.Aathi Jothi Babu के नाम में उपर्युक्त संख्या और तारीख में कर लिया गया है।

Certified that the design of which a copy is annexed hereto has been registered as of the number and date given above in class **24-99** in respect of the application of such design to **MEDITATION ARTICLE** in the name of Dr.Aathi Jothi Babu.

डिजाइन अधिनियम, 2000 तथा डिजाइन नियम, 2001 के अध्यधीन प्रावधानों के अनुसरण में।
In pursuance of and subject to the provisions of the Designs Act, 2000 and the Designs Rules, 2001.

INTELLECTUAL PROPERTY INDIA
PATENTS | DESIGNS | TRADE MARKS
GEOGRAPHICAL INDICATIONS

निर्गमन की तारीख/Date of Issue : 09/03/2023

महानियंत्रक पेटेंट डिजाइन और व्यापार चिह्न
Controller General of Patents, Designs and Trade Marks

पारस्परिकता तारीख (यदि कोई हो) जिसकी अनुमति देश के नाम पर की गई है। डिजाइन का सत्वाधिकार पंजीकरण की तारीख से दस वर्षों के लिए होगा जिसका विस्तार, अधिनियम एवं नियम के निबंधनों के अधीन, पाँच वर्षों की अतिरिक्त अवधि के लिए किया जा सकेगा। इस प्रमाण पत्र का उपयोग विधिक कार्यवाहियों अथवा विदेश में पंजीकरण प्राप्त करने के लिए नहीं हो सकता है।

*The reciprocity date (if any) which has been allowed and the name of the country.Copyright in the design will subsist for ten years from the date of Registration, and may under the terms of the Act and Rules, be extended for a further period of five years.This Certificate is not for use in legal proceedings or for obtaining registration abroad.

INDIA DESIGN PATENT: 4

(Applied)

USA COPYRIGHT

Certificate of Registration

SEAL OF THE UNITED STATES COPYRIGHT OFFICE 1870

This Certificate issued under the seal of the Copyright Office in accordance with title 17, *United States Code*, attests that registration has been made for the work identified below. The information on this certificate has been made a part of the Copyright Office records.

Maria A. Pallante

Register of Copyrights, United States of America

Registration Number

TXu 1-930-019

Effective Date of Registration:
June 17, 2014

Title

Title of Work: Acupressure with pulse point healing by Dr. Aathi Jothi Babu.

Completion/Publication

Year of Completion: 2014

Author

- **Author:** Aathi Jothi Babu
  Author Created: text, artwork
  Citizen of: India
  Domiciled in: India

Copyright Claimant

Copyright Claimant: Aathi Jothi Babu
94/C-23, Fifth Cross, Rajaram Nagar, Salem, 636 007, India

Rights and Permissions

Organization Name: Alprin Law Offices, P.C.
Address: 5 Pinehurst Circle, N.W.
Washington, DC 20015 United States

Certification

Name: Laura Smith
Date: June 17, 2014
Applicant's Tracking Number: ALO-0069037

Correspondence: Yes

Page 1 of 1

INDIA COPYRIGHT : 1

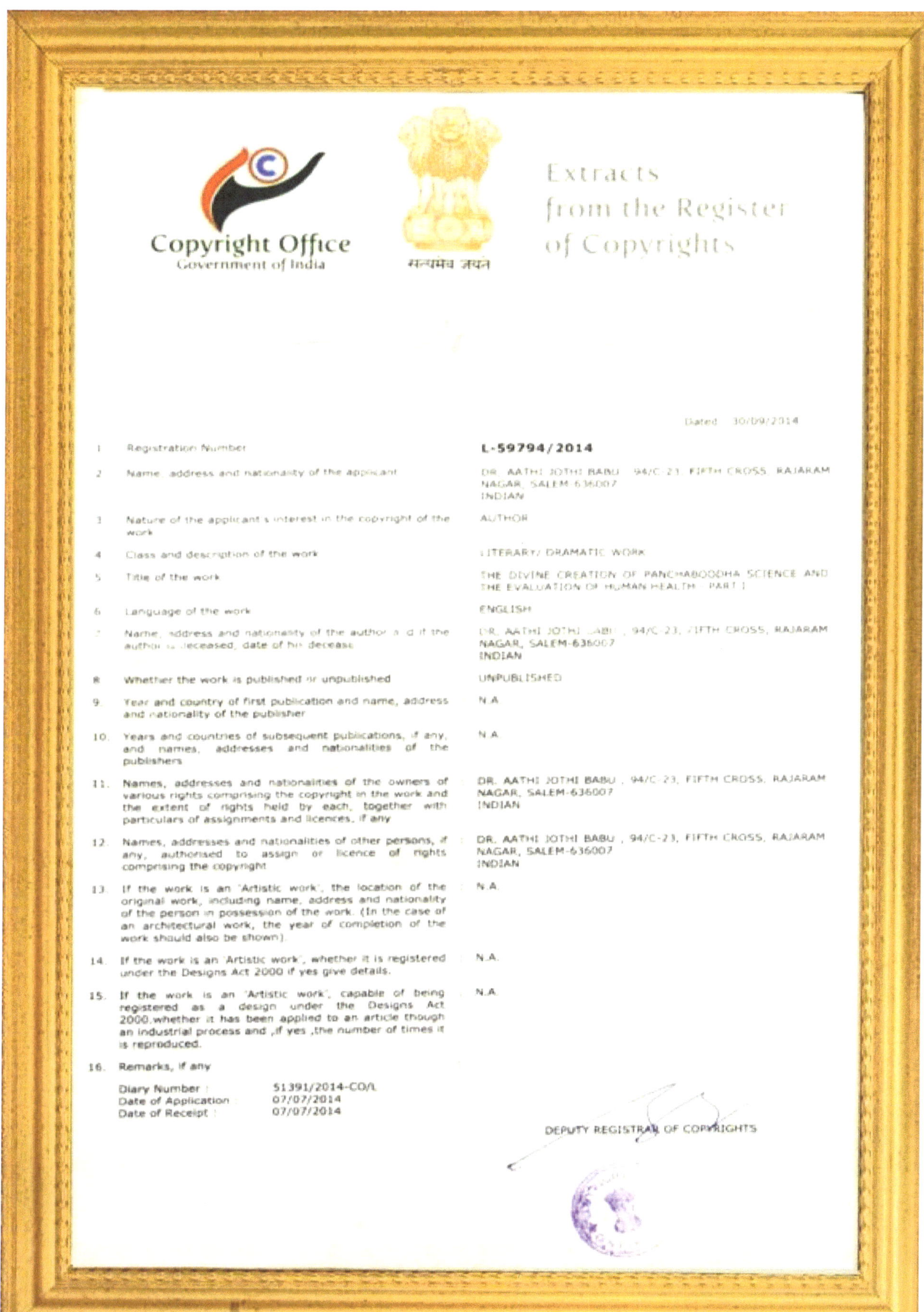

Copyright Office
Government of India

सत्यमेव जयते

Extracts from the Register of Copyrights

Dated 30/09/2014

1	Registration Number	L-59794/2014
2	Name, address and nationality of the applicant	DR. AATHI JOTHI BABU , 94/C-23, FIFTH CROSS, RAJARAM NAGAR, SALEM-636007 INDIAN
3	Nature of the applicant's interest in the copyright of the work	AUTHOR
4	Class and description of the work	LITERARY/ DRAMATIC WORK
5	Title of the work	THE DIVINE CREATION OF PANCHABOODHA SCIENCE AND THE EVALUATION OF HUMAN HEALTH - PART 1
6	Language of the work	ENGLISH
7	Name, address and nationality of the author and if the author is deceased, date of his decease	DR. AATHI JOTHI BABU , 94/C-23, FIFTH CROSS, RAJARAM NAGAR, SALEM-636007 INDIAN
8	Whether the work is published or unpublished	UNPUBLISHED
9.	Year and country of first publication and name, address and nationality of the publisher	N.A
10.	Years and countries of subsequent publications, if any, and names, addresses and nationalities of the publishers	N.A
11.	Names, addresses and nationalities of the owners of various rights comprising the copyright in the work and the extent of rights held by each, together with particulars of assignments and licences, if any	DR. AATHI JOTHI BABU , 94/C-23, FIFTH CROSS, RAJARAM NAGAR, SALEM-636007 INDIAN
12.	Names, addresses and nationalities of other persons, if any, authorised to assign or licence of rights comprising the copyright	DR. AATHI JOTHI BABU , 94/C-23, FIFTH CROSS, RAJARAM NAGAR, SALEM-636007 INDIAN
13.	If the work is an 'Artistic work', the location of the original work, including name, address and nationality of the person in possession of the work. (In the case of an architectural work, the year of completion of the work should also be shown).	N.A.
14.	If the work is an 'Artistic work', whether it is registered under the Designs Act 2000 if yes give details.	N.A.
15.	If the work is an 'Artistic work', capable of being registered as a design under the Designs Act 2000,whether it has been applied to an article though an industrial process and ,if yes ,the number of times it is reproduced.	N.A.
16.	Remarks, if any	

Diary Number : 51391/2014-CO/L
Date of Application : 07/07/2014
Date of Receipt : 07/07/2014

DEPUTY REGISTRAR OF COPYRIGHTS

INDIA COPYRIGHT : 2

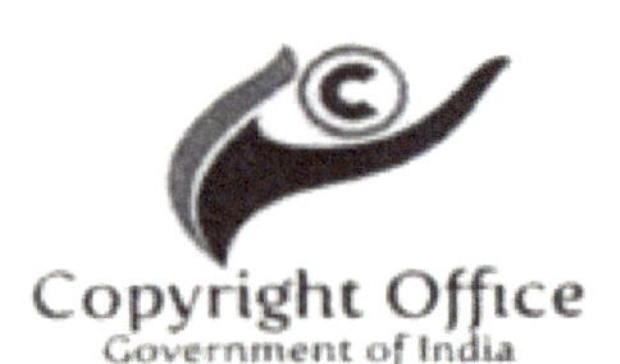

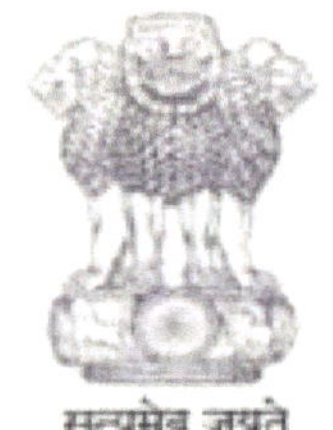

Extracts from the Register of Copyrights

Dated : 22/09/2014

1	Registration Number	**L-59713/2014**
2	Name, address and nationality of the applicant	DR. AATHI JOTHI BABU , 94/C-23, FIFTH CROSS, RAJARAM NAGAR, SALEM-636007 INDIAN
3	Nature of the applicant's interest in the copyright of the work	OWNER
4	Class and description of the work	LITERARY/ DRAMATIC WORK
5	Title of the work	THE DIVINE CREATION OF PANCHABOODHA SCIENCE AND THE EVALUATION OF HUMAN HEALTH- PART II
6	Language of the work	ENGLISH
7	Name, address and nationality of the author and if the author is deceased, date of his decease	DR. AATHI JOTHI BABU , 94/C-23, FIFTH CROSS, RAJARAM NAGAR, SALEM-636007 INDIAN
8	Whether the work is published or unpublished	UNPUBLISHED
9	Year and country of first publication and name, address and nationality of the publisher	N.A.
10	Years and countries of subsequent publications, if any, and names, addresses and nationalities of the publishers	N.A.
11	Names, addresses and nationalities of the owners of various rights comprising the copyright in the work and the extent of rights held by each, together with particulars of assignments and licences, if any	DR. AATHI JOTHI BABU , 94/C-23, FIFTH CROSS, RAJARAM NAGAR, SALEM-636007 INDIAN
12	Names, addresses and nationalities of other persons, if any, authorised to assign or licence of rights comprising the copyright	DR. AATHI JOTHI BABU , 94/C-23, FIFTH CROSS, RAJARAM NAGAR, SALEM-636007 INDIAN
13	If the work is an 'Artistic work', the location of the original work, including name, address and nationality of the person in possession of the work. (In the case of an architectural work, the year of completion of the work should also be shown).	N.A.
14	If the work is an 'Artistic work', whether it is registered under the Designs Act 2000 if yes give details	N.A.
15	If the work is an 'Artistic work', capable of being registered as a design under the Designs Act 2000 whether it has been applied to an article though an industrial process and ,if yes ,the number of times it is reproduced	N.A.
16	Remarks, if any	

Diary Number: 51655/2014-CO/L
Date of Application: 26/06/2014
Date of Receipt: 14/07/2014

DEPUTY REGISTRAR OF COPYRIGHTS

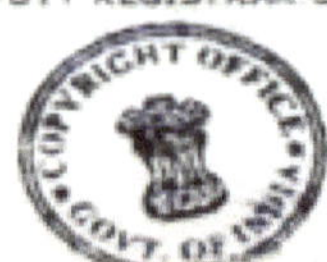

INDIA COPYRIGHT : 3

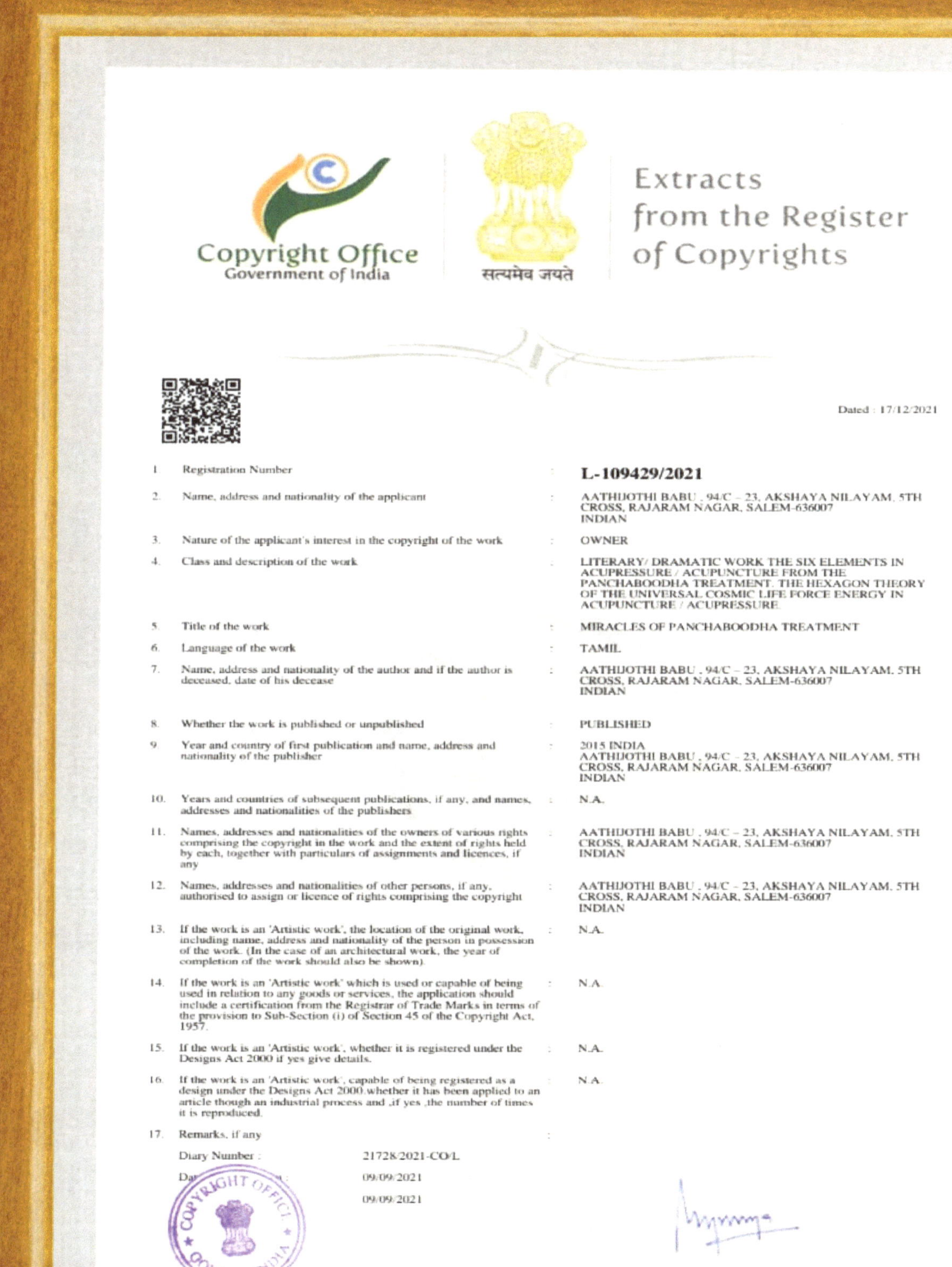

Copyright Office
Government of India

सत्यमेव जयते

Extracts from the Register of Copyrights

Dated : 17/12/2021

1.	Registration Number	:	**L-109429/2021**
2.	Name, address and nationality of the applicant	:	AATHIJOTHI BABU , 94/C – 23, AKSHAYA NILAYAM, 5TH CROSS, RAJARAM NAGAR, SALEM-636007 INDIAN
3.	Nature of the applicant's interest in the copyright of the work	:	OWNER
4.	Class and description of the work	:	LITERARY/ DRAMATIC WORK THE SIX ELEMENTS IN ACUPRESSURE / ACUPUNCTURE FROM THE PANCHABOODHA TREATMENT. THE HEXAGON THEORY OF THE UNIVERSAL COSMIC LIFE FORCE ENERGY IN ACUPUNCTURE / ACUPRESSURE
5.	Title of the work	:	MIRACLES OF PANCHABOODHA TREATMENT
6.	Language of the work	:	TAMIL
7.	Name, address and nationality of the author and if the author is deceased, date of his decease	:	AATHIJOTHI BABU , 94/C – 23, AKSHAYA NILAYAM, 5TH CROSS, RAJARAM NAGAR, SALEM-636007 INDIAN
8.	Whether the work is published or unpublished	:	PUBLISHED
9.	Year and country of first publication and name, address and nationality of the publisher	:	2015 INDIA AATHIJOTHI BABU , 94/C – 23, AKSHAYA NILAYAM, 5TH CROSS, RAJARAM NAGAR, SALEM-636007 INDIAN
10.	Years and countries of subsequent publications, if any, and names, addresses and nationalities of the publishers	:	N.A.
11.	Names, addresses and nationalities of the owners of various rights comprising the copyright in the work and the extent of rights held by each, together with particulars of assignments and licences, if any	:	AATHIJOTHI BABU , 94/C – 23, AKSHAYA NILAYAM, 5TH CROSS, RAJARAM NAGAR, SALEM-636007 INDIAN
12.	Names, addresses and nationalities of other persons, if any, authorised to assign or licence of rights comprising the copyright	:	AATHIJOTHI BABU , 94/C – 23, AKSHAYA NILAYAM, 5TH CROSS, RAJARAM NAGAR, SALEM-636007 INDIAN
13.	If the work is an 'Artistic work', the location of the original work, including name, address and nationality of the person in possession of the work. (In the case of an architectural work, the year of completion of the work should also be shown).	:	N.A.
14.	If the work is an 'Artistic work' which is used or capable of being used in relation to any goods or services, the application should include a certification from the Registrar of Trade Marks in terms of the provision to Sub-Section (i) of Section 45 of the Copyright Act, 1957.	:	N.A.
15.	If the work is an 'Artistic work', whether it is registered under the Designs Act 2000 if yes give details.	:	N.A.
16.	If the work is an 'Artistic work', capable of being registered as a design under the Designs Act 2000,whether it has been applied to an article though an industrial process and ,if yes ,the number of times it is reproduced.	:	N.A.
17.	Remarks, if any	:	

Diary Number : 21728/2021-CO/L

Da[illegible] : 09/09/2021

09/09/2021

COPYRIGHT OFFICE ★ GOVT OF INDIA ★

DEPUTY REGISTRAR OF COPYRIGHTS

TRADEMARKS

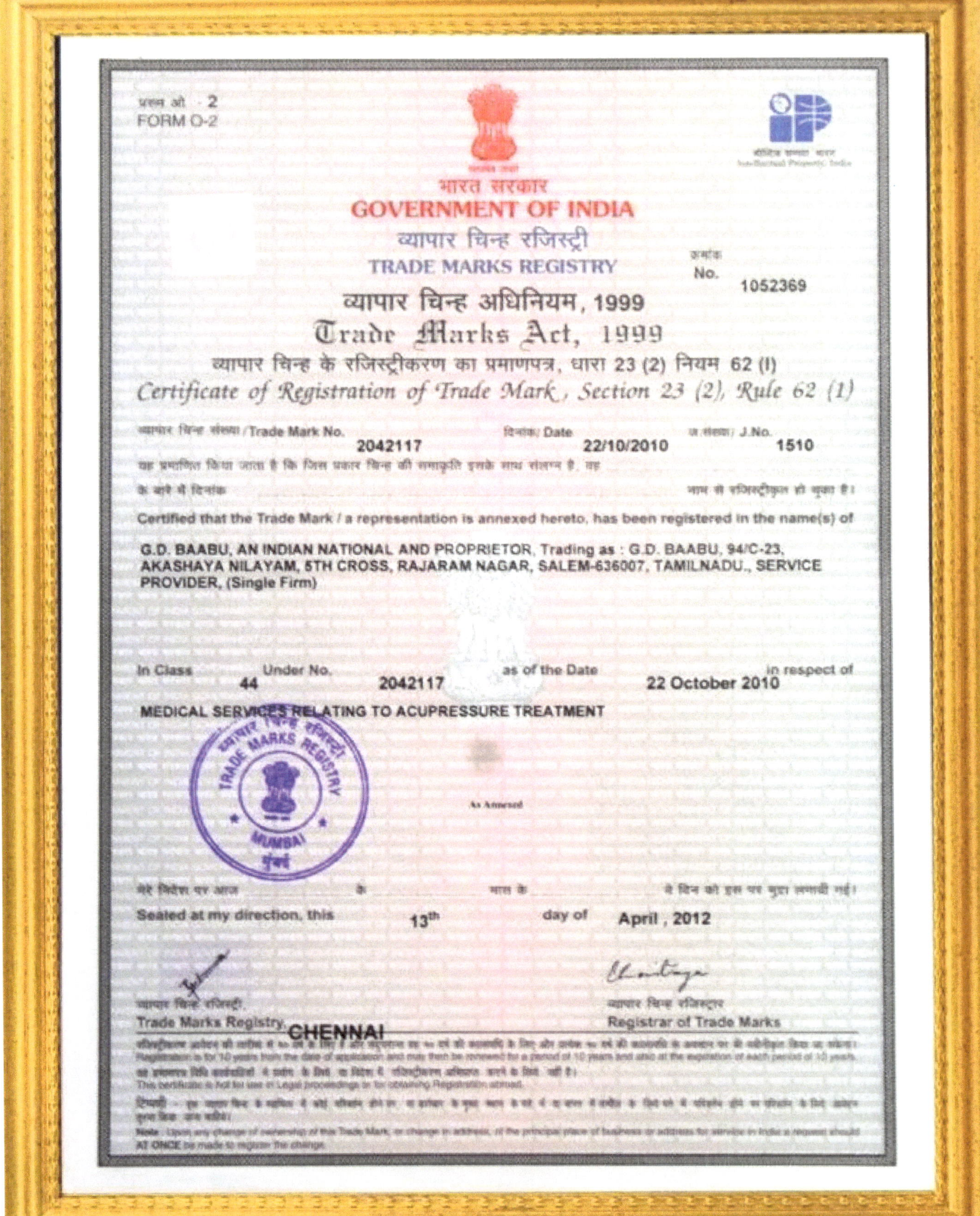

FORM O-2

भारत सरकार

GOVERNMENT OF INDIA

व्यापार चिन्ह रजिस्ट्री

TRADE MARKS REGISTRY

क्रमांक No. 1052369

व्यापार चिन्ह अधिनियम, 1999

Trade Marks Act, 1999

व्यापार चिन्ह के रजिस्ट्रीकरण का प्रमाणपत्र, धारा 23 (2) नियम 62 (I)

Certificate of Registration of Trade Mark, Section 23 (2), Rule 62 (1)

Trade Mark No. 2042117 — Date 22/10/2010 — J.No. 1510

Certified that the Trade Mark / a representation is annexed hereto, has been registered in the name(s) of

G.D. BAABU, AN INDIAN NATIONAL AND PROPRIETOR, Trading as : G.D. BAABU, 94/C-23, AKASHAYA NILAYAM, 5TH CROSS, RAJARAM NAGAR, SALEM-636007, TAMILNADU., SERVICE PROVIDER, (Single Firm)

In Class 44 Under No. 2042117 as of the Date 22 October 2010 in respect of

MEDICAL SERVICES RELATING TO ACUPRESSURE TREATMENT

TRADE MARKS REGISTRY MUMBAI

As Annexed

Sealed at my direction, this 13th day of April, 2012

Trade Marks Registry, CHENNAI

Registrar of Trade Marks

Registration is for 10 years from the date of application and may then be renewed for a period of 10 years and also at the expiration of each period of 10 years.

This certificate is not for use in Legal proceedings or for obtaining Registration abroad.

Note : Upon any change of ownership of this Trade Mark, or change in address, of the principal place of business or address for service in India a request should AT ONCE be made to register the change.

प्रारूप ओ - 2
Form O - 2

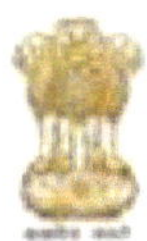

भारत सरकार
Government of India
व्यापार चिन्ह रजिस्ट्री
Trade Marks Registry

क्रमांक
No. 1462351

व्यापार चिन्ह अधिनियम, 1999

Trade Marks Act, 1999

व्यापार चिन्ह के रजिस्ट्रीकरण का प्रमाणपत्र, धारा 23 (2), नियम 62 (1)

Certificate of Registration of Trade Mark, Section 23 (2), Rule 62 (1)

Trade Mark No. 2042115 | **Date** 22/10/2010 | **J. No.** 1762

Certified that Trade Mark / a representation is annexed hereto, has been registered in the name(s) of
G.D. BAABU, 94/C-23, AKASHAYA NILAYAM, 5TH CROSS, RAJARAM NAGAR, SALEM-636007, TAMILNADU , AN INDIAN NATIONAL AND PROPRIETOR, Trading as G.D. BAABU, SERVICE PROVIDER, (Single Firm)

In Class 44 Under No. 2042115 as of the date 22 October 2010 in respect of

MEDICAL SERVICES RELATING TO ACUPRESSURE TREATMENT

THE PANCHABOODHA TREATMENT

Sealed at my direction, this 07th day of February , 2017

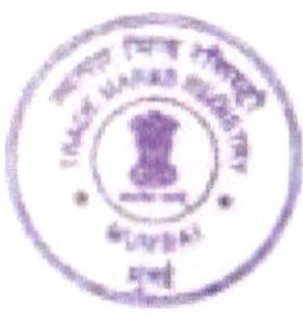

व्यापार चिन्ह रजिस्ट्री
Trade Marks Registry MUMBAI

व्यापार चिन्ह रजिस्ट्रार
Registrar of Trademarks

Registration is for 10 years from the date of application and may then be renewed for a period of 10 years and also at the expiration of each period of 10 years.

This certificate is not for use in legal proceedings or for obtaining Registration abroad.

Note: Upon any change of ownership of this Trademark, or change in address, of the principal place of business or address for service in India a request should AT ONCE be made to register the change.

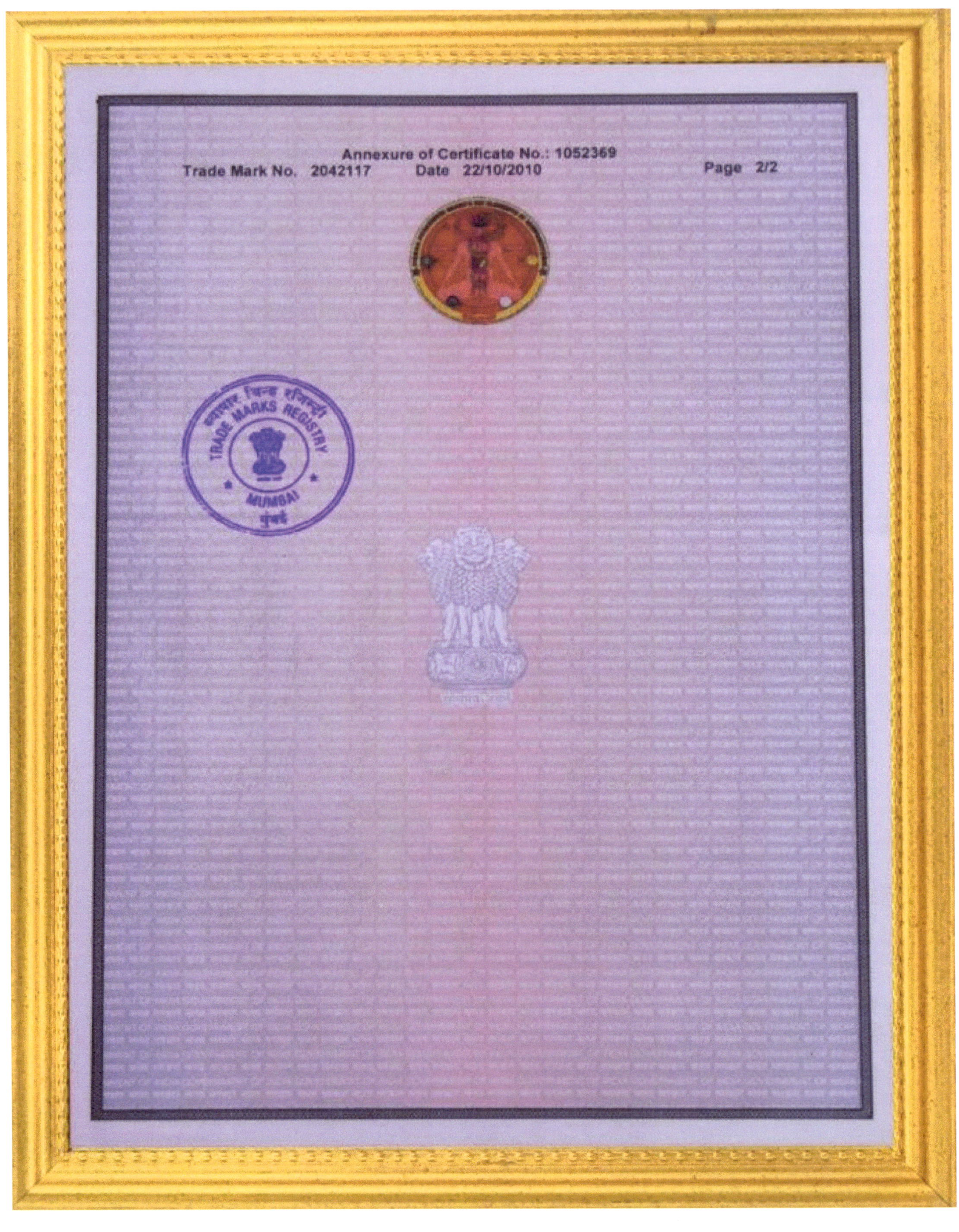

Annexure of Certificate No.: 1052369

Trade Mark No. 2042117 Date 22/10/2010 Page 2/2

TRADE MARKS REGISTRY

MUMBAI

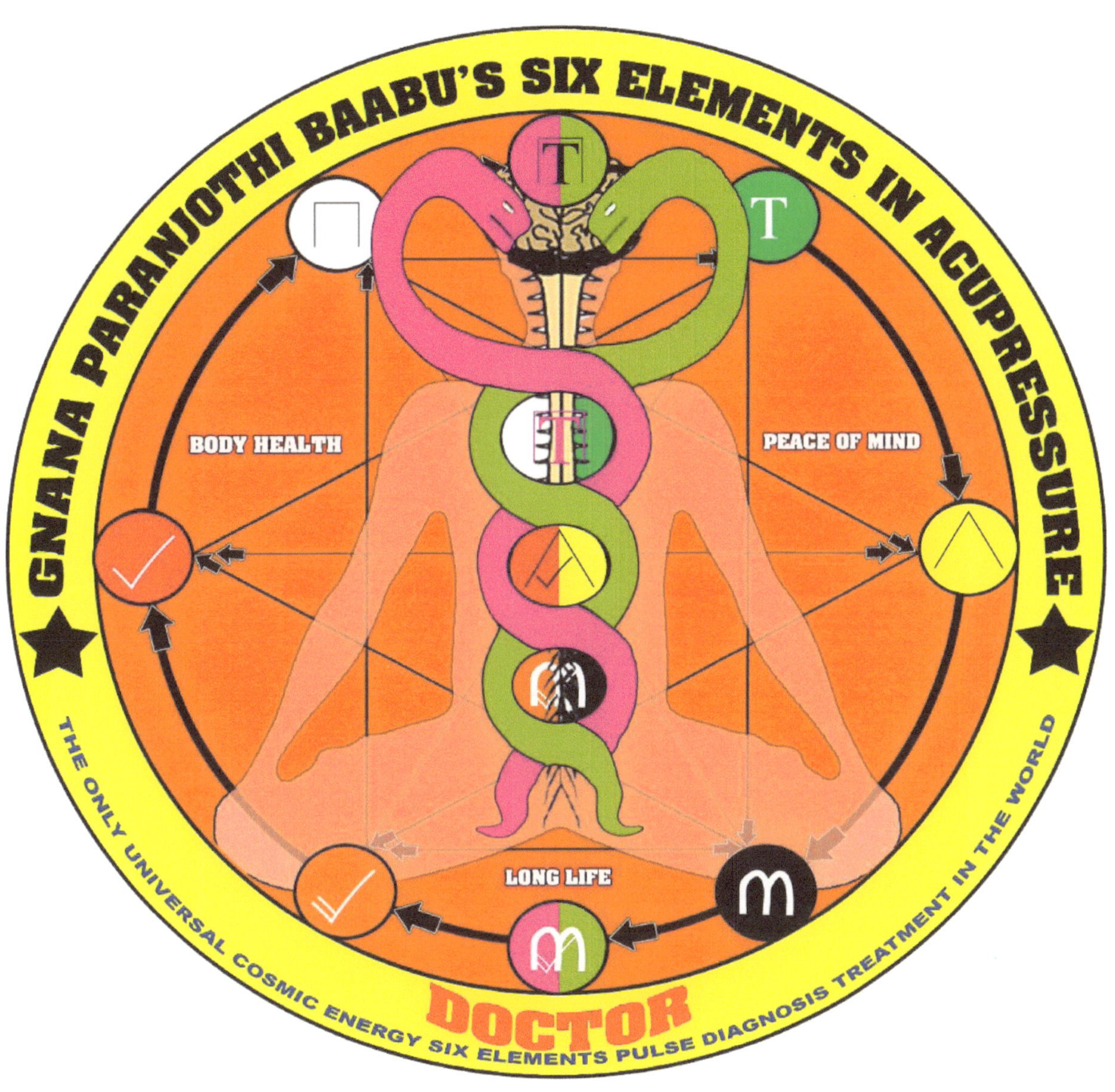
GNANA PARANJOTHI BAABU'S SIX ELEMENTS IN ACUPRESSURE
BODY HEALTH
PEACE OF MIND
LONG LIFE
DOCTOR
THE ONLY UNIVERSAL COSMIC ENERGY SIX ELEMENTS PULSE DIAGNOSIS TREATMENT IN THE WORLD

TRADEMARKS

प्रारूप आरजी - 2
Form RG - 2

भारत सरकार
Government of India
व्यापार चिन्ह रजिस्ट्री
Trade Marks Registry

क्रमांक
No. 1899832

व्यापार चिन्ह अधिनियम, 1999

Trade Marks Act, 1999

व्यापार चिन्ह के रजिस्ट्रीकरण का प्रमाणपत्र, धारा 23 (2), नियम 56 (1)

Certificate of Registration of Trade Mark, Section 23 (2), Rule 56 (1)

Trade Mark No. 2042118 **Date** 22/10/2010 **J. No.** 1835

Certified that Trade Mark / a representation is annexed hereto, has been registered in the name(s) of :
G.D. BAABU, 94/C-23, AKASHAYA NILAYAM, 5TH CROSS, RAJARAM NAGAR, SALEM-636007, TAMILNADU, AN INDIAN NATIONAL AND PROPRIETOR, Trading as : G.D. BAABU, SERVICE PROVIDER, (Single Firm)

In Class 44 Under No 2042118 as of the date 22 October 2010 in respect of

MEDICAL SERVICES RELATING TO ACUPRESSURE TREATMENT

Trade Mark as annexed

Sealed at my direction, this 27th day of June, 2018

व्यापार चिन्ह रजिस्ट्री
Trade Marks Registry MUMBAI

व्यापार चिन्ह रजिस्ट्रार
Registrar of Trademarks

Registration is for 10 years from the date of application and may then be renewed for a period of 10 years and also at the expiration of each period of 10 years.

This certificate is not for use in legal proceedings or for obtaining Registration abroad.

Note: Upon any change of ownership of this Trademark, or change in address, of the principal place of business or address for service in India a request should **AT ONCE** be made to register the change.

Page1 of 2

Trade Mark No. 2042118

Annexure of Certificate No.: 1899832
Date 22/10/2010

Page2 of 2

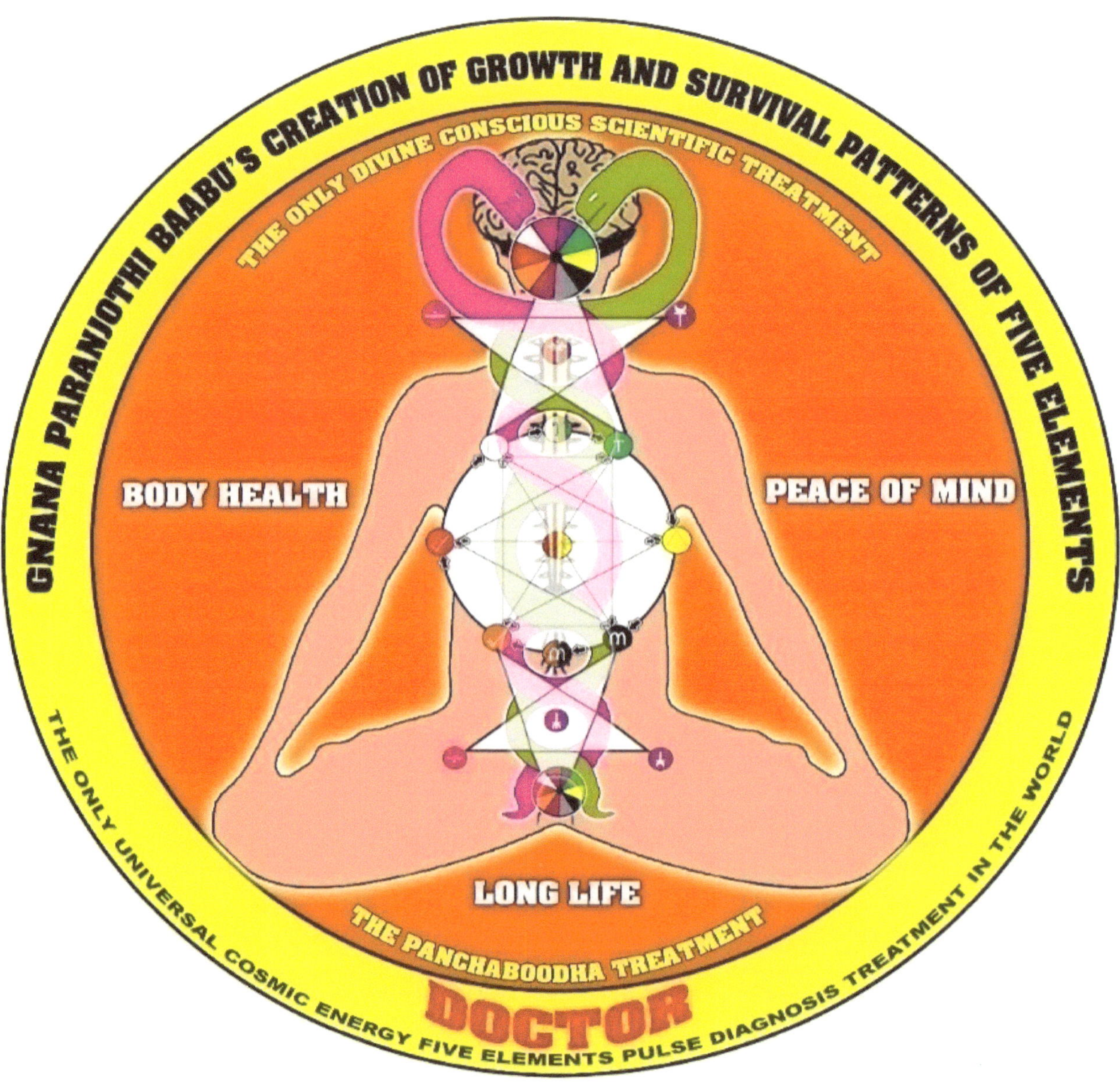
GNANA PARANJOTHI BAABU'S CREATION OF GROWTH AND SURVIVAL PATTERNS OF FIVE ELEMENTS
THE ONLY DIVINE CONSCIOUS SCIENTIFIC TREATMENT
BODY HEALTH
PEACE OF MIND
LONG LIFE
THE PANCHABOODHA TREATMENT
DOCTOR
THE ONLY UNIVERSAL COSMIC ENERGY FIVE ELEMENTS PULSE DIAGNOSIS TREATMENT IN THE WORLD

प्रारूप आरजी - 2
Form RG - 2

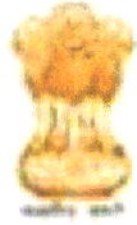

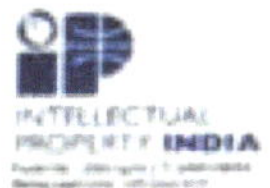

भारत सरकार
Government of India
व्यापार चिन्ह रजिस्ट्री
Trade Marks Registry

क्रमांक
No. 1900223

व्यापार चिन्ह अधिनियम, 1999
Trade Marks Act, 1999

व्यापार चिन्ह के रजिस्ट्रीकरण का प्रमाणपत्र, धारा 23 (2), नियम 56 (1)
Certificate of Registration of Trade Mark, Section 23 (2), Rule 56 (1)

Trade Mark No. 2042120 Date 22/10/2010 J. No. 1835

Mark a representation is annexed hereto, has been registered in the name(s) of -
C-23 AKASHAYA NILAYAM, 5TH CROSS, RAJARAM NAGAR, SALEM-636007, TAMILNADU., AN INDIAN NATIONAL
Trading as G.D BAABU, SERVICE PROVIDER, (Single Firm)

44 Under No 2042120 as of the date 22 October 2010 in respect of

MEDICAL SERVICES RELATING TO ACUPRESSURE TREATMENT

Trade Mark as annexed

Sealed at my direction, this 28th day of June, 2018

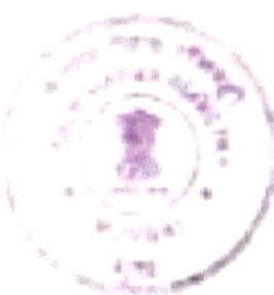

व्यापार चिन्ह रजिस्ट्री
Trade Marks Registry MUMBAI

व्यापार चिन्ह रजिस्ट्रार
Registrar of Trademarks

Registration is for 10 years from the date of application and may then be renewed for a period of 10 years and also at the expiration of each period of 10 years.

This certificate is not for use in legal proceedings or for obtaining Registration abroad.

Note: Upon any change of ownership of this Trademark, or change in address, of the principal place of business or address for service in India a request should AT ONCE be made to register the change.

Trade Mark No. 2042120

Annexure of Certificate No. 1900223
Date 22/10/2010

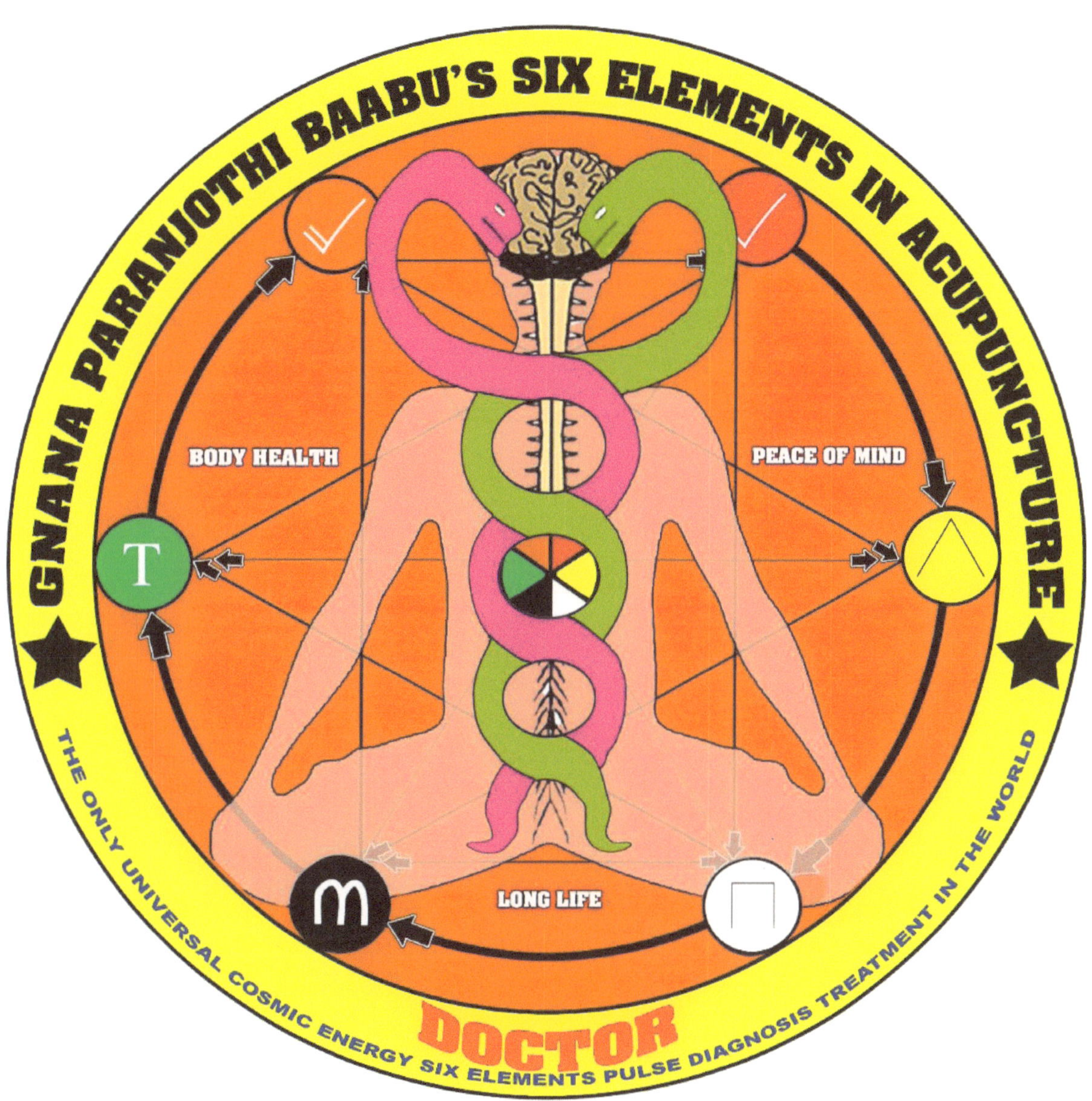
GNANA PARANJOTHI BAABU'S SIX ELEMENTS IN ACUPUNCTURE
BODY HEALTH
PEACE OF MIND
LONG LIFE
T
m
THE ONLY UNIVERSAL COSMIC ENERGY SIX ELEMENTS PULSE DIAGNOSIS TREATMENT IN THE WORLD
DOCTOR

7/25/2018 E-Register - Main Page

(NOT FOR LEGAL USE)

As on Date : 25/07/2018
Status : Registered

View TM Application | View Examination Report

TM Application No.	2042123
Class	44
Date of Application	22/10/2010
Appropriate Office	CHENNAI
State	TAMIL NADU
Country	India
Filing Mode	Branch Office
TM Applied For	A.G.COSMIC CLINIC
TM Category	TRADE MARK
Trade Mark Type	WORD
User Detail	01/01/2000
Certificate Detail	Certificate No. 1056173 Dated : 30/04/2012
Valid upto/ Renewed upto	22/10/2020
Proprietor name	(1) G.D. BAABU Trading As : G.D. BAABU Single Firm
Proprietor Address	94/C-23, AKASHAYA NILAYAM, 5TH CROSS, RAJARAM NAGAR, SALEM-636007, TAMILNADU.
Email Id	
Agent name	R.K. DEWAN & CO.[527]
Agent Address	PODAR CHAMBERS, S.A. BRELVI ROAD, FORT, MUMBAI - 400 001.
Goods & Service Details	[CLASS : 44] MEDICAL SERVICES RELATING TO ACUPRESSURE TREATMENT.
Publication Details	Published in Journal No. : 1515-0 Dated : 19/12/2011
History/PR Details	PURSUANT TO A REQUEST ON FORM TM-50 DATED 07/09/2016 AND ORDER THEREON DATED 01/11/2016 THE ADDRESS FOR SERVICE IS ALTERED TO R.K.DEWAN & CO.,PODAR CHAMBERS, S.A. BRELVI ROAD, FORT, MUMBAI - 400 001.
Uploaded Documents	

Sr No.	Document description	Document Date	
1	TM-1	22/10/2010	View

WARNING/DISCLAIMER : THE DATA OF TRADE MARKS REGISTRY IS UNDER THE PROCESS OF DIGITISATION, IF ANY DISCREPANCY IS OBSERVED IN THE DATA PLEASE CONTACT OR SUBMIT AT APPROPRIATE TRADE MARKS REGISTRY ALONGWITH SUPPORTING DOCUMENTS. THIS WILL HELP IN UPDATION OF ELECTRONIC RECORDS.

PRINT EXIT

http://ipindiaonline.gov.in/eregister/eregister.aspx 1/1

फ़ारूप आरजी - 2
Form RG - 2

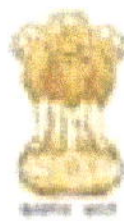

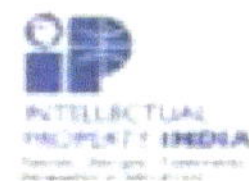

भारत सरकार
Government of India
व्यापार चिन्ह रजिस्ट्री
Trade Marks Registry

क्रमांक
No. 1799718

व्यापार चिन्ह अधिनियम, 1999
Trade Marks Act, 1999

व्यापार चिन्ह के रजिस्ट्रीकरण का प्रमाणपत्र, धारा 23 (2), नियम 56 (1)
Certificate of Registration of Trade Mark, Section 23 (2), Rule 56 (1)

Trade Mark No. 2042124 **Date** 22/10/2010 **J. No.** 1819

Certified that Trade Mark / a representation is annexed hereto, has been registered in the name(s) of -
G.D. BAABU, 94/C-23, AKASHAYA NILAYAM, 5TH CROSS, RAJARAM NAGAR, SALEM-636007, TAMILNADU , AN INDIAN NATIONAL AND PROPRIETOR, Trading as G.D. BAABU, SERVICE PROVIDER (Single Firm)

In Class 44 Under No 2042124 as of the date 22 October 2010 in respect of

MEDICAL SERVICES RELATING TO ACUPRESSURE TREATMENT

GNANAPARANJOTHI BAABU'S SIX ELEMENTS IN ACUPUNCTURE (ACUPRESSURE)

Sealed at my direction, this 07th day of March , 2018

व्यापार चिन्ह रजिस्ट्री
Trade Marks Registry MUMBAI

व्यापार चिन्ह रजिस्ट्रार
Registrar of Trademarks

Registration is for 10 years from the date of application and may then be renewed for a period of 10 years and also at the expiration of each period of 10 years.

This certificate is not for use in legal proceedings or for obtaining Registration abroad.

Note: Upon any change of ownership of this Trademark, or change in address, of the principal place of business or address for service in India a request should AT ONCE be made to register the change.

Page 1 of 1

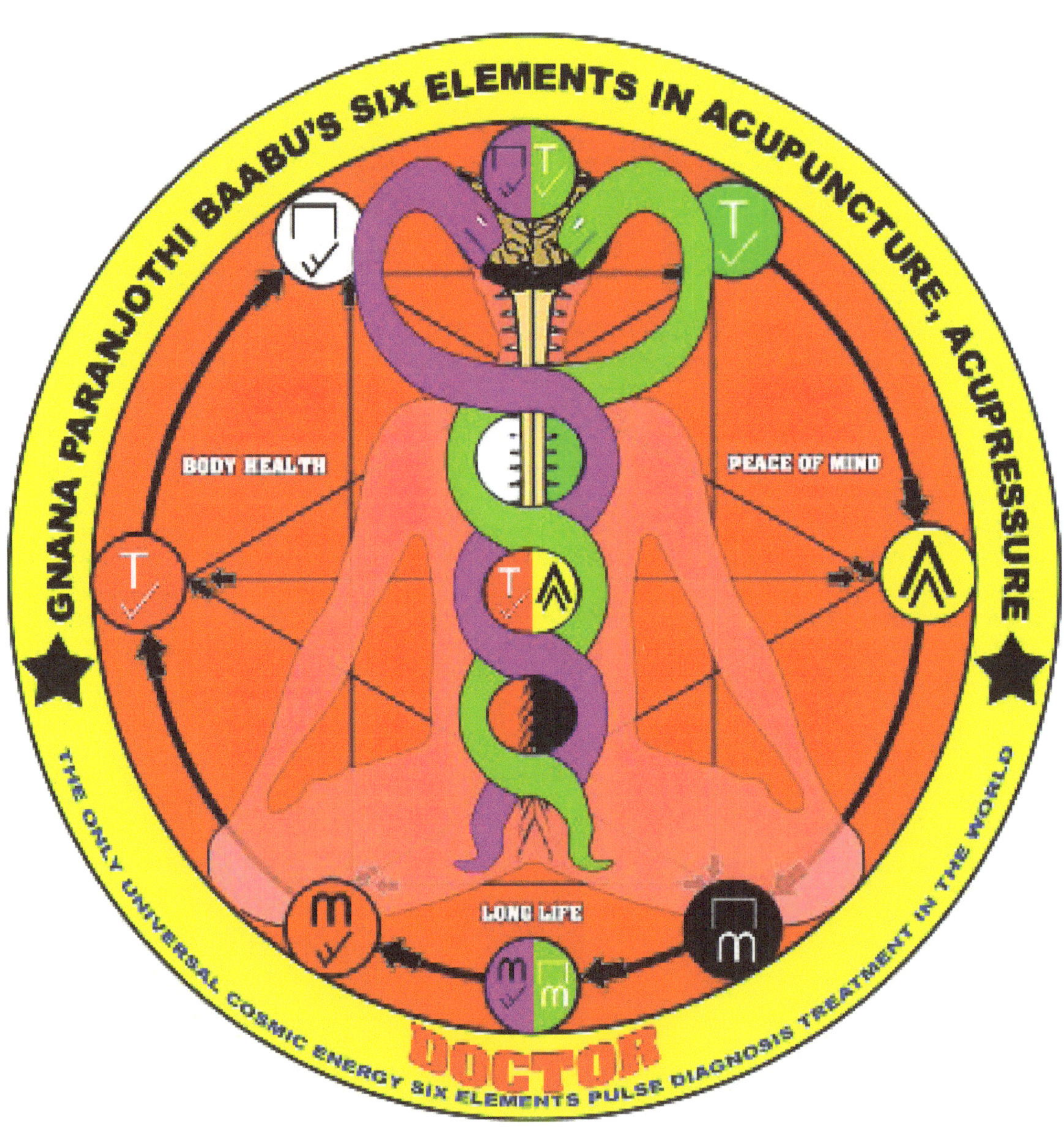
GNANA PARANJOTHI BAABU'S SIX ELEMENTS IN ACUPUNCTURE, ACUPRESSURE
BODY HEALTH
PEACE OF MIND
LONG LIFE
THE ONLY UNIVERSAL COSMIC ENERGY SIX ELEMENTS PULSE DIAGNOSIS TREATMENT IN THE WORLD
DOCTOR

ASIA BOOK OF RECORDS

ASIA
BOOK OF
RECORDS
www.asiabookofrecords.com
CERTIFICATE
The inventor for the unique patented non-medicine treatment therapy based on elements and their energies is Prof. Dr. Aathi Jothi Babu (born on July 29, 1972) at Salem, Tamil Nadu, India. The therapy is practiced at the Cosmic Clinic and Research Institute Salem, Tamil Nadu as on October 27, 2018.
ASIA
BOOK OF
RECORDS
Date: October 27, 2018
NEPAL
BOOK
OF RECORDS
ASIA
BOOK OF
RECORDS
IPSA

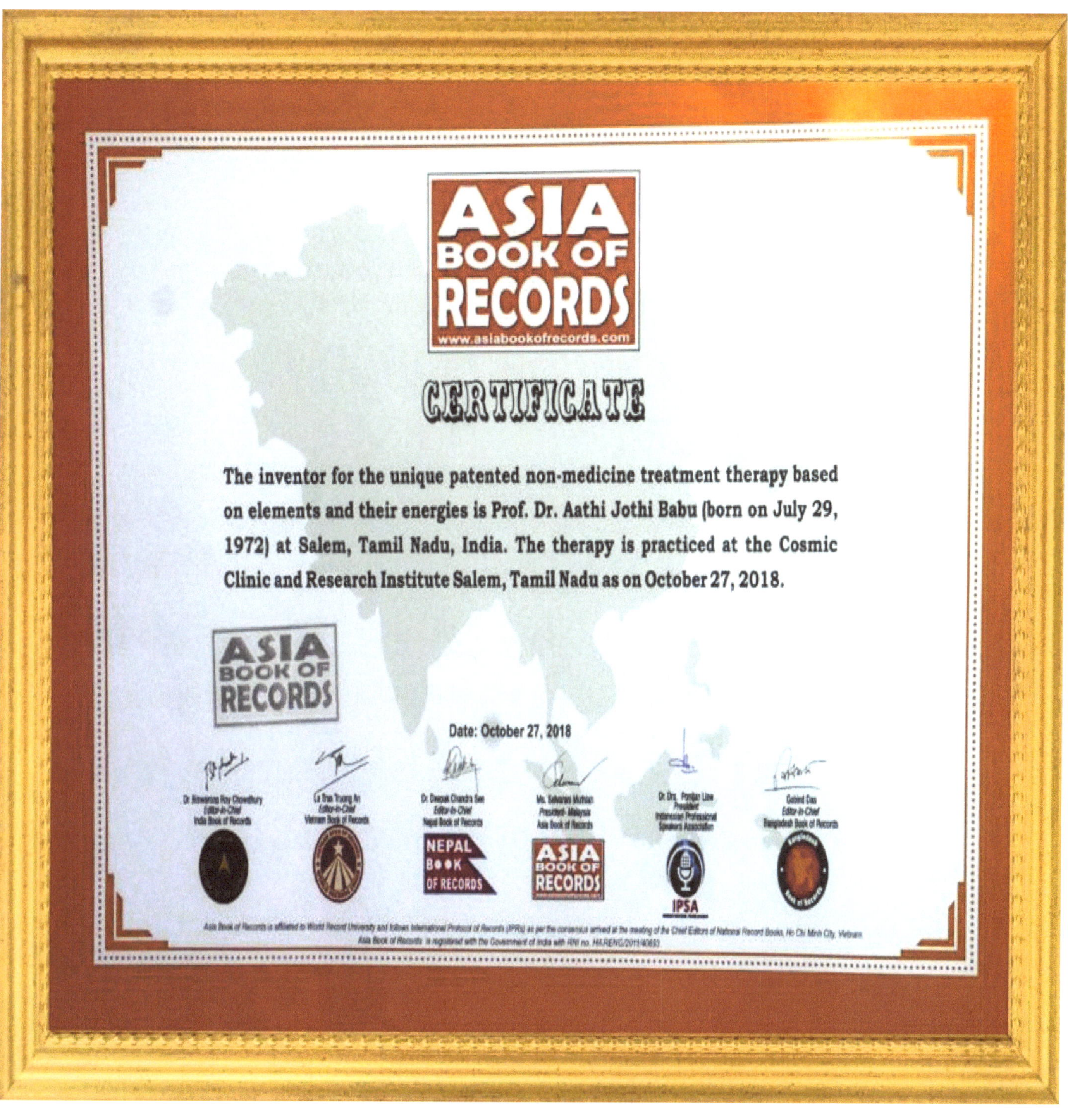

WORLD RECORD

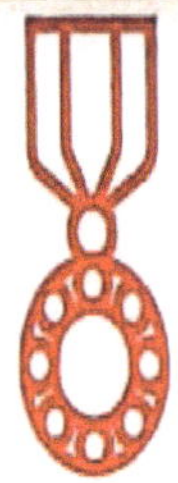

WORLD RECORDS UNION

An Official Registrar of World Records

CERTIFICATE

The record for the patented non-medicine treatment 'The Panchaboodha Treatment' was invented by Prof Dr. Aathi Jothi Babu from India, as confirmed on 26th January 2022. This one-of-a-kind treatment is a non-medicinal treatment therapy as claimed.

www.worldrecordsunion.com

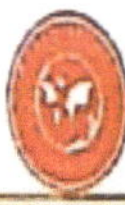

INDIA BOOK OF RECORDS

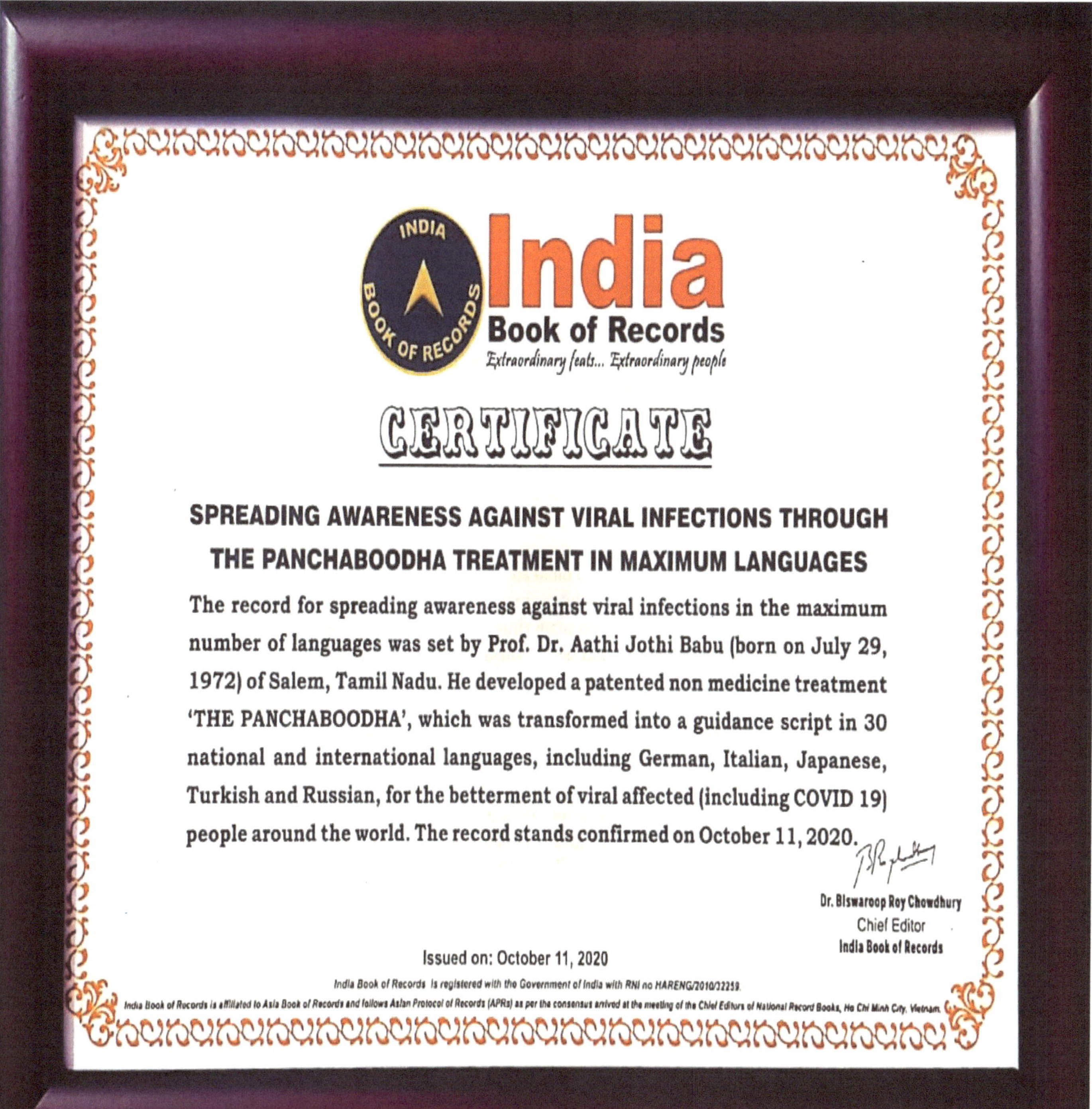

INDIA BOOK OF RECORDS

India Book of Records

Extraordinary feats... Extraordinary people

CERTIFICATE

SPREADING AWARENESS AGAINST VIRAL INFECTIONS THROUGH THE PANCHABOODHA TREATMENT IN MAXIMUM LANGUAGES

The record for spreading awareness against viral infections in the maximum number of languages was set by Prof. Dr. Aathi Jothi Babu (born on July 29, 1972) of Salem, Tamil Nadu. He developed a patented non medicine treatment 'THE PANCHABOODHA', which was transformed into a guidance script in 30 national and international languages, including German, Italian, Japanese, Turkish and Russian, for the betterment of viral affected (including COVID 19) people around the world. The record stands confirmed on October 11, 2020.

Dr. Biswaroop Roy Chowdhury
Chief Editor
India Book of Records

Issued on: October 11, 2020

India Book of Records is registered with the Government of India with RNI no HARENG/2010/32259.

India Book of Records is affiliated to Asia Book of Records and follows Asian Protocol of Records (APRs) as per the consensus arrived at the meeting of the Chief Editors of National Record Books, Ho Chi Minh City, Vietnam.

ASIA BOOK OF RECORDS

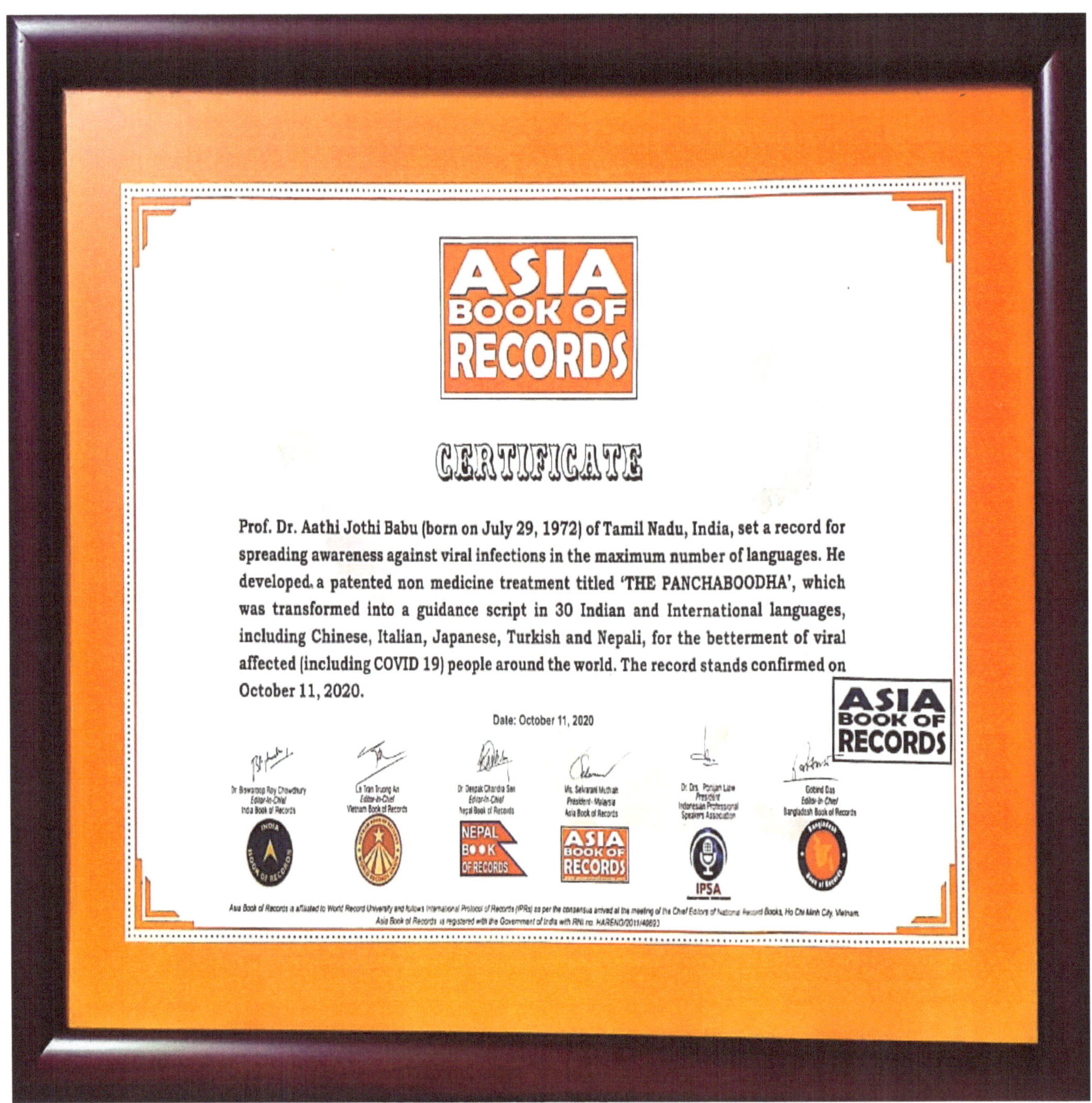

ASIA BOOK OF RECORDS

CERTIFICATE

Prof. Dr. Aathi Jothi Babu (born on July 29, 1972) of Tamil Nadu, India, set a record for spreading awareness against viral infections in the maximum number of languages. He developed a patented non medicine treatment titled 'THE PANCHABOODHA', which was transformed into a guidance script in 30 Indian and International languages, including Chinese, Italian, Japanese, Turkish and Nepali, for the betterment of viral affected (including COVID 19) people around the world. The record stands confirmed on October 11, 2020.

ASIA BOOK OF RECORDS

Date: October 11, 2020

Dr Biswaroop Roy Chowdhury
Editor-In-Chief
India Book of Records

Le Tran Truong An
Editor-In-Chief
Vietnam Book of Records

Dr Deepak Chandra Sen
Editor-In-Chief
Nepal Book of Records

Ms. Selvarani Muthiah
President - Malaysia
Asia Book of Records

Dr. Drs. Ponjan Liaw
President
Indonesian Professional Speakers Association

Gobind Das
Editor-In-Chief
Bangladesh Book of Records

INDIA BOOK OF RECORDS

NEPAL BOOK OF RECORDS

ASIA BOOK OF RECORDS

IPSA

Asia Book of Records is affiliated to World Record University and follows International Protocol of Records (IPRs) as per the consensus arrived at the meeting of the Chief Editors of National Record Books, Ho Chi Minh City, Vietnam.
Asia Book of Records is registered with the Government of India with RNI no. HARENG/2011/40693

Conclusion

There are many methods by which acupuncture treatment is administered. All these methods have their limitations because they are applied based on the symptoms of the patients and/or the allopath reports. Hence, the method of selecting the points is also based either on the symptoms or the experience of the doctors. There are very few doctors who diagnose the five elements' pulse methodically and select the five elements' points. This is because only a few people know how to diagnose the pulses. Moreover, not all the 60 points are in use because some of these points are said to be very dangerous and must be handled carefully when one is needling because there are practical difficulties in needling them. Even if the doctors use these points, the after-effects of needling these points frighten them. This is because they do not have control over these points and do not know whether these aftereffects are doing good or bad to the patients. Since the existing acupuncture doctors do not know the connections between the five elements and the five elements' points, this scenario exists.

Because of the above reason, acupuncture doctors are not able to utilise the five elements' points properly and cure ailments. In most cases, they are not able to cure the ailments because though the symptoms look alike, the reasons and the energy levels, as well as the pattern of energy travelling is unique and they differ from patient to patient.

When the patients are treated with the ***Panchaboodha*** Pulse Diagnosis Method (five elements diagnosis method), the diseases/disorders are cured with even a single point. This method has been used on 6000 patients and their symptoms and diseases have been cured. All the ailments from head to toe of the patients can be cured with one or two points if diagnose accurately based on the ***Panchaboodha*** Pulse Diagnosis Method, the Five Element Energy Cycles and the relevant points.

References

1. *Clinical Acupuncture* by Prof. Dr. Anton Jayasurya (Sri Lanka)
2. *Chinese Acupuncture* by Dr. Wu-Wei-Ping
3. *Acupuncture Therapy* by Dr. Mary Austin.
4. *The Treatment of Disease* *by Acupuncture* by Dr. Felix Mann.
5. *The Way to Locate Acupoints* by Hang Jiasan
6. *Acupressure* by Dr. Dhiran Gala
7. *Selecting the right Acupuncture* by GengJuninget.al
8. *Health Time Magazine* by Dr. Siddiq Jamal and Dr. Fazlur Rahman
9. *Feather Touch Method in Acupuncture/Acupressure* by Dr. Siddiq Jamal and Dr. Fazlur Rahman
10. *Acupuncture in Tamil* by Dr. Ethiraj, M.D (Acu) Dr. R. K. Panneer Selvam, M.D (Acu) Dr. P. Saraswathy Panneer Selvam, M.D (Acu) Dr. M. Ranganathan, M.D (Acu)
11. *Reiki Acupuncture* by Prof. Dr. Abdulla Segu, M.D, PhD (Acu)
12. *Clinical Acupuncture* by Prof. Dr. Anton Jayasurya (Sri Lanka)
13. *Clinical Practice of Acupuncture* by Arjun Lal Agarwal
14. *Peoples China Today* by Bruce Jonson and Others
15. *I GOD* by His Holiness Gnana Vallal Paranjothi Mahan

www.ingramcontent.com/pod-product-compliance
Ingram Content Group UK Ltd.
Pitfield, Milton Keynes, MK11 3LW, UK
UKHW061028310726
14090UKWH00026B/257

9798889099635